AF316745

USEFULNESS OF MEASURING TOTAL 12-LEAD QRS VOLTAGE FOR DIAGNOSING CARDIOVASCULAR DISEASE

Collected Reprints (1982-2018)

By

WILLIAM C. ROBERTS, MD

and

COLLEAGUES

ISBN: 979-8-88680-090-6
Printed in the United States of America on acid-free paper.

Preface

When in medical school (1954–1958), I became interested in the electrocardiogram.
I wondered why the definition of "low QRS voltage" included only three leads (I, II, III)
when the electrocardiograms at the time included 12 leads. I learned that the definition
of "low QRS voltage" was created when the standard electrocardiogram consisted of only
three leads (I, II, III) and it was defined as total QRS voltage as ≤ 15 mm (using 10 mm as
the standard). In the early 1980s my colleagues and I began measuring QRS voltage in all 12
leads in patients with a variety of cardiac conditions. All patients included in our studies had
come to necropsy or to heart transplantation and thus we could compare the total 12-lead
QRS voltage to heart weight in all the patients studied. We learned that the patients with the
biggest hearts (>1000 g) had the highest QRS voltage, and patients with the smallest hearts,
in general, had the lowest 12-lead QRS voltage. Total 12-lead QRS voltage was particularly
helpful in diagnosing cardiac sarcoidosis, arrhythmogenic right ventricular cardiomyopathy,
the carcinoid syndrome, and, of course, cardiac amyloidosis. The obesity epidemic has
reduced total QRS voltage in many of us.

—William C. Roberts, MD

Table of Contents

*Articles are numbered based on WCR's CV.

Electrocardiographic observations in severe aortic valve stenosis: Correlative necropsy study to clinical, hemodynamic, and ECG variables demonstrating relation of 12-lead QRS amplitude to peak systolic transaortic pressure gradient

Most ECG studies in patients with aortic valve stenosis (AS) have involved living patients in whom the status of the left ventricular (LV) myocardium, epicardial coronary arteries, and mitral valve was not precisely known. We examined the 12-lead ECG recorded within 2 months of death in 50 patients aged 16 to 65 years (mean 48) with peak systolic pressure gradients (PSPG) across the aortic valve ranging from 52 to 180 mm Hg (mean 98) and anatomically normal mitral valves. Excluding four patients with complete left bundle branch block (LBBB), 44 (96%) of the other 46 patients had the usual voltage criteria for LV hypertrophy (LVH). Measurement of the total 12-lead QRS amplitude, which ranged from 144 to 417 mm (10 mm = 1 mV), (mean 257) proved useful for it correlated directly with PSPG across the aortic valve and, when the four LBBB patients were excluded, with the peak LV systolic pressure. The total 12-lead QRS amplitude (mm) was similar in most patients to the LV systolic pressure (mm Hg). Thus, subtraction of the indirect systemic arterial systolic pressure (mm Hg) from the total 12-lead QRS amplitude (mm) provides a reasonable noninvasive prediction of the PSPG across the aortic valve in patients with moderate to severe AS. Additionally, the mean of the total 12-lead QRS amplitude was significantly ($p < 0.05$) greater in the 11 younger (≤ 40 years) than in the 39 older patients (278 mm vs 257 mm), in the 14 women than in the 36 men (277 mm vs 249 mm), in the 22 patients with heavier (> 600 gm) hearts (274 mm vs 244 mm), in the 34 patients without compared to the 16 with significant coronary arterial narrowing (270 mm vs 238 mm), and in the 22 patients without compared to the 24 with ECG myocardial damage patterns (269 mm vs 236 mm). (Am Heart J 103:210, 1982.)

Robert J. Siegel, M.D., and William C. Roberts, M.D. *Bethesda, Md.*

The usual ECG findings in patients with aortic valve stenosis (AS) are well recognized, the most characteristic one being excessive voltage indicative of left ventricular hypertrophy (LVH). Among adults with AS and ECG criteria of LVH, the latter correlate poorly with the presence of symptoms of cardiac dysfunction, the amount of obstruction across the aortic valve, or prognosis in the absence of symptoms. Adults with AS frequently also have associated atherosclerotic coronary disease (CAD) which also may alter the ECG. In most ECG studies in adults with AS, the status of the coronary arteries, LV myocardium and mitral valve (MV), and the weight of the heart have not been known. In studies before 1950, the pressure gradient across the aortic valve was not available.

In an attempt to determine the ECG finding attributable only to AS, with or without aortic regurgitation (AR), we analyzed the ECG in 50 necropsy patients aged 16 to 65 years with severe or moderately severe AS, all of whom had ECG and cardiac catheterization performed within 2 months of death, and thorough examination of the major coronary arteries, LV myocardium and MV at necropsy. The total amplitude of the QRS complexes in all 12 leads was measured in each patient

From the Pathology Branch, National Heart, Lung and Blood Institute, National Institutes of Health.

Received for publication Sept. 4, 1981; accepted Sept. 28, 1981.

Reprint requests: William C. Roberts, M.D., Pathology Branch, NHLBI-NIH, Bldg. 10A, Room 3E-30, Bethesda, MD 20205.

Table I. Clinical and necropsy finding in severe isolated aortic valve stenosis

Parameter	Number
1. Age (years)	16-65 (mean 48)
2. Male: female (pts)	36:14
3. Angina pectoris (pts)	34
4. Pressures (mm Hg)	
Left ventricle (LV) peak systolic	149-270 (avg 210)
Systemic artery (SA) systolic	63-180 (avg 112)
LV-SA peak systolic gradient	52-180 (avg 98)
LV end-diastolic	4-45 (avg 18)
SA end-diastolic	34*-88 (avg 62)
Cardiac index (L/min/m²)	1.3-4.5 (mean 2.7)
Aortic valve area (cm²)	0.16-0.89 (mean 0.53)
Aortic valve area index (cm²/BSA)	0.16-0.44 (mean 0.29)
5. Aortic regurgitation murmur (pts)	24
6. Heart weight (Gm)	380-880 (mean 606)
7. Narrowed (> 75%) coronary artery (pts)	16
8. Gross LV scar (pts)	7

*LVSP only 63 mm in this patient.

pts = patients.

Table II. ECG observations in severe isolated aortic valve stenosis

Finding	Number
1. Rhythm (pts)	
Sinus	45
Atrial fibrillation	5
2. Atrial abnormality (pts)	
Left only	16
Right only	0
Both	1
3. Ventricular premature complexes (pts)	7
4. PR interval > 0.20 sec (pts)	7
5. Left axis deviation (pts)	12
6. Left ventricular hypertrophy and strain without BBB (pts)	44
7. Left bundle branch block (BBB) (pts)	4
8. QRS amplitude (mm)	
All 12 leads	144-417 (mean 257)
Leads I-III only	12-78 (mean 39)
9. Myocardial damage pattern (without BBB) (pts)	24
A. Poor precordial R-wave progression	18
B. Q waves > 30 ms in $\geq$ 2 leads	2
1. II, III, AVF = 2	
2. I, AVL, V_{4-6} = 0	
C. A + B1	2
D. A + B2	2

and correlated with the age, sex, pressure gradient across the aortic valve, LV peak systolic pressure, heart weight, and the presence of angina pectoris, CAD, LV scarring, and ECG myocardial damage pattern.

METHODS

Patient criteria. Criteria for patient inclusion in this study included the following: (1) peak systolic pressure gradient across the aortic valve of > 50 mm Hg demonstrated at catheterization within 2 months of death; (2) age of death > 15 years and < 66 years; (3) ECG recorded within 2 months of death and available for reexamination, and recorded before an operation was performed on the aortic valve; and (4) anatomically normal MV, tricuspid, and pulmonic valves at necropsy. The first 50 patients in the files of the Pathology Branch, NHLBI, fulfilling these above four criteria form the basis of this study.

ECG criteria. ECG criteria utilized for LVH were the point-score system of Romhilt and Estes.[1] Four or more points were considered evidence of LVH. A LV strain pattern was diagnosed when the ST segment was displaced and the T wave was directed 180 degrees away from the major QRS axis at least in leads V_5 and V_6. Left atrial (LA) abnormality was diagnosed when the P wave in lead V_1 was diphasic with the negative component reaching at least 1 mm in amplitude and at least 120 msec in width, and when the P wave in leads I, II_L or aV_L was notched and at least 120 msec in width. Right atrial (RA) abnormality was diagnosed when the P wave amplitude in leads II, III, of aV_F was 3 mm or greater. Left axis deviation (LAD) was diagnosed when the QRS axis in the frontal plane was −30 degrees or less and right axis deviation (RAD) when it was 110 degrees or greater. Left bundle branch block (LBBB) was defined by: (1) QRS duration > 12 seconds in the extremity leads; (2) presence of broad monophasic R wave in leads I, V_5 and V_6, and (3) displacement of the ST segment and T wave 180 degrees away from the major QRS defection. Two myocardial damage patterns were diagnosed: type A, when the R wave in V_1 was absent and < 5 mm in amplitude in lead V_2; type B, when Q waves > 30 msec were present in two or more leads posteriorly (leads II, III, aV_F) or laterally (leads I, aV_L, V_4 to V_6).

Clinical observations. The 50 patients ranged in age from 16 to 65 years (mean 48); 36 (72%) were male and 14 (28%) were female (Table I). The peak systolic pressure gradient between LV and systemic artery ranged from 52 to 180 mm Hg (mean 98), the aortic valve area (AVA) from 0.16 to 0.89 cm² (mean 0.53), the AVA indices from 0.16 to 0.44 cm²/m² (mean 0.29) and the cardiac index (CI) from 1.3 to 4.7 L/min/m² (mean 2.7). Precordial murmurs of AR were recorded in 24 patients (48%) and AR was observed by angiography in 4 of the 13 patients in whom contrast material was injected into the proximal portion of ascending aorta. Of the 50 patients, 34 (68%) had angina pectoris; none had had a clinical event compatible with acute myocardial infarction. An operation on the aortic valve was performed in 38 (76%) patients: 20 died within 24 hours of operation, 11 others within 2 weeks, and seven

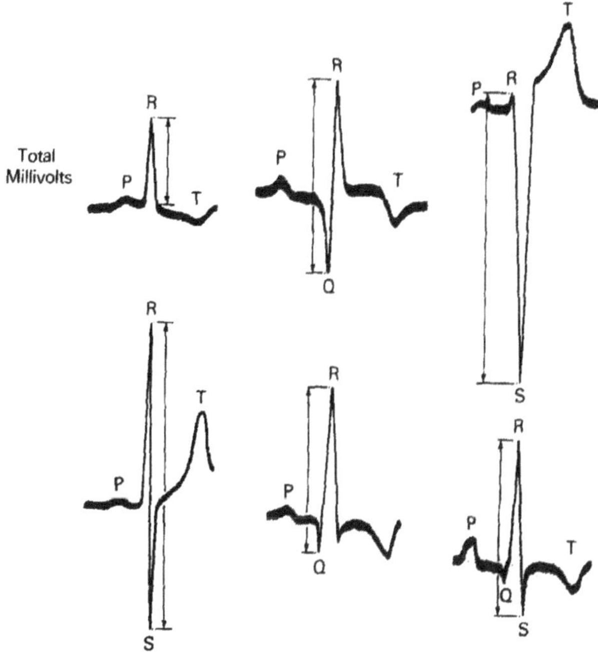

Fig. 1. Various QRS complexes showing how each was measured.

others from 2 to 6 weeks postoperatively. Two other patients died during induction of anesthesia or during the skin incision for planned aortic valve operation. All 50 patients were in functional classes III or IV (New York Heart Association classification). In the 10 unoperated patients, aortic valve operations had been planned or recommended in each, but death occurred, usually suddenly, before they were performed.

Necropsy observations. The hearts ranged in weight from 380 to 880 gm (mean 606). All were examined by one of us (WCR) and most by RJS as well (Table I). The number of cusps in the aortic valve (identified at operation by the surgeon, by examination of the excised valve by one of us [WCR] or from examination of the heart at necropsy) were the following: one cusp (unicuspid unicommissural) = five patients (10%); two cusps (bicuspid) = 29 patients (58%); three cusps (tricuspid) = 15 patients (30%); and uncertain structure = one patient. One or more of the four major epicardial coronary arteries was narrowed > 75% in cross-sectional area by atherosclerotic plaques in 16 patients (32%). LV scars were present at necropsy in seven patients (14%) and in each they were relatively small: subendocardial (inner one half of wall) only in two patients and transmural (> the inner one half of the wall) in five patients. Only one patient had gross evidence of LV necrosis and this patient died 33 days after the ring of a caged-ball prosthesis had severely narrowed the ostium of his right coronary artery.

RESULTS

General ECG observations. These are summarized in Table II. Sinus rhythm was present in 45 patients and chronic atrial fibrillation in five. None had atrial premature contractions or supraventricular tachycardia recorded; seven patients had ventricular premature complexes recorded. Abnormal configuration of the P wave was recorded in 16 patients, of the LA type in 15. The PR interval was greater than 0.20 second in seven patients. LAD was present in 12 patients and none had RAD. Four patients had LBBB and none had right bundle branch block or complete heart block. Excluding the four patients with LBBB, 44 (99%) of the remaining 46 patients had ECG evidence of LVH, with a LV strain pattern in 43. Although all 50 patients at necropsy had right ventricular hypertrophy (RVH), none had ECG evidence of RVH.[1] Myocardial damage patterns were present in 24 patients: poor precordial R-wave progression only in 18 patients, Q waves > 30 msec in width in two or more leads only in two patients, and combinations of the two in four patients. In each of the 12 leads in all 50 patients, the amplitude of the QRS complexes were measured from the peak of the R wave to the maximal dip of the S or Q wave, whichever was greatest (Fig. 1). The sum of the amplitude of the QRS complexes in all 12 leads in the 50 patients ranged from 144 to 417 mm (mean 257) (10 mm = 1 mV) and the sum of the amplitude of the QRS complexes in leads I, II, and III in all patients ranged from 12 to 78 mm (mean 39).

Correlation of age and gender to clinical, hemodynamic, ECG, and necropsy findings. Compared to the 11 patients aged 40 years and under, the 39 patients over age 40 had a higher frequency of angina pectoris (30 of 39 [77%] vs 4 of 11) ($p < 0.005$), lower average peak systolic pressure gradients across the aortic valve (94 mm Hg vs 113 mm Hg) ($p < 0.025$), more frequent significant CAD (16 of 39 [41%] vs 0 of 11) and LV scarring (7 of 39 [18%] vs 0 of 12) ($p < 0.025$), and lower average total QRS amplitude in the 12 leads (257 mm vs 278 mm) ($p < 0.05$). (Table III). Compared to the 14 women, the 36 men had lower average peak systolic pressure gradients between LV and a systemic artery (91 mm Hg vs 144 mm Hg) ($p < 0.01$), higher mean heart weights (639 gm vs 521 gm) ($p < 0.01$), and lower total QRS amplitude in the 12 leads (249 mm vs 277 mm) ($p < 0.05$) (Table IV).

Correlation of transaortic pressure gradient, LV systolic pressure and heart weight to clinical, hemodynamic, ECG, and necropsy findings. The total amplitude of the QRS complexes in the 12 leads in the 33 patients with LV to systemic arterial peak systolic pressure gradients ≤ 100 mm Hg (mean 82) averaged 244 mm and in the 17 patients with higher gradients, 281 mm ($p < 0.05$) (Table V). The average LV peak systolic pressure in the patients with

Table III. Comparison of 12 patients aged 16 to 40 years to 38 patients aged 41 to 65 years with isolated severe aortic valve stenosis

Age (years)	16-40 (n = 11)	41-65 (n = 39)	p value
Mean age (years)	31	53	< 0.0005
Male:Female (pts)	6:5	30:9	ns
Angina pectoris (pts)	4	30 (77%)	< 0.005
LV-SA psg (mm Hg)	70-180 (113)	52-145 (94)	< 0.025
LVSP (mm Hg)	175-270 (220)	149-260 (208)	ns
Aortic valve area (cm²)	0.40-0.58 (.44)	0.16-0.89 (0.54)	ns
CI (L/min/m²)	2.0-4.3 (2.9)	1.6-4.8 (2.5)	ns
Heart weight (gm)	380-880 (593)	400-880 (614)	ns
CA narrowing > 75% (pts)	0	16 (41%)	< 0.025
LV scar (pts)	0	7 (18%)	ns
Electrocardiogram			
VPC (pts)	1 (9%)	6 (15%)	ns
LAD (pts)	1 (9%)	11 (28%)	ns
MDP (pts)	6 (55%)	18 (46%)	ns
QRS amplitude (mm)			
12 leads	193-395 (278)	144-417 (257)	< 0.05
I-III	26-58 (40)	12-78 (38)	ns

Abbreviations: CA = coronary artery; LAD = left axis deviation; LV = left ventricular; LVSP = left ventricular systolic pressure; MDP = myocardial damage pattern; psg = peak systolic pressure gradient; SA = systemic artery, VPC = ventricular premature complex; ns = $p > 0.05$.

Table IV. Comparison of 35 men to 15 women with severe isolated aortic valve stenosis

Sex	Men (n = 36)	Women (n = 14)	p value
Age (years)	16-64 (48)	16-65 (47)	ns
Angina pectoris (pts)	23 (64%)	11 (79%)	ns
LV-SA psg (mm Hg)	52-160 (91)	70-180 (107)	< 0.01
LVSP (mm Hg)	149-260 (203)	192-270 (228)	< 0.01
Aortic valve areas (cm²)	0.16-0.89 (0.59)	0.28-0.54 (0.42)	< 0.0025
CI (L/min/m²)	1.2-4.8 (2.7)	2.0-4.2 (2.7)	ns
Heart weight (gm)	440-880 (639)	380-700 (521)	< 0.01
CA narrowing > 75% (pts)	11 (31%)	5 (36%)	ns
LV scar (pts)	6 (17%)	1 (7%)	ns
Electrocardiogram			
VPC (pts)	5 (14%)	2 (14%)	ns
LAD (pts)	10 (28%)	2 (14%)	ns
MDP (pts)	19 (53%)	5 (40%)	ns
QRS amplitude (mm)			
12 leads	144-417 (249)	193-376 (277)	< 0.05
I-III	12-78 (36)	27-72 (47)	< 0.002

Abbreviations as in Table III.

gradients ≤ 100 mm Hg was 198 mm Hg and in those with higher gradients, 234 mm Hg ($p < 0.0005$).

The 22 patients with peak LV systolic pressure ≤ 200 mm Hg had smaller peak systolic pressure gradients across the aortic valve (80 mm Hg vs 122 mm Hg) ($p < 0.0005$) and lower total QRS amplitudes (247 mm vs 265 mm) ($p < 0.05$) than did those with higher pressures (Table VI). Compared to the 28 patients with smaller hearts, the 22 patients with hearts weighing over 600 gm were more often men (20 of 22 [91%] vs 16 of 28 [57%]) ($p < 0.025$), had lower average LV peak systolic pressures (205 mm Hg vs 214 mm Hg) ($p < 0.05$), more commonly had LAD (39% vs 7%) ($p < 0.01$), and higher average total QRS amplitude (274 mm vs 244 mm) ($p < 0.025$) (Table VII).

Correlation of angina, CAD, and LV scarring to clinical, hemodynamic, ECG, and necropsy findings. The 34 patients with angina had smaller mean heart

Table V. Comparison of 33 patients with transaortic peak systolic pressure gradients (psg) of 51 to 100 mm Hg to 17 patients with gradients >100 mm Hg in isolated severe aortic valve stenosis

LV-SA psg (mm Hg)	51-100 (n = 33)	>100 (n = 17)	p value
Age (years)	16-65 (50)	18-63 (46)	ns
Male:female (pts)	28:5	8:9	< 0.005
Angina pectoris (pts)	24 (73%)	10 (59%)	ns
LV-SA psg (mm Hg)	52-100 (82)	105-180 (135)	< 0.0005
LVSP (mm Hg)	149-255 (198)	192-270 (234)	< 0.0005
Aortic valve areas (cm²)	0.30-0.67 (0.54)	0.28-0.89 (0.50)	ns
CI (L/min/m²)	1.3-4.3 (2.49)	2.0-4.5 (2.79)	ns
Heart weight (gm)	380-880 (583)	400-770 (612)	ns
CA narrowing > 75% (pts)	12 (36%)	4 (23%)	ns
LV scar (pts)	6 (18%)	1 (6%)	ns
Electrocardiogram			
VPC (pts)	6 (18%)	1 (6%)	ns
LAD (pts)	9 (27%)	3 (3%)	ns
MDP (pts)	15 (45%)	9 (53%)	ns
QRS amplitude (mm)			
12 leads	144-417 (244)	216-370 (281)	< 0.05
I-III	12-78 (37)	25-58 (41)	ns

Abbreviations as in Table III.

Table VI. Comparison of 22 patients with peak left ventricular systolic pressure (LVSP) ≤ 200 mm Hg to 28 patients with LVSP > 200 mm Hg in isolated severe aortic valve stenosis

LVSP (mm Hg)	≤200 (n = 22)	>200 (n = 28)	p value
Age (years)	18-65 (49)	16-64 (48)	ns
Male:female (pts)	19:3	17:11	ns
Angina pectoris (pts)	14 (64%)	20 (71%)	ns
LV-SA psg (mm Hg)	52-129 (80)	60-180 (112)	< 0.0005
LVSP (mm Hg)	149-200 (185)	202-270 (230)	< 0.0005
Aortic valve areas (cm²)	0.3-0.7 (0.54)	0.2-0.9 (0.51)	ns
CI (L/min/m²)	1.3-3.7 (2.49)	1.8-4.5 (2.68)	ns
Heart weight (gm)	410-880 (613)	380-880 (600)	ns
CA narrowing > 75% (pts)	8 (36%)	8 (29%)	ns
LV scar (pts)	4 (18%)	3 (11%)	ns
Electrocardiogram	3 (14%)	4 (14%)	ns
VPC (pts)			
LAD (pts)	7 (32%)	5 (18%)	ns
MDP (pts)	11 (50%)	13 (46%)	ns
QRS amplitude (mm)			
12 leads	144-417 (247)	193-395 (265)	< 0.05
I-III	12-78 (38)	20-58 (39)	ns

Abbreviations as in Table III.

weights than the 16 patients without (580 gm vs 661 gm) ($p < 0.025$), more frequent ventricular premature complexes recorded (7 of 34 vs 0 of 16) ($p < 0.05$), less frequent occurrence of LAD (3 of 34 vs 9 of 16) ($p < 0.0005$), and higher QRS amplitude in leads I to III (42 mm vs 32 mm) ($p < 0.005$) (Table VIII). Compared to the 34 patients with lesser degrees of coronary narrowing, the 16 patients with > 75% cross-sectional area coronary narrowing by atherosclerotic plaques of one or more of the four major (right, left main, left anterior descending, left circumflex) epicardial coronary arteries were older (54 years vs 46 years) ($p < 0.01$), had higher frequency of LV scars at necropsy (31% vs 6%) ($p < 0.01$), ECG myocardial damage patterns (81% vs 32%) ($p < 0.025$), and lower total 12-lead QRS amplitude (238 mm vs 270 mm) ($p < 0.05$) (Table IX). No significant differences occurred in the amount of ST segment depression or the depth of T wave inversion between patients with and without significant coronary narrowing. Compared to the 43 patients without, the seven patients with grossly visible LV scars were older (53 years vs 47 years) ($p < 0.05$), had lower average peak systolic gradients across the

Table VII. Comparison of 28 patients with heart weight ≤600 gm to 22 patients with larger hearts in isolated severe aortic valve stenosis

Heart weight (gm)	≤600 (n = 28)	>600 (n = 22)	p value
Age (years)	16-65 (49)	31-64 (48)	ns
Male:female (pts)	16:12	20:2	< 0.025
Angina pectoris (pts)	21 (75%)	13 (59%)	ns
LV-SA psg (mm Hg)	52-180 (97)	52-160 (99)	ns
LVSP (mm Hg)	149-270 (214)	155-255 (250)	< 0.05
Aortic valve areas (cm²)	0.28-0.89 (0.28)	0.4-0.68 (0.32)	ns
CI (L/min/m²)	1.28-4.5 (2.74)	1.8-3.2 (2.46)	ns
Heart weight (gm)	380-600 (517)	610-880 (719)	< 0.0005
CA narrowing > 75% (pts)	10 (36%)	6 (27%)	ns
LV scar (pts)	3 (11%)	4 (18%)	ns
Electrocardiogram			
VPC (pts)	3 (11%)	4 (18%)	ns
LAD (pts)	3 (11%)	9 (41%)	< 0.01
MDP (pts)	16 (57%)	8 (36%)	ns
QRS amplitude (mm)			
12 leads	144-376 (244)	200-417 (274)	< 0.025
I-III	12-72 (39)	21-78 (39)	ns

Abbreviations as in Table III.

Table VIII. Comparison of 34 angina patients to 16 patients without angina in isolated severe aortic valve stenosis

Angina pectoris	Present (n = 34)	Absent (n = 16)	p value
Age (years)	18-65 (50)	16-63 (45)	ns
Male:female (pts)	27:7	9:7	ns
LV-SA psg (mm Hg)	52-180 (97)	70-153 (99)	ns
LVSP (mm Hg)	149-270 (212)	175-255 (203)	ns
Aortic valve areas (cm²)	0.16-0.89 (0.54)	0.30-0.77 (0.05)	ns
CI (L/min/m²)	1.8-4.7 (2.7)	1.2-4.3 (2.5)	ns
Heart weight (gm)	380-840 (580)	410-880 (661)	< 0.025
CA narrowing > 75% (pts)	12 (35%)	4 (25%)	ns
LV scar (pts)	6 (18%)	1 (6%)	ns
Electrocardiogram			
VPC (pts)	7 (21%)	0	< 0.05
LAD (pts)	3 (9%)	9 (56%)	< 0.0005
MDP (pts)	14 (41%)	10 (62%)	ns
QRS amplitude (mm)			
12 leads	144-417 (265)	162-395 (242)	ns
I-III	19-78 (42)	12-50 (32)	< 0.005

Abbreviations as in Table III.

aortic valve (77 mm Hg vs 101 mm Hg) ($p < 0.025$), and more frequent CAD (6 of 7 vs 9 of 43) ($p < 0.001$) (Table X).

Correlation of ECG myocardial damage pattern, QRS amplitude, AF and LBBB to clinical, hemodynamic, ECG, and necropsy findings. Excluding the four patients with LBBB, the mean total 12-lead QRS amplitude was lower in the 24 patients with ECG myocardial damage patterns than in the 24 patients without (243 mm vs 269 mm) ($p < 0.05$) (Table XI). Compared to the 26 patients with total 12-lead QRS amplitude ≤ 250 mm, the 24 patients in whom this amplitude was > 250 mm had a higher frequency of angina pectoris (79% vs 58%) ($p < 0.001$) and a

lower frequency of ECG myocardial damage patterns (33% vs 58%) ($p < 0.01$) (Table XII).

The five patients (four men) with *atrial fibrillation* (AF) ranged in age from 45 to 63 years (mean 53) and the peak systolic pressure gradients across their aortic valves, from 52 to 140 mm Hg (average 75). Three had LAD, three had ventricular premature complexes, and three had ECG myocardial damage patterns (poor R wave progression in precordial leads). The total 12-lead QRS amplitude ranged from 199 to 306 mm (mean 245), and in the other 33 patients over age 40 years with sinus rhythm it averaged 259 mm. The QRS amplitude in leads I to III ranged from 21 to 51 mm (mean 31).

Table IX. Comparison of 15 patients with severe coronary narrowing to 35 patients without CAD in isolated severe aortic valve stenosis

Coronary narrowing	≤75% (n = 16)	>75% (n = 34)	p value
Age (years)	16-65 (46)	41-64 (54)	< 0.01
Male:female (pts)	24:10	12:4	ns
Angina pectoris (pts)	23 (68%)	11 (69%)	ns
LV-SA psg (mm Hg)	52-180 (99)	60-145 (95)	ns
LVSP (mm Hg)	145-270 (209)	149-260 (208)	ns
Aortic valve areas (cm²)	0.28-0.89 (0.47)	0.33-0.77 (0.44)	ns
CI (L/min/m²)	1.28-4.5 (2.7)	1.8-3.2 (2.5)	ns
Heart weight (gm)	380-880 (602)	450-840 (615)	ns
LV scar (pts)	2 (6%)	5 (31%)	< 0.01
Electrocardiogram			
VPC (pts)	6 (18%)	1 (6%)	ns
LAD (pts)	9 (26%)	3 (19%)	ns
MDP (pts)	11 (32%)	13 (81%)	< 0.025
QRS amplitude (mm)			
12 leads	144-329 (270)	162-417 (238)	< 0.05
I-III	12-78 (35)	19-57 (41)	ns
ST segment depression*	0-0.4 (0.17)	0-0.2 (0.13)	ns
T wave inversion depth*	0-13 (4.9)	0-6 (3.8)	ns

*Excludes patients with complete bundle branch block.
Abbreviations as in Table III.

Table X. Comparison of seven patients with grossly visible left ventricular scars to 43 patients without scar in isolated severe aortic valve stenosis

LV scar	Present (n = 7)	Absent (n = 43)	p value
Age (years)	16-65 (47)	41-64 (53)	< 0.05
Male:female (pts)	6:1	30:13	ns
Angina pectoris (pts)	6	28 (65%)	ns
LV-SA psg (mm Hg)	52-111 (77)	52-180 (101)	< 0.025
LVSP (mm Hg)	149-240 (196)	175-270 (212)	ns
Aortic valve areas (cm²)	0.52-0.68 (0.60)	0.16-0.89 (0.50)	ns
CI (L/min/m²)	1.8-2.6 (2.2)	1.3-4.5 (2.3)	ns
Heart weight (gm)	450-840 (646)	380-880 (599)	ns
CA narrowing >75% (pts)	6	9 (21%)	< 0.001
Electrocardiogram			
VPC (pts)	2	5 (12%)	ns
LAD (pts)	2	13 (30%)	ns
MDP (pts)	5	19 (44%)	ns
QRS amplitude (mm)			
12 leads	144-417 (259)	162-395 (257)	ns
I-III	19-78 (37)	12-72 (39)	ns

Abbreviations as in Table III.

The hearts ranged in weight from 520 to 750 gm (mean 645). The aortic valves were tricuspid in four and bicuspid in one. Two of the five patients had one or more major coronary arteries narrowed > 75% in cross-sectional area by atherosclerotic plaques and one of them had a small transmural LV scar. Four patients had no grossly visible LV scarring.

The four patients with *complete LBBB* were aged 19 to 56 years (mean 42); three were over age 40 years. Two were women and two were men. All four had sinus rhythm, three had LAD, one had prolonged PR interval, and two had LA abnormality. The peak systolic pressure gradients were 75, 75, 102, and 145 mm Hg (average 100) and the total 12-lead QRS amplitude was 256, 417, 376, and 216 mm (mean 316), respectively. In the other 46

Table XI. Comparison of 24 patients with myocardial damage pattern (in absence of bundle branch block) to 22 patients without in isolated severe aortic valve stenosis

Myocardial damage pattern	Present (n = 24)	Absent (n = 22)	p value
Age (years)	16-63 (48)	31-65 (50)	ns
Male:female (pts)	19:5	15:7	ns
Angina pectoris (pts)	14 (58%)	15 (68%)	ns
LV-SA psg (mm Hg)	52-180 (102)	52-160 (94)	ns
LVSP (mm Hg)	149-270 (213)	175-255 (209)	ns
Aortic valve areas (cm^2)	0.16-0.89 (0.58)	0.23-0.66 (0.52)	ns
CI (L/min/m^2)	1.28-4.5 (2.64)	2.8-3.6 (2.58)	ns
Heart weight (gm)	380-880 (590)	410-780 (621)	ns
CA narrowing >75% (pts)	12 (50%)	13 (59%)	ns
LV scar (pts)	5 (21%)	1 (4%)	ns
Electrocardiogram			
VPC (pts)	2 (8%)	4 (18%)	ns
LAD (pts)	6 (25%)	4 (18%)	ns
QRS amplitude (mm)			
12 leads	144-353 (236)	199-395 (269)	< 0.05
I-III	12-72 (37)	20-72 (39)	ns

Abbreviations as in Table III.

Table XII. Comparison of 26 patients with total (12-lead) QRS amplitude ≤250 to 24 patients with amplitude >250 mm in isolated severe aortic valve stenosis

Total QRS amplitude (mm)	≤250 (n = 26)	>250 (n = 24)	p value
Age (years)	32-63 (50)	16-65 (46)	ns
Male:female (pts)	20:6	16:8	ns
Angina pectoris (pts)	15 (58%)	19 (79%)	< 0.001
LV-SA psg (mm Hg)	52-158 (93)	52-180 (105)	ns
LVSP (mm Hg)	149-260 (205)	155-270 (215)	ns
Aortic valve areas (cm^2)	0.28-0.89 (0.54)	0.39-0.66 (0.51)	ns
CI (L/min/m^2)	1.3-4.5 (2.6)	1.8-4.2 (2.7)	ns
Heart weight (gm)	380-880 (595)	400-880 (614)	ns
CA narrowing >75% (pts)	10 (38%)	6 (25%)	ns
LV scar (pts)	3 (12%)	4 (17%)	ns
Electrocardiogram			
VPC (pts)	3 (12%)	4 (17%)	ns
LAD (pts)	7 (27%)	5 (21%)	ns
MDP (pts)	15 (58%)	8 (33%)	< 0.01
QRS amplitude (mm)			
12 leads	144-250 (207)	252-417 (305)	< 0.001
I-III	12-55 (42)	28-78 (46)	< 0.01

Abbreviations as in Table III.

patients in whom the QRS width was < 0.12 seconds, the 12-lead amplitude averaged 252 mm. The sum of the QRS amplitude in leads I to III in the four patients ranged from 36 to 51 mm (mean 42). The hearts ranged in weight from 400 to 880 gm (mean 615). The aortic valves were congenitally malformed in each. None had significant narrowing of any of the major epicardial coronary arteries, and only one had a LV scar which was small and subendocardial.

DISCUSSION

Initial substantive necropsy study of abnormal ECG correlations in hemodynamically documented isolated severe AS. Although there are many reports on ECG observations in patients with pressure overloaded left ventricles (systemic hypertension,[2-6] aortic valve stenosis,[4, 7-29] hypertrophic cardiomyopathy,[30, 31] and discrete subaortic stenosis[14]), virtually none have focused on necropsy patients in whom direct hemodynamic data were obtained shortly before death.

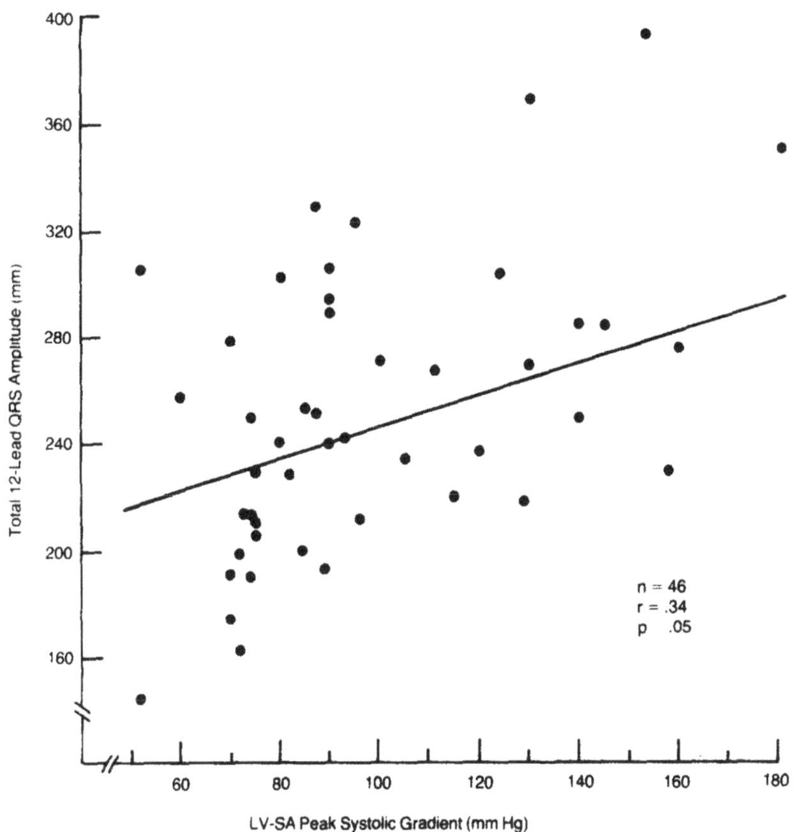

Fig. 2. Relation between the total 12-lead QRS amplitude (in mm) and the peak left ventricular *(LV)* systemic arterial *(SA)* pressure gradient in 46 necropsy patients with aortic valve stenosis without bundle branch block.

All 50 patients included herein had isolated AS, i.e., anatomically normal tricuspid, pulmonic, and mitral valves, with peak systolic pressure gradients between LV and a systemic artery of > 50 mm Hg (average = 98) and all had necropsy examination of the heart. Of the 15 parameters analyzed in each patient (Tables III to XII), 10 were further analyzed to compare patients with to those without, or those with greater than to those with less than a certain figure. Of these 10 categories in which the 15 parameters were compared, excluding the factor analysed, 33 (22%) of the 150 were significantly ($p < 0.05$) different between the two groups.

Total 12-lead QRS amplitude best single predictor of most marked AS without CAD in young adult males in severe AS patients. Of the 15 parameters analyzed, the one most often showing significant differences between the 10 groups compared was total 12-lead QRS amplitude. The mean of the total 12-lead QRS amplitude was significantly greater in the younger (≤ 40 years) than in the older patients (278 mm vs 257 mm); in the women than in the men (277 mm vs 249 mm), in the patients with higher (> 100 mm Hg) peak systolic pressure gradients across the aortic

valve (281 mm vs 244 mm); in the patients with heavier (> 600 gm) hearts (274 mm vs 244 mm); in the patients without versus those with significant CAD (270 mm vs 238 mm), and in those without compared to those with ECG myocardial damage patterns (269 mm vs 236 mm). Although the mean values of the total QRS amplitude were significantly different between these six groups, comparison of patients with total 12-lead QRS amplitude of ≤ 250 mm to those with higher amplitude disclosed the frequency of angina pectoris and of ECG myocardial damage patterns to be the only factors significantly different. Although the mean values of the total 12-lead QRS amplitude was not significantly different in the groups of patients with and without angina pectoris, the sum of the QRS amplitude in leads I, II, and III was significantly greater in the patients with compared to those without angina (42 mm vs 32 mm). In contrast to the significant mean differences between total 12-lead QRS amplitude in 6 of the 10 groups compared and in QRS amplitude in leads I to III in 2 of the 10 groups compared, the frequency of the usual ECG criteria of LVH was similar in all 10 groups compared because all but 2 of

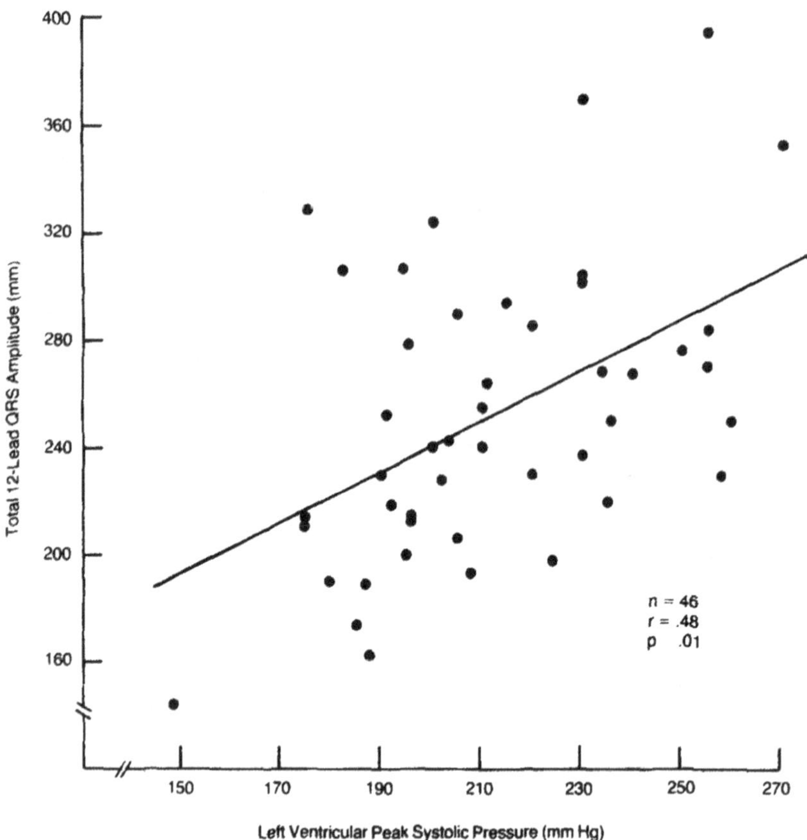

Fig. 3. Relation between the total 12-lead QRS amplitude (in mm) and the left ventricular peak systolic pressure (in mm Hg) in 46 necropsy patients with aortic valve stenosis without bundle branch block.

the 46 patients without LBBB had LVH by ECG utilizing common criteria.[1]

Total QRS amplitude (peak LV systolic pressure) minus peak systolic systemic arterial pressure implies peak systolic transaortic pressure gradient in severe AS patients. Using regression analysis, the total 12-lead QRS amplitude correlated directly with the peak systolic pressure gradient across the aortic valve ($p < 0.05$, $r = 0.31$) and when the four patients with LBBB were excluded, this correlation improved ($r = 0.34$) (Fig. 2). When the four patients with LBBB were excluded, the total 12-lead QRS amplitude correlated directly with the LV peak systolic pressure ($p < 0.01$, $r = 0.48$) (Fig. 3). Indeed, the LV systolic pressure (in mm Hg) was generally similar to the total 12-lead QRS amplitude (in mm) (Fig. 4). Thus measurement of the total 12-lead amplitude (in mm) appears to allow a reasonable prediction of LV systolic pressure and subtraction of the systemic arterial systolic pressure from the total 12-lead amplitude (in mm) appears to provide a reasonable noninvasive means of predicting the peak systolic pressure gradient across the aortic valve among patients with moderate to severe AS and without LBBB (Fig. 4).

We found no previous reports describing amplitude of the QRS complexes in all 12 precordial leads in patients with AS. Simonson,[32] however, has provided data on the upper and lower limits of amplitude of the QRS complexes in each of the 12 leads in normal men and women aged 20 to 59 years. (The mean for the normals is not available.) The upper and lower limits of normal for men aged 50 to 59 years was 277 and 36 mm, and for the women 248 and 27 mm, respectively. The upper and lower limits of amplitude in all 12 leads in our 50 patients with AS was 417 and 144 mm, respectively, and averaged 260 mm. For the 36 men in our study, the total QRS voltage (all 12 leads) averaged 249 mm and for the 14 women, 277 mm.

Only three other ECG findings differed significantly between any of the 10 groups analyzed. LAD occurred in 3 (11%) of the 28 patients with hearts weighing < 600 gm and in 9 (41%) of the 22 patients with larger hearts ($p < 0.01$). Additionally, LAD occurred in 9 (56%) of the 16 patients without angina pectoris and in only 3 (9%) of the 34 patients with angina ($p < 0.0005$). Ventricular premature complexes were recorded on routine ECG in 7 (20%) of the 34 patients with angina and in none of the 16

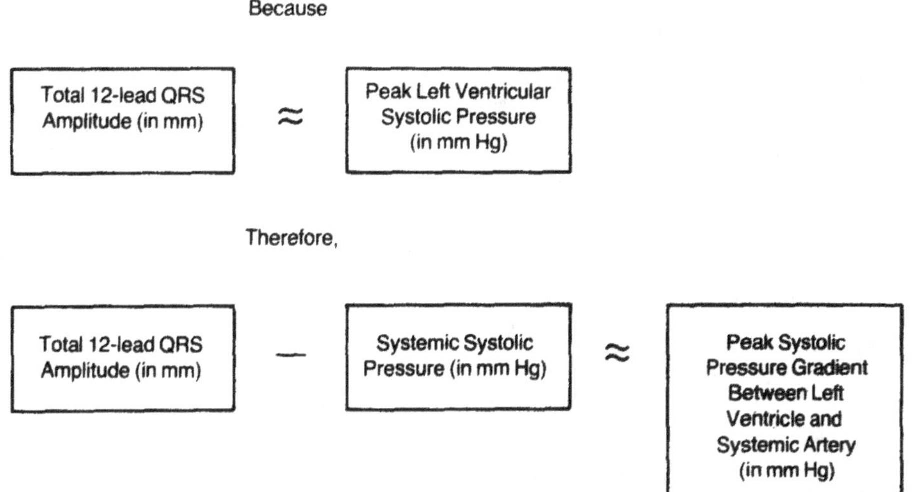

Fig. 4. Usefulness of measuring the total 12-lead QRS amplitude in predicting left ventricular–systemic arterial pressure gradient in valvular aortic stenosis unassociated with bundle branch block.

patients without angina ($p > 0.05$). Finally, ECG myocardial damage patterns were significantly more frequent in the 16 patients with CAD at necropsy compared to the 34 patients without (81% vs 32%) ($p < 0.025$). The frequency of myocardial ischemic changes (ST segment depression and depth of T wave inversion) was not significantly different in the patients with and without coronary narrowing.

Concomitant CAD suggested by ECG myocardial damage patterns and less increased QRS amplitude in older adults, but not by angina. Certain factors did suggest the presence of significant ($> 75\%$ in cross-sectional area) CAD. All 16 patients with narrowing of one or more major coronary arteries were over 40 years of age (mean 54); it occurred in 16 (41%) of the 39 patients over age 40 years and in none of the 11 aged 40 years or under. ECG myocardial damage patterns occurred in 13 (81%) of the 16 patients with CAD and in 11 (32%) of the 34 patients without significant narrowing. The patients with CAD also had lower total amplitude of QRS complexes in the 12 leads compared to those without coronary narrowing (238 mm vs 270 mm) and also a much higher frequency of grossly visible myocardial scarring: in 5 (31%) of the 16 patients with CAD and in 2 (6%) of the 34 patients without CAD ($p < 0.001$). As demonstrated by others,[33-37] the frequency of angina pectoris was similar in the patients with and without significant CAD (69% and 68%).

The presence of grossly visible LV scars did not alter the ECG finding in our patients with AS. All seven with scars, however, were among the 39 patients over age 40 years (mean 53), six of the seven had significantly ($> 75\%$) narrowed coronary arteries ($p < 0.001$) and the average peak transaortic gradient in the seven patients with compared to the 43 patients without scars was smaller (77 mm Hg vs 101 mm Hg) ($p < 0.025$).

REFERENCES

1. Romhilt DW, Estes EH: A point-score system for the ECG diagnosis of left ventricular hypertrophy. Am Heart J **75**:752, 1968.
2. Sokolow M, Lyon TP: The ventricular complex in left ventricular hypertrophy as obtained by unipolar precordial and limb leads. Am Heart J **37**:161, 1949.
3. Sannersdedt R, Bjure J, Varnauskas E: Correlation between electrocardiographic changes and systemic hemodynamics in human arterial hypertension. Am J Cardiol **26**:117, 1970.
4. Kini PM, Eddelman EE, Pipberger HV: Electrocardiographic differentiation between left ventricular hypertrophy and anterior myocardial infarction. Circulation **42**:875, 1970.
5. McCaughan D, Littmann D, Pipberger HV: Computer analysis of the orthogonal electrocardiogram and vectorcardiogram in 939 cases with hypertensive cardiovascular disease. Am Heart J **85**:467, 1973.
6. Toshima H, Koga Y, Kimura N: Correlations between electrocardiographic, vectorcardiographic, and echocardiographic findings in patients with left ventricular overload. Am Heart J **94**:547, 1977.
7. Mitchell AM, Sackett CH, Hunzicker WJ, Levine SA: The clinical features of aortic stenosis. Am Heart J **48**:684, 1954.
8. Bergeron J, Abelmann WH, Vazquez-Milan H, Ellis LB: Aortic stenosis—clinical manifestations and course of the disease. Review of one hundred proved cases. Arch Intern Med **94**:911, 1954.
9. Wood P: Aortic stenosis. Am J Cardiol **1**:553, 1958.
10. Hancock EW, Fleming PR: Aortic stenosis. Q J Med **29**:209, 1960.
11. Reynolds JL, Nadas AS, Rudolph AM, Gross RE: Critical congenital aortic stenosis with minimal electrocardiographic changes. N Engl J Med **262**:276, 1960.
12. Björk VO, Cullhed I, Lodin H: Aortic stenosis. Correlations between pressure gradient and left ventricular angiography. Circulation **23**:509, 1961.
13. Hugenholtz PG, Lee MM, Nadas AS: The scalar electrocardiogram, vectorcardiogram, and exercise electrocardiogram in the assessment of congenital aortic stenosis. Circulation **26**:79, 1962.

14. Braunwald E, Goldblatt A, Aygen MM, Rockoff SD, Morrow AG: Congenital aortic stenosis. I. Clinical and hemodynamic findings in 100 patients. Circulation **27**:426, 1963.

15. Morris JJ Jr, Estes WH Jr, Whalen RE, Thompson HK Jr, McIntosh HD: P-wave analysis in valvular heart disease. Circulation **27**:242, 1964.

16. Cullhed I: Aortic stenosis. A clinical study of aortic stenosis, isolated or combined with aortic insufficiency, with special reference to hemodynamic and angiographic observations. Stockholm, 1964, Alxqvist & Wiksell, pp 154.

17. Gamboa R, Hugenholtz PG, Nadas AS: Comparison of electrocardiograms and vectorcardiograms in congenital aortic stenosis. Br Heart J **27**:344, 1965.

18. Fowler RS: Ventricular repolarization in congenital aortic stenosis. AM HEART J **70**:603, 1965.

19. Gooch AS, Calatayud JB, Rogers JB, Corman PA: Analysis of the P wave in severe aortic stenosis. Dis Chest **49**:459, 1966.

20. Myler RK, Sanders CA: Aortic valve disease and atrial fibrillation. Report of 122 patients with electrographic, radiographic, and hemodynamic observations. Arch Intern Med **121**:530, 1968.

21. Postell WN, Rainey RL, Witham, AC, Edmonds JH Jr: Vectorcardiographic and electrocardiographic manifestations of increasing left ventricular pressure overload. AM HEART J **77**:33, 1969.

22. Holt JH Jr, Barnard ACL, Lynn MS: A study of the human heart as a multiple dipole electrical source. II. Diagnosis and quantitation of left ventricular hypertrophy. Circulation **40**:697, 1969.

23. Hilsenrath J, Hamby RI, Glassman E, Hollman I: Pitfalls in prediction of coronary arterial obstruction from patterns of anterior infarction on electrocardiogram and vectorcardiogram. Am J Cardiol **29**:164, 1972.

24. Kornreich F, Brismee D: II. Diagnosis of left ventricular hypertrophy and myocardial infarction from "total" surface waveform information. Circulation **48**:996, 1973.

25. Bennett DH, Evans DW: Correlation of left ventricular mass determined by echocardiography with vectorcardiographic and electrocardiographic voltage measurements. Br Heart J **36**:981, 1974.

26. Dhingra RC, Amat-y-Leon F, Pietras RJ, Wyndham C, Deedwania PC, Wu D, Denes P, Rosen KM: Sites of conduction disease in aortic stenosis. Significance of valve gradient and calcification. Ann Intern Med **87**:275, 1977.

27. Yankopoulos NA, Haisty W, Pipberger HV: Computer analysis of the orthogonal electrocardiogram and vectorcardiogram in 257 patients with aortic valve disease. Am J Cardiol **40**:707, 1977.

28. Friedman HS, Zaman Q, Haft JI, Melendez S: Assessment of atrioventricular conduction in aortic valve disease. Br Heart J **40**:911, 1978.

29. Thompson R, Mitchell A, Ahmed M, Towers M, Yacoub M: Conduction defects in aortic valve disease. AM HEART J **98**:3, 1979.

30. Estes EH Jr, Whalen RE, Roberts SR Jr, McIntosh HD: The electrocardiographic and vectorcardiographic findings in idiopathic hypertrophic subaortic stenosis. AM HEART J **65**:155, 1963.

31. Savage DD, Seides SF, Clark CE, Henry WL, Maron BJ, Robinson FC, Epstein SE: Electrocardiographic findings in patients with obstructive and nonobstructive hypertrophic cardiomyopathy. Circulation **58**:402, 1978.

32. Simonson F: Differentiation between normal and abnormal in electrocardiography. St. Louis, Mo, 1961, The CV Mosby Co, p 328.

33. Moraski RE, Russell RO Jr, Mantle JA, Rackley CE: Aortic stenosis, angina pectoris, coronary artery disease. Cathet Cardiovasc Diagn **2**:157, 1976.

34. Paquay PA, Anderson G, Diefenthal H, Nordstrom L, Richman HG, Gobel FL: Chest pain as a predictor of coronary artery disease in patients with obstructive aortic valve disease. Am J Cardiol **38**:863, 1976.

35. Graboys TB, Cohn PF: The prevalence of angina pectoris and abnormal coronary arteriograms in severe aortic valvular disease. AM HEART J **93**:683, 1977.

36. Miller DC, Stinson EB, Oyer PE, Rossiter SJ, Reitz BA, Shumway NE: Surgical implications and results of combined aortic valve replacement and myocardial revascularization. Am J Cardiol **43**:494, 1979.

37. Storstein O, Enge I: Angina pectoris in aortic valvular disease and its relation to coronary pathology. Acta Med Scand **205**:275, 1979.

Cardiac Amyloidosis Causing Cardiac Dysfunction: Analysis of 54 Necropsy Patients

WILLIAM C. ROBERTS, MD and BRUCE F. WALLER, MD

Clinical and morphologic findings are described in 54 necropsy patients (32 men [59%]) aged 21 to 97 years (mean 64) with cardiac amyloid deposits extensive enough to cause fatal cardiac dysfunction. Chronic congestive heart failure (CHF) was present in 46 (85%). The duration of CHF, known in 39 patients, ranged from 1 to 108 months (mean 18) and lasted ≤12 months in 25 patients (64%). All 8 patients without CHF died suddenly and unexpectedly. Systemic arterial pressures were recorded in the last 3 months of life in 43 patients: the peak indirect systolic pressure was ≤130 mm Hg and the diastolic pressure <90 mm Hg in all. Electrocardiograms, recorded in the last 6 months of life in 40 patients, were abnormal in each: low voltage in 35 (63%); "myocardial infarction pattern" in 33 (83%); abnormal QRS axis in 29 (73%); arrhythmias in 29 (73%); first, second, or third degree heart block in 28 (45%); and complete bundle branch block in 7 (18%). In 30 patients, the QRS amplitude in all 12 leads was measured: in the 15 men it ranged from 60 to 197 mm (mean 99) (10 mm = 1 mV) and in the 15 women from 58 to 199 mm (mean 109). Diagnosis of amyloidosis was established by biopsy of noncardiac organs or tissues during life in only 18 (33%) patients. During life the condition simulated hypertrophic cardiomyopathy in 5 patients, constrictive pericardial disease in 3, and coronary heart disease (because of angina pectoris) in 4.

At necropsy, the hearts ranged in weight from 300 to 900 g (mean 554), and all but 1 had a "rubbery," noncompliant consistency. In addition to their presence in myocardial interstitium (53 patients) and in intramural coronary arteries (54 patients), amyloid deposits were present grossly in mural endocardium in all 54 patients and in valvular endocardium in 46 (85%). The cardiac ventricles were not dilated in 43 patients (80%), but both atria were dilated in all 54 patients. Intracardiac thrombi were present in 14 patients (26%). Cardiac amyloidosis must be considered in any elderly patient with chronic CHF unassociated with chest pain when blood pressure is normal and the electrocardiogram discloses low voltage and a pattern of "healed myocardial infarction."

In 1970, clinical and necropsy findings in 15 patients with cardiac dysfunction secondary to cardiac amyloidosis were reported from this laboratory.[1] During the past 13 years we have studied at necropsy an additional 39 patients with fatal cardiac amyloidosis. This report summarizes clinical and morphologic findings in these 54 patients with cardiac amyloid deposits extensive enough to cause cardiac dysfunction, with particular emphasis on electrocardiographic observations.

Patients Studied and Findings

Clinical findings: The 54 patients ranged in age at death from 21 to 97 years (mean 64). The 32 men (59%) ranged in age from 32 to 97 years (mean 65) and the 22 women (41%) from 21 to 93 years (mean 62) (Fig. 1). Thirty-eight (70%) were white and 16 (30%) were black. Of the 54 patients, 46 (85%) had clinical evidence of congestive heart failure (CHF) at some time. The duration of CHF was discernible in 39 of the 46 patients and ranged from 1 to 108 months (mean 18): for ≤12 months in 25 patients (64%), from >12 to 24 months in 6 patients (15%), from >24 to 36 months in 3 patients (8%), and from 60 to 108 months (mean 82) in 5 patients (13%). The duration of CHF in 18 women ranged from 1 to 72 months (mean 18) and in 25 men from 2 to 108 months (mean 22). Each of the 8 patients (15%) without clinical evidence of CHF died suddenly and unexpectedly: in 3 sudden death was the first evidence of amyloidosis, 2 had familial amyloidosis, 2 had multiple myeloma, and 1 clinically had presumed alcoholic cirrhosis (which at necropsy actually was massive hepatic amyloid infiltration). The 8 patients dying suddenly without ever having clinical evidence of CHF ranged in age from 21 to 88 years (mean 56) and the 46 patients with CHF from 32 to 97 years (mean 65). Chest pain was present at some time during amyloid illness in 8 patients (15%), 4 of whom were considered to have angina pectoris.[2,3] Of the 4 patients (aged

From the Pathology Branch, National Heart, Lung, and Blood Institute, National Institutes of Health, Bethesda, Maryland. Manuscript received and accepted April 12, 1983.

Address for reprints: William C. Roberts, MD, Building 10A, Room 3E30, National Institutes of Health, Bethesda, Maryland 20205.

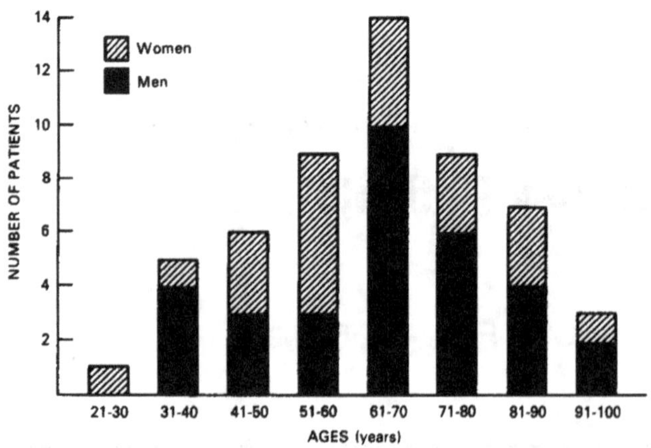

FIGURE 1. Age and sex distribution in the 54 necropsy patients with cardiac amyloidosis extensive enough to cause cardiac dysfunction.

67 to 89 years [mean 80]) with angina, 2 at necropsy had 1 or more of the 4 major (right, left main, left anterior descending, and left circumflex) epicardial coronary arteries narrowed 76 to 100% in cross-sectional area by atherosclerotic plaques.

Seven patients (13%) had histories of illnesses considered compatible with acute myocardial infarction that healed, but electrocardiographic and enzymatic documentation of myocardial necrosis at the time was unavailable. Grossly visible left ventricular scars, however, were absent at necropsy in all 7 patients, indicating that the histories of acute myocardial infarction in them were fallacious.

Four patients (7%) had 1 or more episodes of syncope. One patient was among the 4 with familial amyloidosis with peripheral neuropathy and postural hypotension. The mechanism of the syncope in the other 3 patients was not determined.

Systemic arterial pressure recordings during the last 3 months of life were available in 43 (80%) of the 54 patients. Although 24 (44%) of the 54 patients had a history of "hypertension," in none of the 43 patients (including the 24) with indirect blood pressure recordings available during the last 3 months of life was the systolic pressure >130 mm Hg or the diastolic pressure >90 mm Hg. The range of systolic arterial

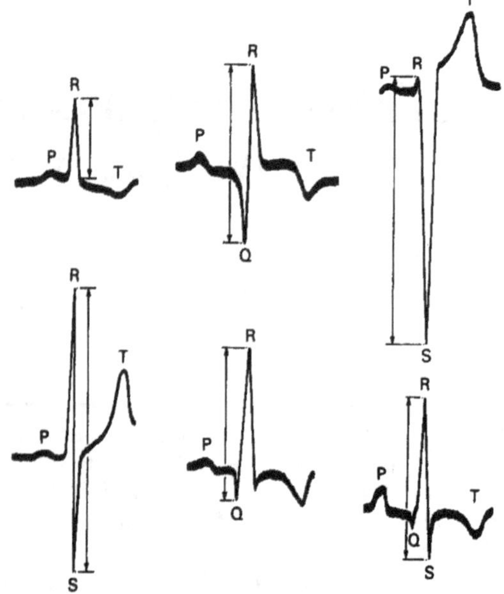

FIGURE 2. Various QRS complexes showing how each was measured.

pressures during the last 3 months of life was 80 to 130 mm Hg (average 102) and of diastolic pressures 40 to 90 mm Hg (average 66).

The cardiac silhouette was enlarged on chest roentgenogram during the last few months of life in 39 (72%) of 54 patients. In several patients, however, earlier radiographs had shown the cardiac silhouette to be of normal size.

Adequate information on precordial examinations during the last few months of life was available in 44 of the 54 patients, 36 (82%) of whom had precordial murmurs. They were of a blowing type and consistent with mitral or tricuspid regurgitation, or both, in 35 (97%): grade 1 to 2/6 in 26, grade 3/6 in 7, and grade 4/6 in 2 patients. In addition, 1 patient had a murmur typical of valvular aortic stenosis (grade 3/6), which was confirmed to be present and was the type typically observed in the elderly.[4] At least 22 patients had third heart sounds (S_3) and at least 8 patients had fourth heart sounds (S_4).

Reports of 1 or more electrocardiograms recorded in the last 6 months of life were available in 40 patients, and all were abnormal (Table I). Of the 40 patients, electrocardiograms, recorded 0 to 160 days (mean 41) before death, were available for reexamination in 30 (Table II). In each of these 30 patients (15 women and 15 men), the QRS amplitude in all 12 leads was measured (Fig. 2). The total 12-lead QRS amplitude in the 15 men (mean age 52 years) ranged from 60 to 197 mm (mean 99) (10 mm = 1 mV) and in the 15 women (mean age 65 years) from 58 to 199 mm (mean 109). The heart weights in the 15 men ranged from 410 to 750 g (mean 570), and in the 15 women from 370 to 900 g (mean (494) (p <0.01). Some electrocardiograms are illustrated in Figures 3 to 6.

Information regarding digitalis therapy was available in 40 patients, and 31 of them received this drug. At least 12 (39%) of the 31 patients developed physical or electrical signs, or both, considered typical of digitalis toxicity.

M-mode echocardiograms were performed in the last few months of life in 11 patients. The findings are summarized in Table III and illustrated in Figures 6 and 7.

Cardiac catheterization was performed in the last few months of life in 10 patients (19%), and the findings are summarized in Table IV.

TABLE I Cardiac Amyloid Causing Cardiac Dysfunction: Electrocardiographic Observations in 40 Patients*

Abnormality [No. (%)]	No. of Patients (%)
1. Low voltage (QRS ≤ 15 mm in I + II + III)	25 (63)
2. Myocardial infarct pattern	33 (83)
Anterior = 26 (79)	
Posterior = 2 (6)	
Both = 5 (15)	
3. Abnormal QRS axis	29 (73)
Right (+111 to +210°) = 6 (21)	
Left (−30 to −90°) = 23 (79)	
4. Arrhythmias	29 (73)
Atrial fibrillation = 9 (31)	
Atrial or junctional tachycardia = 10 (34)	
Ventricular premature complexes = 21 (72)	
5. Heart block	18 (45)
P-R interval >0.20 = 9 (50)	
2° AV block = 4 (22)	
3° AV block = 5 (28)	
6. Complete bundle branch block (QRS ≥0.12)	7 (18)
Right = 5	
Left = 2	

AV = atrioventricular.
* Numbers in parentheses represent percentages.

Of the 54 patients, the amyloidosis was primary in 42 (78%), associated with multiple myeloma in 7 (13%), and familial in 5 (9%). None of the 54 patients had "secondary" amyloidosis.

Diagnosis of amyloidosis was established by biopsy of noncardiac organs or tissues during life in 18 patients (33%), including 5 of the 8 patients without and in 13 (28%) of the 46 patients with chronic CHF. Of the 21 patients having undergone biopsy of noncardiac organs or tissues, findings in 18 were positive for amyloid: rectum, 6 of 6; gingiva, 3 of 4; liver, 3 of 3; tongue, 2 of 3; kidney, 1 of 2; and each of prostate gland, thyroid gland, and lymph node, 1 of 1. In addition, endomyocardial biopsy of the right ventricular aspect of the ventricular septum was performed in 1 patient, but amyloid was not observed on histologic examination.

Of the 46 patients with chronic CHF, biopsy of a noncardiac organ or tissue was performed in 10 and all findings were positive for amyloid. In addition to these 10 patients, amyloidosis was considered the most likely cause of chronic CHF in 9 other patients. The cause of chronic CHF was never established during life in the remaining 27 patients (59%). Of the 11 patients having undergone M-mode echocardiography, the maximal thickness of the ventricular septum was greater than that of the left ventricular free wall in 5, and as a consequence hypertrophic cardiomyopathy was the suspected diagnosis clinically in each of them (Fig. 8 and 9). One of these 5 patients also had undergone cardiac catheterization, and hypertrophic cardiomyopathy continued to be the most likely clinical cardiac diagnosis after that procedure. Inability to differentiate clinically between constrictive pericardial disease and restrictive cardiomyopathy led to thoracotomy in 3 patients. At operation, all 3 had normal visceral and parietal pericardia and normal amounts of pericardial fluid. Each of these 3 patients died within 5 days of thoracotomy.

Eight patients had transient episodes of chest pain. In 4 the pain was consistent with angina pectoris, and a diagnosis of coronary heart disease was made in each. At necropsy, however, only 2 of the 4 patients had significant narrowing of an epicardial coronary artery by atherosclerotic plaque. Of the 4 patients with chest pain not consistent with myocardial ischemia, 1 had significant narrowing of 1 or more epicardial coronary arteries by atherosclerotic plaques. One of the latter 4 patients was 1 of the 3 with clinical pericardial constriction syndrome. The cause of chest pain in the other 2 was unclear. All 8 patients with chest pain had chronic CHF, and 2 had a history of acute myocardial infarction in the remote past. All 8 patients had luminal narrowing of many intramural coronary arteries by amyloid deposits.

Morphologic findings: The hearts in all 54 patients were examined initially by 1 of us (WCR), and 40 were reexamined together by both of us. Heart weights, available in 50 of the 54 patients, ranged from 300 to 900 g (mean 554). Of the 22 women, heart weights, available in 19, ranged from 300 to 900 g (mean 484) and 17 (89%) of the 19 weighed >350 g (a weight considered the upper limit of normal in adult women). Of the 32 men, heart weights (available in 31) ranged from 410 to 900 g (mean 596) and all 31 weighed >400 g (a weight considered the upper limit of normal in men).

TABLE II Electrocardiographic QRS Voltage (mm) in Each of 12 Leads in 15 Men and 15 Women With Cardiac Amyloidosis Causing Fatal Cardiac Dysfunction

Case	Necropsy Number	Age (yr) at Death	Interval (Days) ECG to Death	I	II	III	R	L	F	V₁	V₂	V₃	V₄	V₅	V₆	Total QRS 12-Lead	Heart Weight (g)
								Men									
1	A63-125	32	88	6	10	6	8	4	7	11	23	16	14	11	9	125	700
2	Vt. MCV A75-174	35	56	4	4	3	4	3	4	5	9	9	11	13	8	77	750
3	A65-159	38	10	2	4	6	2	5	6	5	19	11	6	9	7	82	410
4	A70-254	38	2	2	2	5	1	3	3	4	18	16	16	9	5	84	600
5	A79-25	45	2	5	4	8	2	6	6	12	27	21	22	30	15	158	780
6	A81-6	46	13	5	5	5	4	4	3	2	10	17	19	19	13	106	545
7	NNMC 80A-15	49	107	6	3	4	3	6	3	14	20	15	12	9	4	99	850
8	A60-19	54	0	4	4	1	4	3	3	10	10	3	10	8	5	65	550
9	A56-81	55	23	2	3	2	2	1	3	5	9	11	11	7	4	60	480
10	A61-190	55	2	2	4	5	3	4	5	3	15	14	12	12	6	85	535
11	GT 74A-259	62	9	2	3	3	2	2	3	1	6	23	21	11	2	79	470
12	A65-232	65	103	7	20	12	11	3	15	8	15	24	32	27	23	197	560
13	A69-187	68	5	5	5	7	3	6	6	13	16	11	9	8	6	95	550
14	A67-241	68	35	9	5	6	7	7	3	11	7	13	15	12	6	101	420
15	A66-151	69	59	4	3	5	3	5	4	7	10	11	8	5	4	69	450
Mean		52	34	4.3	5.3	5.2	3.9	4.1	4.9	7.4	14.3	14.3	14.5	12.7	7.8	99	570
								Women									
1	A65-25	21	58	5	5	5	5	5	3	11	28	30	16	10	12	135	530
2	A68-23	48	50	4	3	3	3	3	3	5	7	9	8	9	8	65	450
3	GT 80A-262	50	91	4	3	3	2	3	3	11	24	20	18	11	14	116	460
4	A68-277	53	15	3	2	3	1	3	3	6	10	10	10	4	3	58	370
5	HU A77-19	54	51	5	2	8	2	7	6	7	15	15	4	7	6	84	420
6	Wil., D. WMC A79-24	55	8	1	8	9	4	5	9	14	21	17	9	9	5	110	430
7	SH A81-47	61	0	2	6	6	5	3	6	6	19	21	16	9	8	107	385
8	GT 71A-67	67	76	8	8	8	7	6	7	7	19	18	17	14	8	127	650
9	GT 81A-90	70	42	3	4	2	3	1	3	3	11	14	9	8	7	68	485
10	GT 71A-435	72	70	5	14	12	9	6	12	3	4	12	24	12	8	121	480
11	SH A79-76	75	30	7	10	7	6	12	5	16	18	17	17	15	15	145	510
12	GT 79A-127	78	49	3	5	4	4	2	3	4	9	16	17	21	9	97	520
13	WHC A82-120	82	6	5	8	12	4	7	10	8	18	34	41	25	27	199	900
14	GT 79A-195	89	160	3	5	1	4	2	3	3	9	14	18	20	9	91	440
15	Sibley A80-99	93	3	10	6	12	5	10	10	9	10	11	14	14	6	117	380
Mean		65	47	4.5	5.9	6.3	4.3	5.0	5.7	7.5	14.8	17.2	15.8	12.5	9.7	109	494
Total (mean)		58	41	4.4	5.6	5.8	4.1	4.6	5.3	7.5	14.5	15.8	15.2	12.6	8.7	104	532

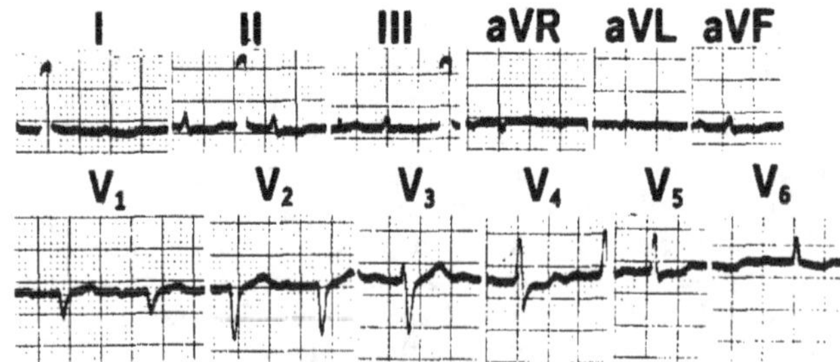

FIGURE 3. Electrocardiogram in a 55-year-old man (A56-81) recorded 23 days before death. The patient never had congestive heart failure. The heart weighed 480 g. The total 12-lead QRS voltage is only 60 mm. R waves are absent in leads V_1 and V_2 and small in V_3.

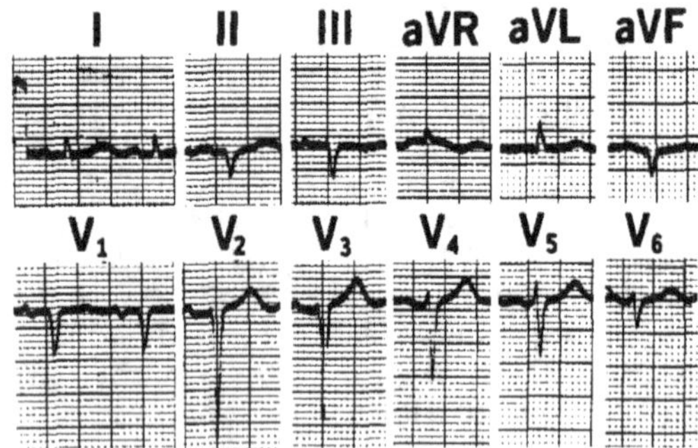

FIGURE 4. Electrocardiogram in a 55-year-old man (A61-190) recorded 2 days before death. The heart weighed 535 g and the total 12-lead QRS voltage is 85 mm. The voltage is decreased. The axis is leftward, Q waves are present in leads II, III, and aVF, and R waves are absent or small in the precordial leads.

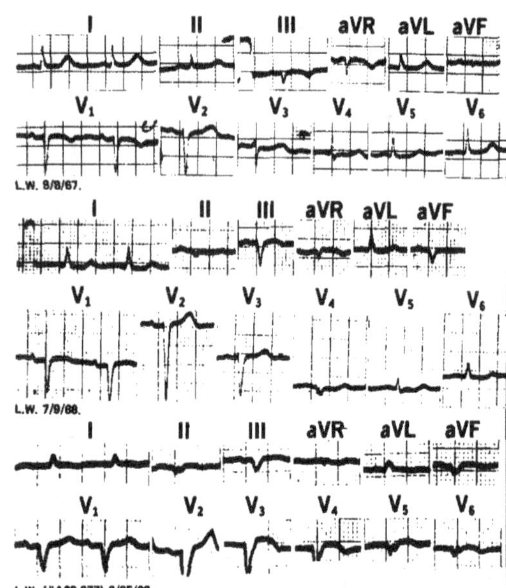

FIGURE 5. Electrocardiograms recorded over a 13-month period in a 53-year-old woman (A68-277) who had congestive heart failure for 5 months. The heart weighed 370 g. She died October 9, 1968. She had low voltage, left axis deviation, and absent R waves in the precordium. On the final electrocardiogram, the total 12-lead QRS voltage is 58 mm.

The hearts in 53 of the 54 patients were firm and rubbery, and this noncompliant consistency of the walls of all 4 cardiac chambers usually allowed the diagnosis of cardiac amyloidosis to be made immediately at necropsy without knowledge of clinical findings (Fig. 7 to 10). Both atria in all 54 patients on gross inspection were dilated, usually to a moderate degree. In contrast, the cardiac ventricles on gross inspection were of normal size in 43 patients (80%) and dilated in 11 (20%). The patients with dilated ventricles usually had other conditions that probably caused the dilatation: coronary heart disease

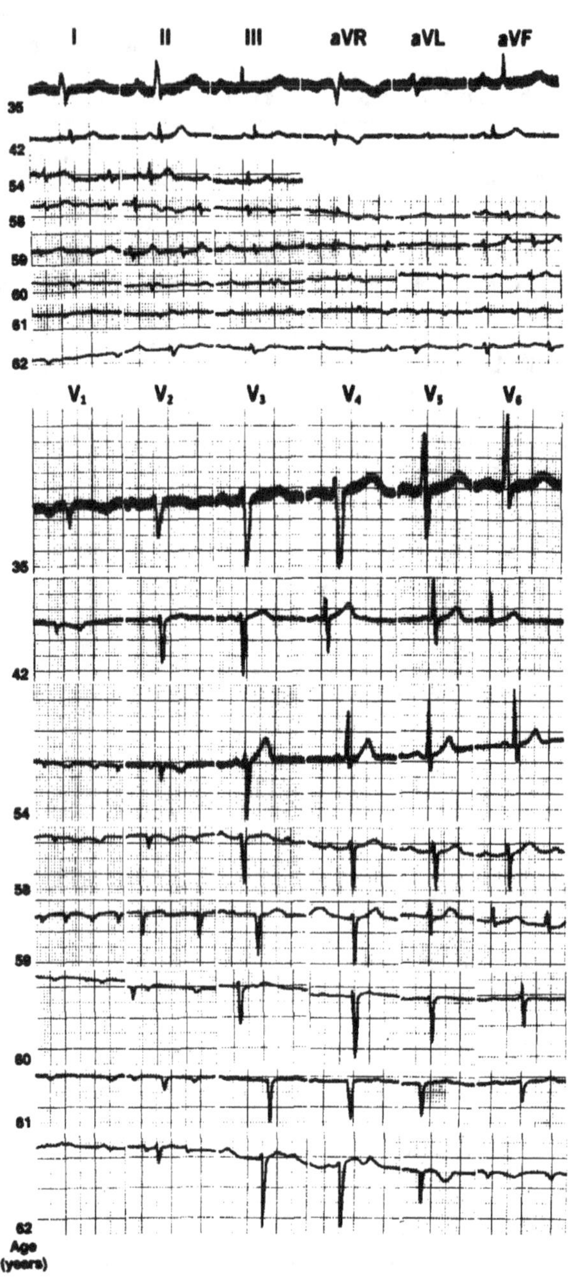

FIGURE 6. Electrocardiograms over a 27-year period in a 62-year-old man (GT 74A-259) who had congestive heart failure for 96 months and, at necropsy, a heart weighing 470 g. The QRS voltage progressively diminished, the axis changed, and R waves disappeared from the precordial leads. While taking digitalis, he developed atrial tachycardia with 2:1 block. The total 12-lead QRS voltage on the final electrocardiogram recorded 9 days before death was 79 mm.

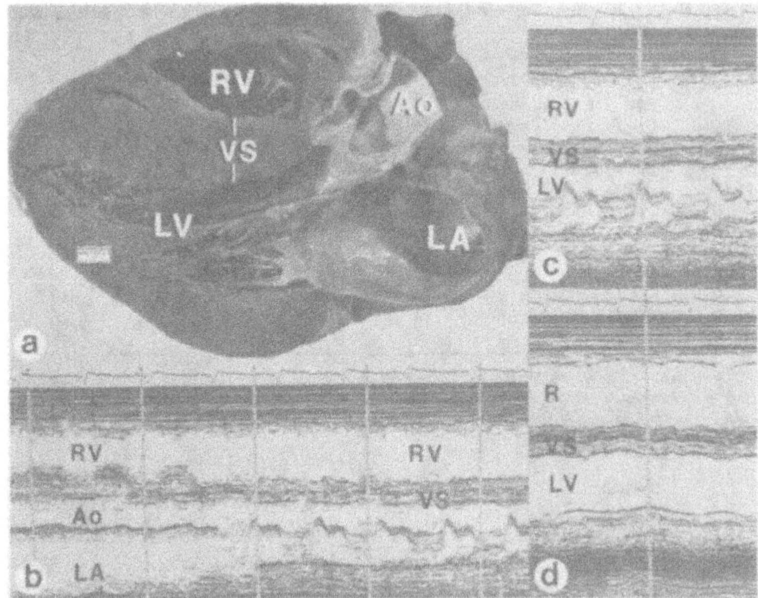

FIGURE 7. Cardiac amyloid with anasarca and pulmonary emboli. Longitudinal view of heart, weighing 545 g, in a 46-year-old man (A81-6) who had been well until 25 months before death, when parathesias and shoulder pain were noted. During his last 3 months he had severe congestive heart failure. When hospitalized 8 days before death, he had anasarca and third and fourth cardiac sounds. Electrocardiography showed a left atrial abnormality, right axis deviation, and poor R-wave progression over the precordium. Echocardiograms (b, c, and d) disclosed the ventricular septum (VS) and left ventricular (LV) free walls to be of similar thickness and each moved hardly at all. Both the left atrium (LA) and right ventricle (RV) were dilated. The pressures in mm Hg were: mean pulmonary artery wedge pressure, 27; pulmonary artery, 60/30; RV, 60/16; left ventricle, 90/26; and brachial artery, 90/60. He died from ventricular tachyarrhythmias. The heart in a longitudinal axis view is shown in a. The myocardium had the typical firm, rubbery appearance of extensive amyloidosis. Several pulmonary emboli may be the explanation of the right ventricular dilatation. Ao = aorta.

with left ventricular transmural scarring or chronic lung disease. The maximal thickness of the ventricular septum was identical or nearly so to the maximal thickness of the left ventricular free wall in 50 patients (93%); in the other 4 (7%) the septum was >1.3 times thicker than the free wall.

By gross examination, amyloid deposits (focal, tan, and waxy-appearing) were observed (and confirmed histologically) in the mural endocardium of 1 or both atria in all 54 patients and in valvular endocardium of 1 or more cardiac valves in 46 patients (85%) (Fig. 11): in the leaflets of the tricuspid valve in 45 patients (83%), the mitral valve in 43 patients (80%), the pulmonic valve in 29 patients (54%), and the aortic valve in 29 patients (54%). In 27 patients (50%), amyloid deposits were observed grossly in the leaflets of all 4 cardiac valves.

Focal transmural left ventricular lesions were observed grossly in 9 patients (17%) (Fig. 8); on histologic examination the lesions consisted entirely of fibrous tissue in 7 patients (13%) and of amyloid deposits in 2 (4%).

At least 3 histologic sections of heart were examined in each patient. In every patient, at least 1 section of left ventricular wall and at least 1 section of atrial wall were examined. Amyloid deposits, readily identified on hematoxylin-eosin stains, were confirmed by either congo red or crystal violet stains or both. In the chamber walls, the amyloid deposits were located in (1) interstitium, that is, between myocardial fibers, not within them in all but 1 patient,[4] (2) endocardium, often of all 4 chambers but always of 1 or both atria in all patients, and (3) within the walls of several intramural coronary arteries in all patients (Fig. 12). Additionally, amyloid deposits often were found in the lumina of some intramural coronary arteries, causing severe (>75% in cross-sectional area) narrowing of some lumina. Despite numerous sections of the major epicardial coronary arteries, no amyloid deposits were observed. At least 1 and usually multiple cardiac valves contained amyloid deposits, but none were judged to have deposits of sufficient quantity to cause valvular dysfunction. In several patients in whom histologic sections included coronary sinus, amyloid deposits were visible histologically in the wall of this structure.

In all 54 patients, amyloid deposits were observed in 1 or more other body organs. No patient had amyloid limited to the heart.

TABLE III   M-Mode Echocardiographic Observations in 11 Necropsy Patients With Fatal Cardiac Amyloidosis*

		Interval (Days) Cath to Death	VS		LV Wall		VS/LV Ratio		LV Cavity		LA Cavity		Ascending Aorta	
Case	Age (yr) & Sex		ES	ED	ES	ED	ES	ED	ES	ED	ES	ED	ES	ED
1	21F	90	14	12	21	14	0.7	0.9	20	36	28	22	24	20
2	40M	...	...	20	...	20	...	1.0	...	...	...	36	...	41
3	45M	15	28	24	18	15	1.6	1.6	24	32	...	58	...	...
4	46M	62	14	14	18	14	0.7	1.0	36	40	36	40	34	30
5	54F	...	...	20	...	20	...	1.0	...	...	...	36	...	41
6	55F	334	30	26	18	15	1.7	1.7	26	36	...	30	...	27
7	55F	150	25	24	26	20	0.9	1.2	29	33	35	30	40	38
8	62M	300	19	19	22	18	0.9	1.1	38	42	20	18	38	30
9	63M	15	35	25	25	16	1.4	1.6	...	...	...	...	...	...
10	78F	169	12	9	13	8	0.9	1.1	36	48	45	40	35	31
11	89F	13	20	19	18	10	1.1	1.9	55	65	45	42	35	32

* All measurements in millimeters.
Cath = catheterization; ED = end-diastole; ES = end-systole; LV = left ventricular; VS = ventricular septum.

TABLE IV Hemodynamic Data in 9 Necropsy Patients With Fatal Cardiac Amyloidosis

Case	Age (yr) & Sex	Interval (Days) Cath to Death	Right Atrium*			PAW*			RV* (s/d)	PA* (s/d)	LV* (s/d)	SA* (s/d)	CI (liters/min/m²)
			a	v	m	a	v	m					
1	35M	90	...	...	11	...	...	25	52/16	48/28	100/24	100/70	...
2	38M	4	24	22	21	...	...	34	56/18	61/34	110/12	110/65	1.3
3	45M	14	12	13	11	28	38	30	60/11	65/33	100/28	100/64	1.7
4	46F	180	10	8	7	...	42	28	50/9	65/33	98/28	98/70	1.6
5	46M	360	...	...	20	...	...	27	60/16	60/30	90/26	90/65	...
6	47F	90	15	14	12	21	28	20	36/12	36/17	110/20	110/80	2.2
7	70M	7	...	...	...	...	...	30	50/	50/30	...	110/60	...
8	78F	150	14	11	10	...	30	26	70/2	70/30	100/20	100/60	2.3
9	96M	7	...	...	17	...	...	34	60/18	60/30	...	90/70	...

a = peak of a wave averaged for several beats; Cath = cardiac catheterization procedure; CI = cardiac index; LV = left ventricle; m = mean; PA = pulmonary artery; PAW = pulmonary arterial wedge; RV = right ventricle; SA = systemic artery; s/d = systolic/diastolic; v = peak of v wave averaged for several beats.

* Measurements in mm Hg.

Thrombi were observed grossly in 1 or more of the 4 cardiac chambers in 14 (26%) of the 54 patients: in 1 chamber only in 8 patients, in 2 chambers in 3 patients, in 3 chambers in 1 patient, and in all 4 chambers in 1 patient. Of the 22 cardiac chambers that contained thrombi (mainly fibrin in all) in the 14 patients, the right atrial appendage contained thrombi in 10 patients (isolated in 5); the left atrial appendage contained thrombi in 7 patients (isolated in 2); the right ventricle con-

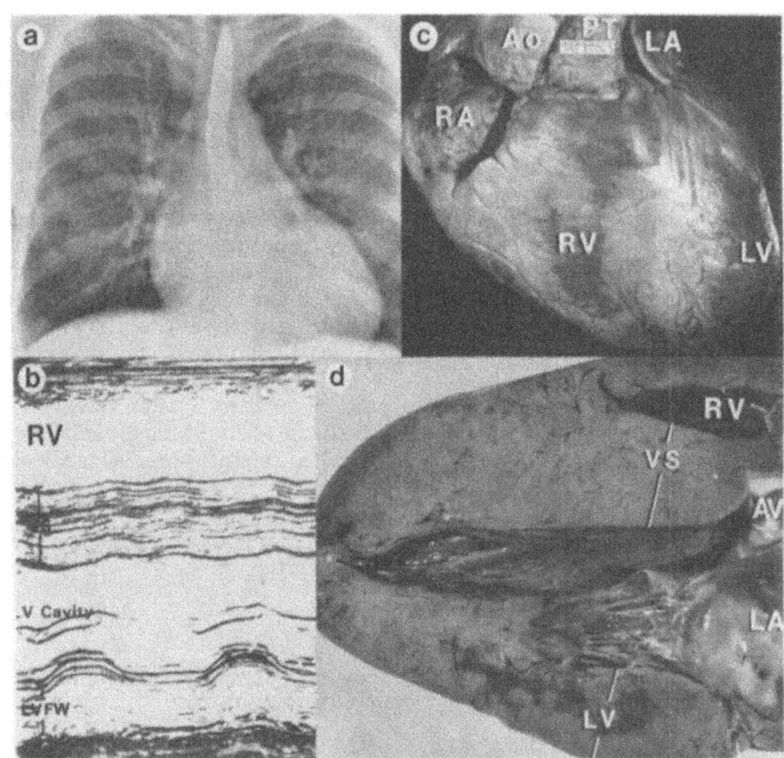

FIGURE 8. Cardiac amyloidosis simulating hypertrophic cardiomyopathy. Chest radiograph (**a**), M-mode echocardiogram just caudal to the tips of the mitral leaflets (**b**), exterior view of heart (**c**), and longitudinal axis view of heart (**d**) in a 46-year-old man (A79-25) who noted dyspnea while walking 24 months before death. M-mode echocardiography 1 month later disclosed the ventricular septum (VS) to be 1.7 times thicker than the left ventricular free wall (LVFW). The anterior mitral leaflet moved anteriorly during ventricular systole. The left atrial cavity was 30 mm in diameter. The pressures in mm Hg were: mean pulmonary arterial wedge, 5; pulmonary artery, 17/6; right ventricle (RV), 17/3; left ventricle (LV), 130/11; and aorta (Ao), 115/70. Clinically, the patient at that time was considered to have hypertrophic cardiomyopathy. Nine months before death, he had transient sudden left-sided weakness with slurred speech, worsened dyspnea, transient chest pain, and the carpal-tunnel syndrome was noted. Now the mean pulmonary arterial wedge pressure was 23; right ventricular pressure, 47/7; LV, 95/25; and Ao, 95/65 mm Hg. Echocardiogram now showed the ventricular septum to be 2.0 cm and the LVFW 1.5 cm; SAM now was absent. The left atrium (LA) now was 55 mm in diameter. A third catheterization performed 10 days before death showed the mean pulmonary wedge pressure to be 32 and that in the RV 65/11 mm Hg. The cardiac index was 1.4 liters/min/m². The heart was enlarged (**a**). M-mode echocardiogram (**b**) now showed the VS to be 2.6 cm and the LVFW 1.5 cm thick. Cardiac amyloidosis was never diagnosed clinically. At necropsy, the heart weighed 780 g. In addition to the usual interstitial myocardial amyloid, large deposits of amyloid were visible grossly on the LVFW (**d**). The VS is thicker than the free wall. The epicardial coronary arteries were virtually free of atherosclerotic plaques. AV = aortic valve; PT = pulmonary trunk; RA = right atrium; SAM = systolic anterior motion of the anterior mitral leaflet.

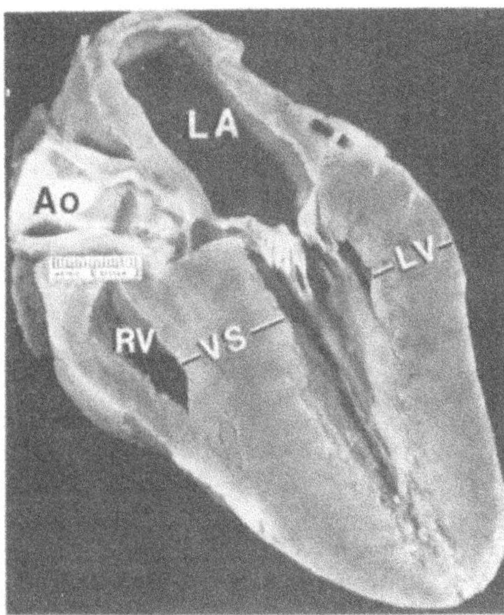

FIGURE 9. Cardiac amyloidosis simulating hypertrophic cardiomyopathy. Long-axis view of heart in a 55-year-old woman (WMC#A79-24) who had been well until 6 months before death when she developed periorbital purpura, pedal edema, and right-arm pain. When syncope occurred a month later, she was hospitalized and found to have multiple myeloma. Electrocardiography disclosed both atrial and ventricular arrhythmias and electrophysiologic studies disclosed distal H-V block. She never had congestive heart failure. On the day of death at home she fainted and soon thereafter had fatal cardiac arrest. The heart weighed 430 g and it had the typical amyloid consistency. A long-axis view is shown. The ventricular septum (VS) is thicker than the left ventricular (LV) free wall. The left atrium (LA) is dilated. Ao = aorta; RV = right ventricular cavity.

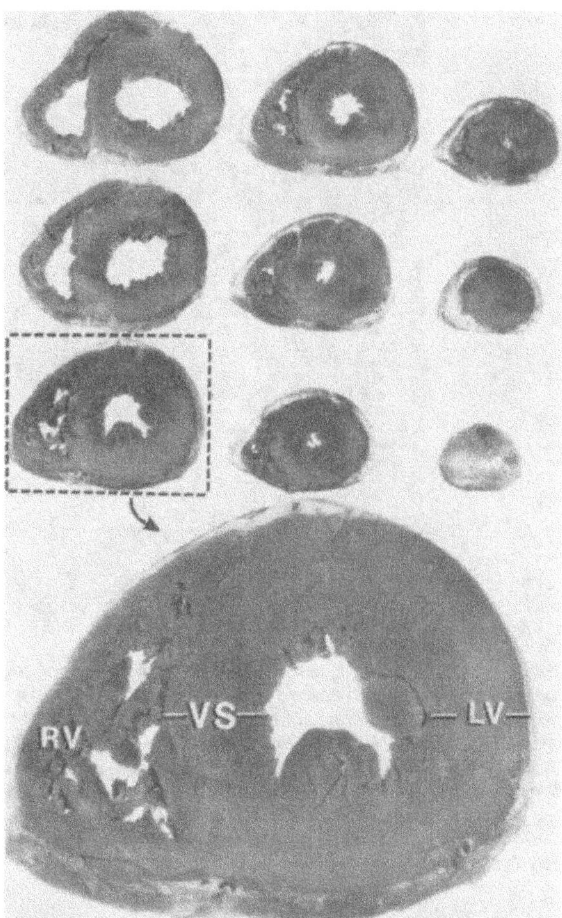

FIGURE 10. Massive ventricular amyloid deposits. Transverse cuts of the ventricles in the 49-year-old man (NNMC#A80-15), described in detail in Figure 3. This uniform appearance of the ventricular walls is the most common finding in extensive cardiac amyloidosis. LV = left ventricle; RV = right ventricle; VS = ventricular septum.

tained thrombi in 2 patients (none isolated), and the left ventricle contained thrombi in 3 patients (isolated in 2). Thus, of the 22 chambers with thrombi, 17 were atrial appendages and 5 were ventricles. None of the 5 ventricles containing thrombi appeared dilated by gross inspection. Of the 14 patients with intracardiac thrombi, 13 had clinical evidence of CHF and 1 died suddenly without evidence at any time of CHF: 2 (of 13) had chronic atrial fibrillation; 2 had clinical evidence of either pulmonary or systemic emboli, and 5 had severe narrowing of 1 or more epicardial cardiac arteries by either atherosclerotic plaque (4 patients) or fibrin-platelet embolus (1 patient). The latter patient was reported on previously.[2]

In addition to the extensive cardiac amyloid deposits, 8 patients (15%) had narrowing >75% in cross-sectional area by atherosclerotic plaques of 1 or more of the 4 major (right, left main, left anterior descending, and left circumflex) epicardial coronary arteries: in 5 patients, 3 of the 4 major arteries were so narrowed; in 1 patient 2 arteries, and in 2 patients 1 artery. The ages of these 8 patients ranged from 65 to 96 years (mean 78); 6 were men and 2 were women. Four had had periodic chest pain, considered angina pectoris in 2. One patient died suddenly and unexpectedly. At necropsy none had foci of myocardial necrosis, but 4 had healed transmural left ventricular infarcts, all of which had been clinically silent.

Calcific deposits were present in the mitral anulus in 7 patients (13%) and in 1 or more aortic valve cusps in 9 patients (17%). In 6 patients, the calcific deposits were present in both mitral anulus and in aortic valve cusps, in 3 patients they were limited to aortic valve cusps, and in 1 patient they were limited to mitral anulus. In 2 of the 9 patients with aortic valve calcium, the deposits appeared extensive enough to cause nar-

rowing of the aortic valve orifice. In none of the 7 patients with mitral anulus calcium did the calcific deposits appear to cause clinically significant mitral dysfunction. All 10 patients (19%) with either mitral anular or aortic valve cuspal calcific deposits, or both, had calcific deposits in 1 or more of the 4 major epicardial coronary arteries, and in each patient they were within atherosclerotic plaques.

Discussion

Patients with cardiac amyloid deposits may readily be separated into 2 major groups: (1) those with amyloid deposits too small to produce cardiac dysfunction, and (2) those with amyloid deposits large enough to produce cardiac dysfunction which eventually is fatal. The finding of minute cardiac amyloid deposits in the heart in elderly persons at necropsy is common,[5–13] but patients with minute cardiac deposits, whether they be young or old, are not included in the present analysis. Each of our 54 patients had heavy cardiac amyloid deposits that caused fatal cardiac dysfunction. All but 1 had firm, rubbery ventricular and usually atrial walls with amyloid deposits in the interstitium (between myocardial cells) of the walls of all 4 chambers, in mural and usually in valvular endocardium, and in the in-

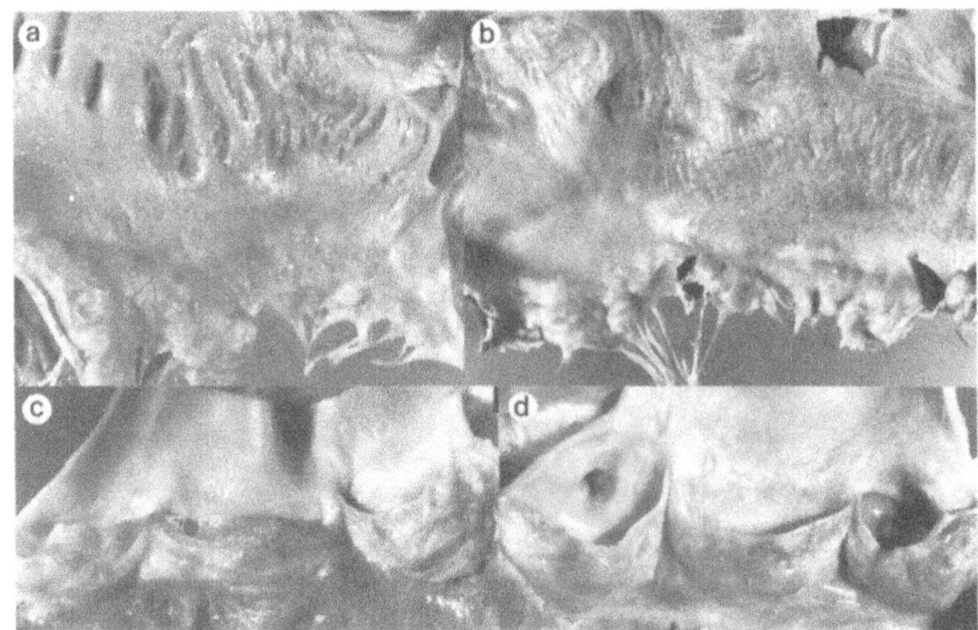

FIGURE 11. Endocardial amyloidosis. Opened right atrium and tricuspid valve (**a**), opened left atrium and mitral valve (**b**), opened pulmonic valve and pulmonary trunk (**c**), and opened aortic valve and aorta (**d**). The mural endocardium of each chamber and the cusps of all 4 cardiac valves contain amyloid deposits. The ventricular myocardium (shown in Figure 4) also contained massive quantities of amyloid, as did the pulmonary trunk. This 49-year-old man (NNMC#A80-15) had been well, but an automobile accident prompted an examination 10 months before death. Both pedal edema and hepatomegaly were found, the blood pressure was elevated (160/100 mm Hg), the heart was enlarged (cardiothoracic ratio 0.55), and electro-cardiogram disclosed no R waves in leads V_1–V_3, nonspecific ST-T wave abnormalities, and low voltage. Echocardiogram was normal. Hepatic biopsy yielded amyloid. He remained asymptomatic until 4 months before death, when extensive subcutaneous edema appeared and pericardial effusion (700 ml) was found. The systemic blood pressure was then 120/80 mm Hg. His condition progressively worsened thereafter. He became acutely dyspneic at home and died.

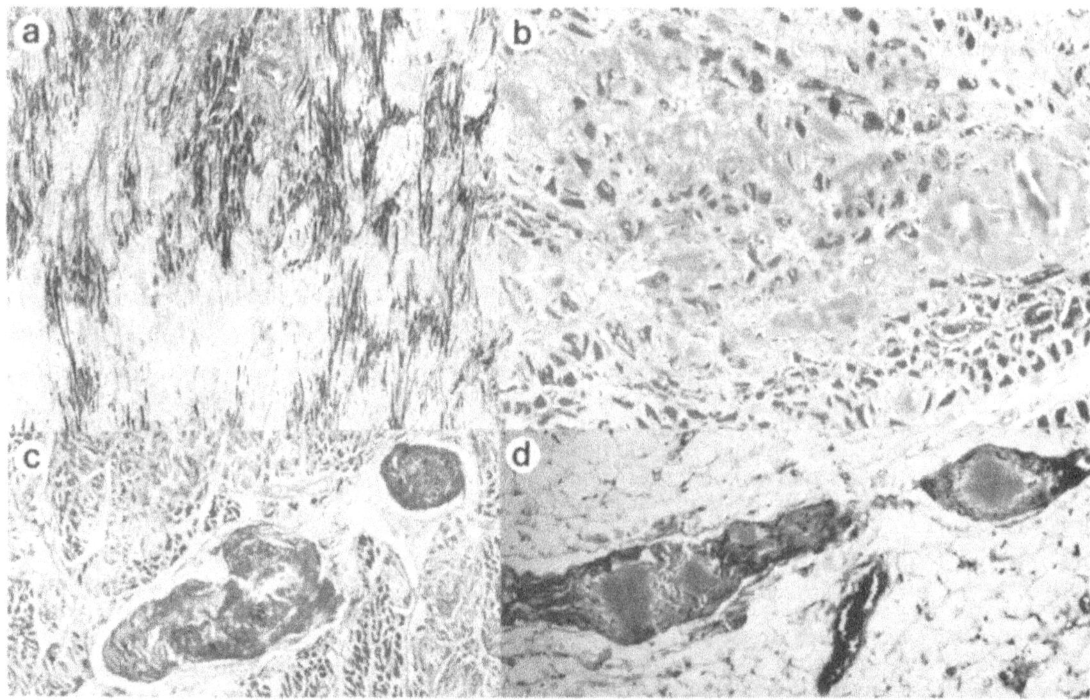

FIGURE 12. Location of amyloid in myocardium (**a** and **b**), intramural coronary artery (**c**) and epicardial nerve (**d**). **a**, massive interstitial myocardial amyloid observed in a longitudinal section in an 89-year-old man (A69-259) with chronic congestive heart failure (CHF) and a heart weighing 520 g. In this section, more amyloid than myocardial fibers are present. **b**, massive interstitial myocardial amyloid observed in cross section in a 68-year-old man (H-A76-143) who had CHF for 36 months. **c**, amyloid occluding the lumens of intramural coronary arteries in a 67-year-old man (A69-187) with chronic CHF and a heart weighing 550 g. **d**, amyloid in epicardial nerves in a 74-year-old man (A58-190) who died suddenly from familial amy-loidosis and had a heart weighing 700 g. (Hematoxylin-eosin stain [**a**] ×25 and [**d**] ×100; Movat stain [**b**] ×100; Masson stain [**c**] ×39, all reduced 25%.)

tramural coronary arteries. The 1 patient without interstitial myocardial amyloid had amyloid filling the lumina of most intramural coronary arteries.[3] Additionally, several patients had amyloid in the epicardium but never in the walls or lumina of the major epicardial coronary arteries. All our 54 patients with cardiac amyloid had amyloid deposits in 1 or more noncardiac body organs. We suspect that cardiac amyloid severe enough to cause clinical evidence of cardiac dysfunction is never limited exclusively to the heart.

Although a diagnosis of cardiac amyloidosis was established clinically in less than half of our 54 patients, most were studied clinically before echocardiography and radionuclide angiography became commonly performed procedures. Echocardiography is now often one of the first clues to the diagnosis of cardiac amyloidosis,[14–19] and myocardial technetium-99m pyrophosphate scintigraphy may be diagnostic of this condition.[20–23] Thus, cardiac amyloidosis severe enough to cause cardiac dysfunction almost surely will be suspected hereafter in a majority rather than in a minority of patients. Clinically, diagnosis of cardiac amyloidosis should be suspected in an older patient with evidence of CHF, poorly responsive and/or particularly sensitive to digitalis, unassociated with chest pain or systemic hypertension, and in the presence of cardiomegaly by chest radiograph but low voltage by electrocardiogram. The echocardiogram, rather than showing dilatation of the left ventricle, shows this chamber to be of normal or near-normal size and the ventricular walls to move poorly, and these findings can be confirmed by hemodynamic and angiographic studies.[24–27] Biopsy of either noncardiac or cardiac[28] tissue is required for absolute diagnosis.

Severe cardiac amyloidosis is 1 of the causes of spontaneous cure of systemic hypertension. Although nearly half of our 54 patients had had either a history of systemic hypertension or recordings of elevated systemic arterial pressures, or both, all had systolic systemic pressures ≤130 mm Hg and diastolic systemic pressures ≤90 mm Hg in the last 3 months of life. The average recorded peak systolic arterial pressure in the last 3 months of life in our patients was 102 mm Hg and the diastolic pressure was 70 mm Hg. Thus, if the systemic arterial pressure is elevated in a patient with CHF, the chance that the CHF is the result of cardiac amyloidosis is minimal. Additionally, none of our patients had evidence of left ventricular hypertrophy by electrocardiogram in their final 3 months, although several had had left ventricular hypertrophy by electrocardiogram >1 year earlier.

The length of time necessary to develop cardiac amyloid deposits extensive enough to cause cardiac dysfunction is uncertain. One clue to the amount of time required can be gained by study of the systemic arterial pressures over several years. We have now observed several patients with systolic systemic pressures in the vicinity of 180 mm Hg; during a period of 4 to 5 years this pressure gradually decreased to about 100 mm Hg without use of antihypertensive agents. Thus, a gradual but spontaneous decrease in systemic arterial pressure also might be a clue to the development of cardiac amyloidosis.

Cardiac amyloidosis needs to be added to the list of great cardiac masqueraders. Initially, it was cardiovascular syphilis that was stated to frequently simulate other cardiac conditions. In recent years, hypertrophic cardiomyopathy has become the most prominent masquerader. The QRS and T-wave changes on the electrocardiogram in cardiac amyloidosis are similar to those produced by healed myocardial infarction secondary to coronary atherosclerosis. The presence of a nondilated left ventricle and the presence of a ventricular septum thicker than the left ventricular free wall by echocardiogram has suggested the presence of hypertrophic cardiomyopathy. Five of our 11 patients with echocardiograms were suspected of having hypertrophic cardiomyopathy because of the combination of these findings. Simulation of cardiac amyloidosis clinically to pericardial constriction has long been recognized.[1,24–27] Three of our 54 patients underwent thoracotomy because of suspected pericardial constriction. Cardiac amyloidosis may present as pericardial tamponade.[29] Its delayed left ventricular filling may simulate mitral stenosis on rare occasions.[30]

Although amyloid deposits are always more extensive in "working" than in "conducting" myocardium,[1,31,32] arrhythmias and conduction disturbances are common (Table I). Some of these disturbances, however, may be the result of aging rather than the result of extensive cardiac amyloidosis.[13,33] In our patients, left-axis deviation (58%), atrial fibrillation (23%), and bundle branch block (18%) were common, but these also are relatively common in elderly patients without cardiac amyloidosis.[13,33] The frequency of low voltage (63%) and a healed myocardial infarction pattern (83%), however, was striking in our patients, and each of these should raise the possibility of cardiac amyloidosis in a patient with CHF of unclear cause.

This report provides for the first time measurements of QRS voltages in each of the 12 leads of an electrocardiogram in patients with cardiac amyloidosis. Simonson[34] provided data on the upper and lower limits of amplitude of the QRS complexes in each of the 12 leads in normal men and women aged 20 to 59 years. (The mean for normal subjects is not available.) The upper and lower limits of normal for men aged 50 to 59 years were 277 and 36 mm and for women 248 and 27 mm, respectively. The upper and lower limits of amplitude in all leads in 30 of our 54 patients (Table II) were 199 and 58 mm, respectively, and averaged 104 mm. For our 15 women from whom the data were available, the total 12-lead QRS voltage ranged from 58 to 199 mm (mean 109) and for our 15 men from 60 to 197 mm (mean 99).

In comparison, Siegel and Roberts[35] determined the total 12-lead QRS voltage in 50 patients (aged 16 to 65 years) with severe and fatal isolated aortic valve stenosis. The upper and lower limits of amplitude in all 12 leads in their 50 patients were 417 and 144 mm, respectively, and averaged 260 mm. In their 14 women with aortic stenosis, the total 12-lead QRS voltage averaged 277 mm and in their 36 men, 249 mm. The average heart weight of their 14 women with aortic stenosis was 521 g, and the heart weight in our 15 women with severe cardiac amyloidosis and available total 12-lead

QRS voltage was 494 g. The difference, however, in average total 12-lead QRS voltage (277 mm versus 109 mm) was a factor of 2.5 times. The mean heart weight of the 36 men with aortic stenosis studied by Siegel and Roberts[35] was 639 g and that of our 15 men with fatal cardiac amyloidosis and available total 12-lead QRS voltage was 570 g. The average total 12-lead QRS voltage in the 36 men with aortic stenosis, however, was 249 mm compared with only 99 mm in our 15 men with fatal cardiac amyloid, again a 2.5-fold difference. Thus, although the sum of the QRS voltage in leads I, II, and III may not fulfill criteria of "low voltage," that is, ≤15 mm, the total QRS voltage in all 12 leads in severe cardiac amyloidosis is usually considerably lower than normal, and particularly small in proportion to the weight of the heart.

References

1. **Buja LM, Khol NB, Roberts WC.** Clinically significant cardiac amyloidosis. Clinicopathologic findings in 15 patients. Am J Cardiol 1970;26:394–405.
2. **Barth RF, Willerson JT, Buja LM, Decker JL, Roberts WC.** Amyloid coronary artery disease, primary systemic amyloidosis and paraproteinemia. Arch Intern Med 1970;127:627–630.
3. **Saffitz JE, Sazama K, Roberts WC.** Amyloidosis limited to small arteries causing angina pectoris and sudden death. Am J Cardiol 1983;51:1234–1235.
4. **Roberts WC, Perloff JK, Costantino T.** Severe valvular aortic stenosis in patients over 65 years of age. A clinicopathologic study. Am J Cardiol 1971;27:497–506.
5. **Brandt K, Cathcart ES, Cohen AS.** A clinical analysis of the course and prognosis of forty-two patients with amyloidosis. Am J Med 1968;44:955–959.
6. **Schwartz P.** Amyloidosis. Cause and manifestation of senile deterioration. Springfield, IL: Charles C Thomas, 1970:395.
7. **Kyle RA, Bayrd ED.** Amyloidosis: review of 236 cases. Medicine 1975;54:271–300.
8. **Hodkinson HM, Pomerance A.** The clinical significance of senile cardiac amyloidosis: a prospective clinico-pathological study. Quart J Med 1977;46:381–387.
9. **Smith RRL, Hutchins GM, Moore GW, Humphrey RL.** Type and distribution of pulmonary parenchymal and vascular amyloid. Correlation with cardiac amyloid. Am J Med 1979;66:96–104.
10. **Westermark P, Johansson B, Natvig JB.** Senile cardiac amyloidosis: evidence of two different amyloid substances in the aging heart. Scand J Immunol 1979;10:303–308.
11. **Cornwell GG III, Westermark P.** Senile amyloidosis: a protean manifestation of the aging process. J Clin Pathol 1980;33:1146–1152.
12. **Wright JR, Calkins E.** Clinical-pathological differentiation of common amyloid syndromes. Medicine 1981;60:429–448.
13. **Waller BF, Roberts WC.** Cardiovascular disease in the very elderly. Analysis of 40 necropsy patients aged 90 years or older. Am J Cardiol 1983;51:403–421.
14. **Child JS, Levisman JA, Abbasi AS, MacAlpin RN.** Echocardiographic manifestations of infiltrative cardiomyopathy. A report of seven cases due to amyloid. Chest 1976;70:726–731.
15. **Borer JS, Henry WL, Epstein SE.** Echocardiographic observations in patients with systemic infiltrative disease involving the heart. Am J Cardiol 1977;39:184–188.
16. **Child JS, Krivokapich J, Abbasi AS.** Increased right ventricular wall thickness on echocardiography in amyloid infiltrative cardiomyopathy. Am J Cardiol 1979;44:1391–1395.
17. **Sigueira-Filho AG, Cunha CLP, Tajik AJ, Seward JB, Schattenberg TT, Giuliani ER.** M-mode and two-dimensional echocardiographic features in cardiac amyloidosis. Circulation 1981;63:188–196.
18. **St John Sutton MG, Reichek N, Kastor JA, Giuliani ER.** Computerized M-mode echocardiographic analysis of left ventricular dysfunction in cardiac amyloid. Circulation 1982;66:790–799.
19. **Bhandari AK, Nanda NC.** Myocardial texture characterization by two-dimensional echocardiography. Am J Cardiol 1983;51:817–825.
20. **Wizenberg TA, Muz J, Sohn YH, Samlowski W, Weissler AM.** Value of positive myocardial technetium-99m-pyrophosphate scintigraphy in the noninvasive diagnosis of cardiac amyloidosis. Am Heart J 1982;103:468–473.
21. **Schiff S, Bateman T, Moffatt R, Davidson R, Berman D.** Diagnostic considerations in cardiomyopathy: unique scintigraphic pattern of diffuse biventricular technetium-99m-pyrophosphate uptake in amyloid heart disease. Am Heart J 1982;130:562–563.
22. **Sobol SM, Brown JM, Bunker SR, Patel J, Lull RJ.** Noninvasive diagnosis of cardiac amyloidosis by technetium-99m-pyrophosphate myocardial scintigraphy. Am Heart J 1982;103:563–566.
23. **Falk RH, Lee VW, Rubinow A, Hood WB Jr, Cohen AS.** Sensitivity of Technetium-99m-pyrophosphate scintigraphy in diagnosing cardiac amyloidosis. Am J Cardiol 1983;51:826–830.
24. **Chew C, Ziady GM, Raphael MJ, Oakley CM.** The functional defect in amyloid heart disese. The "stiff heart" syndrome. Am J Cardiol 1975;36:438–444.
25. **Meaney E, Shabetai R, Bhargava V, Shearer M, Weidner C, Mangiardi, LM, Smalling R, Peterson K.** Cardiac amyloidosis, constrictive pericarditis and restrictive cardiomyopathy. Am J Cardiol 1976;38:547–556.
26. **Swanton RH, Brooksby IAB, Davies MJ, Coltart DJ, Jenkins BS, Webb-Peploe MM.** Systolic and diastolic ventricular function in cardiac amyloidosis. Studies in six cases diagnosed with endomyocardial biopsy. Am J Cardiol 1977;39:658–664.
27. **Tyberg TI, Goodyer AVN, Hurst VW III, Alexander J, Langou RA.** Left ventricular filling in differentiating restrictive amyloid cardiomyopathy and constrictive pericarditis. Am J Cardiol 1981;47:791–796.
28. **Schroeder JS, Billingham ME, Rider AK.** Cardiac amyloidosis. Diagnosis by transvenous endomyocardial biopsy. Am J Med 1975;59:269–273.
29. **Brodarick S, Paine R, Higa E, Carmichael KA.** Pericardial tamponade, a new complication of amyloid heart disease. Am J Med 1982;73:133–135.
30. **Shenoy UA, Peric-Golia L.** Primary cardiovascular amyloidosis manifesting as mitral stenosis. Hum Pathol 1982;13:768–770.
31. **Ridolfi RL, Bulkley BH, Hutchins GM.** The conduction system in cardiac amyloidosis. Clinical and pathologic features of 23 patients. Am J Med 1977;62:677–686.
32. **Bharati S, Lev M, Denes P, Modlinger J, Wyndham C, Bauernfeind R, Greenblatt M, Rosen KM.** Infiltrative cardiomyopathy with conduction disease and ventricular arrhythmia: electrophysiologic and pathologic correlations. Am J Cardiol 1980;45:163–173.
33. **Fisch C.** Electrocardiogram in the aged: an independent marker of heart disease? Am J Med 1981;70:4–6.
34. **Simonson F.** Differentiation between normal and abnormal in electrocardiography. St. Louis: CV Mosby, 1961:328.
35. **Siegel RJ, Roberts WC.** Electrocardiographic observations in severe aortic valve stenosis: correlative necropsy study to clinical, hemodynamic, and ECG variables demonstrating relation of 12-lead QRS amplitude to peak systolic transaortic pressure gradient. Am Heart J 1982;103:210–221.

The Heart in Massive (More Than 300 Pounds or 136 Kilograms) Obesity: Analysis of 12 Patients Studied at Necropsy

CAROLE A. WARNES, MB, BS, MRCP, and WILLIAM C. ROBERTS, MD

Observations are described in 12 massively obese patients (5 women, 7 men), aged 25 to 59 years (mean 37), who weighed 312 to more than 500 pounds (mean 381). Seven patients had had systemic hypertension, 4 hypersomnia or sleep apnea, 2 diabetes mellitus, and 1 patient symptomatic coronary artery disease. Five patients died suddenly from undetermined causes, 2 from right-sided congestive heart failure, 1 patient from acute myocardial infarction; 1 from aortic dissection; 1 from intracerebral hemorrhage; 1 from a drug overdose, and 1 soon after an ileal bypass. The heart weight was increased in all 12 patients. The heart weight to body weight ratio expressed as a percent ranged from 0.22 to 0.61 (mean 0.37) (normal for men 0.42 to 0.46 [mean 0.43], normal for women 0.38 to 0.46 [mean 0.40]). The left ventricular cavity was dilated in 11 patients and the right ventricular cavity in all 12. Only 2 patients (aged 42 and 59 years) had 1 or more major epicardial coronary arteries narrowed >75% in cross-sectional area by atherosclerotic plaque, 1 of whom had no symptoms of myocardial ischemia. Of 664 five-millimeter segments from the 4 major epicardial coronary arteries from 11 patients (mean 60 per patient), 431 (65%) were narrowed 0 to 25% in XSA, 143 (21%) were narrowed 26 to 50%, 73 (11%) were narrowed 51 to 75%, and 17 (3%) were narrowed 76 to 100%. Thus, these extremely obese patients who died prematurely did not have more coronary atherosclerosis than might be expected at their ages.

(Am J Cardiol 1984;54:1087–1091)

Although obesity may predispose to cardiovascular disease, few studies have focused on morphologic cardiac findings in patients who are massively obese. This report describes such findings in 12 patients who weighed more than 300 pounds (>136 kg).

Patients and Findings

Source of patients: Of the 12 patients, 8 died outside the hospital: necropsy in each of the 8 was performed at the Washington, D.C., Medical Examiner's Office. The other 4 patients died in a Washington, D.C., area hospital. The hearts in all 12 patients were submitted to the Pathology Branch, National Heart, Lung, and Blood Institute, and each heart was examined by both investigators. Findings in the 12 patients are summarized in Table I. All 12 patients had been severely obese for several years before death, usually from puberty. The patients weighed 312 to 500 pounds (mean 381), equivalent to 88 to 268% (mean 180) increase over ideal body weight. (The ideal body weight was taken as the average body weight for sex and height from the recommendations of the 1973 Fogarty Center conference data adapted from the Metropolitan Life Insurance Company tables.[1])

Clinical features: Information on the presence or absence of episodes of sleep apnea or hypersomnia was available in 6 patients. Three had sleep apnea, 2 of whom had resting arterial blood gases which were PO_2 63 and PCO_2 43 mm Hg in 1 and PO_2 42 and PCO_2 53 mm Hg in 1; another patient had hypersomnia, but blood gas values were unavailable. Of 7 patients in whom historical information was available, all 7 had had "high blood pressure." Actual systemic arterial recordings were available in 4 patients and all were elevated. Information on diabetes mellitus was available in 3 patients; 2 had it, 1 of whom was treated with insulin and 1 with oral hypoglycemic agents only.

Mode of death: Five patients died suddenly outside the hospital, only 1 of whom had significant narrowing of 1 or more major coronary arteries; the precise cause of the sudden death in the other 4 patients is unclear. One patient had a fatal acute myocardial infarction. Two patients had progressive right-sided congestive heart failure (cor pulmonale), which became intractable and eventually fatal. Two patients died from complications of systemic hypertension: 1 patient from aortic dissection and 1 from intracerebral hemorrhage. One

From the Pathology Branch, National Heart, Lung, and Blood Institute, National Institutes of Health, Bethesda, Maryland 20205. Dr. Warnes' present address: National Heart Hospital, Westmoreland Street, London W1, England. Manuscript received July 16, 1984, accepted July 19, 1984.

Address for reprints: William C. Roberts, MD, Building 10A, Room 3E-30, National Institutes of Health, Bethesda, Maryland 20205.

patient died 2 hours after an ileal bypass operation and 1 died of an overdose of opiates plus alcohol.

Morphologic findings: The heart weight in all 12 patients was increased, ranging from 380 to 990 g (mean 616). The relation of heart weight to body weight is shown in Figure 1; no consistent relation occurred (r = 0.27). The relation of the increase in heart weight above the upper limit of normal (350 g for women, 400 g for men) to the increase in body weight above ideal[1] is shown in Figure 2; no consistent relation occurred (r = 0.05).

The subepicardial adipose tissue by visual inspection appeared to be increased in 9 of the 12 patients: mild in 3, moderate in 4 and severe in 5 patients (Fig. 3 to 6). The fat deposits were graded mild when they were limited to areas adjacent to the epicardial coronary arteries; moderate when they also covered all or a portion of right ventricular wall, and severe when they also covered all or a portion of left ventric-

TABLE I Certain Findings in the 12 Patients with Massive Obesity (More Than 300 Pounds)

Pt	Age (yr) & Sex	Height (in)	Height (cm)	Body Weight (lb)	Body Weight (kg)	Ideal BW (lb)	Ideal BW (kg)	Increase over Ideal Weight (%)	HW (g)*	HW as % of BW†	EF (1 +− 3+)‡	SA and/or H	Hx of SH	BP recording (mm Hg)	Rx of SH	DM	Mode of Death	Narrowing 76–100% of ≥1 Major Coronary Artery	LV N or F
1	25F	70	178	425	193	144	65	195	720	0.37	2	—	+	200/110	+	—	AD	0	0
2	26F	66	168	345	157	128	58	169	625	0.40	3	+	—	—	—	—	Sudden	0	0
3	29F	62	158	375	170	113	51	232	380	0.22	1	+	—	—	—	—	CHF	0	0
4	37F	62	158	319	145	113	51	182	430	0.30	3	—	+	—	—	—	Sudden	0	0
5	40F	63	160	370	168	116	53	219	450	0.27	1	—	+	—	+	—	Sudden	0	0
6	25M	69	175	425	193	149	68	185	620	0.32	1	—	+	—	+	—	PO IB	0	0
7	34M	66	168	>500§	>227§	136	62	268	825	0.36	2	0	+	175/110	+	0	CNS Bleed	0	0
8	35M	74	188	358	162	171	78	109	990	0.61	3	—	+	—	—	—	Overdose	0	0
9	42M	73	185	312	142	166	75	88	665	0.47	2	—	—	—	—	—	Sudden	+	+
10	48M	68	173	450	204	145	66	210	560	0.27	2	+	+	140/95	+	+	CHF	0	0
11	48M	71	180	346	157	158	72	119	720	0.46	3	+	+	180/100	+	—	Sudden	0	0
12	59M	—	—	>350§	>159§	—	—	—	410	—	3	0	—	—	—	+	AMI	+	+

* Normal heart weight: ≤350 g in women; ≤400 g in men.
† Heart weight (g) × 100 ÷ body weight (g).
‡ 1+ = mild; 2+ = moderate; 3+ = severe.
§ Body weight exceeded upper limit of available scales and is therefore an approximation.
AD = aortic dissection; AMI = acute myocardial infarction; BP = blood pressure; BW = body weight; CHF = right-sided congestive heart failure; CNS = central nervous system; DM = diabetes mellitus; EF = epicardial fat; F = fibrosis; H = hypersomnia; HW = heart weight; Hx = history; IB = ileal bypass; LV = left ventricle; N = necrosis; PO = postoperative; RV = right ventricle; Rx = treatment; SA = sleep apnea; SH = systemic hypertension; — = no information available; + = present or positive; 0 = absent or negative.

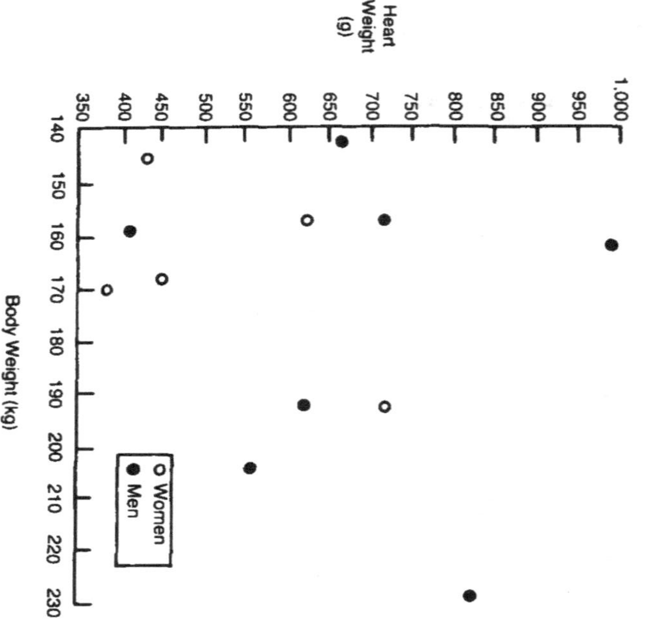

FIGURE 1. Relation of heart weight to body weight in the 12 patients.

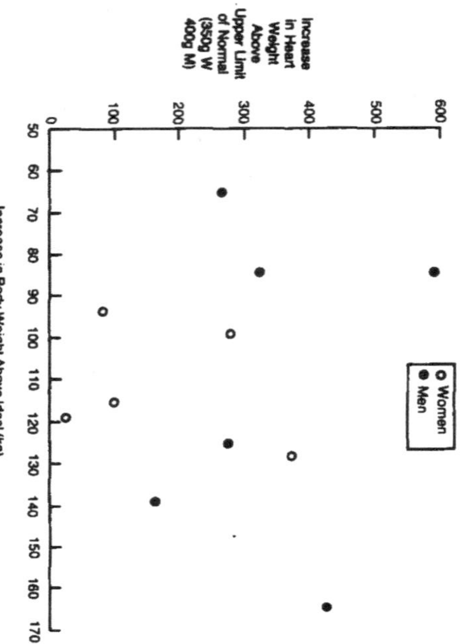

FIGURE 2. Relation of increase in heart weight above upper limit of normal to increase in body weight above ideal in 11 patients who weighed more than 300 pounds. M = men; W = women.

ular wall. In no patient did the heart float in water.[2] On gross examination, 3 patients (nos. 4, 8 and 10) had fatty infiltration of the right ventricular myocardium (confirmed in each by microscopy). The maximal thickness of the atrial septum in all 12 patients was ≤1.6 cm. No patient had lipomatous hypertrophy of the atrial septum.

The thickness of the left ventricular wall (similar in all patients to the thickness of the ventricular septum) ranged from 1.3 to 2.3 cm (mean 1.6). In 4 patients, the maximal thickness of right ventricular wall was more than 5 mm. By gross inspection, the right ventricular cavity appeared dilated in all 12 patients, the left ventricular cavity in 11 patients, the right atrial cavity in 10, and the left atrial cavity in 9. Patient 12 had a transmural acute myocardial infarct and a small subendocardial left ventricular scar; patient 11 also had a healed transmural left ventricular scar. Two patients (nos. 3 and 5) had a valvular incompetent patent foramen ovale associated with a redundant atrial septum. Sections of ventricular myocardium (mean 4 per patient) were studied in each case. Histologic examination showed myocardial fiber hypertrophy of both right and left ventricles in all 12 patients.

The 4 major coronary arteries were excised intact, x-rayed and, if necessary, decalcified. Each artery was then cut transversely into 5-mm segments and labeled sequentially, either from the aortic ostium or from its origin from the left main coronary artery. The segments were then processed for histologic study and a section prepared, stained by the Movat technique,[3] from each segment. The amount of luminal narrowing by atherosclerotic plaque was determined by magnification of the histologic sections 25 to 50 times. The percent of cross-sectional area (XSA) narrowing of each 5-mm segment was categorized into 4 groups: 0 to 25%, 26 to 50%, 51 to 75% and 76 to 100%. All sections were examined by 1 of us (CAW), and the accuracy of the assessment of luminal narrowing was spot-checked by video planimetry. The agreement between these 2 techniques is approximately 95%.[4]

Two patients had 76 to 100% narrowing in XSA by atherosclerotic plaque of 1 or more major coronary arteries: in each, both the right and left anterior descending were narrowed to this degree.

Of the 48 major epicardial coronary arteries in the 12 patients (4 per patient), 4 were narrowed at some point 76 to 100% in XSA by plaque.

A total of 664 five-millimeter segments were examined from 11 hearts (mean 60 per patient). (The coronary arteries in patient 11 had been opened previously in longitudinal fashion and, thus, the arteries in him could not be examined quantitatively.) The percent of 5-mm segments of the 4 major epicardial coronary arteries narrowed to varying degrees of XSA

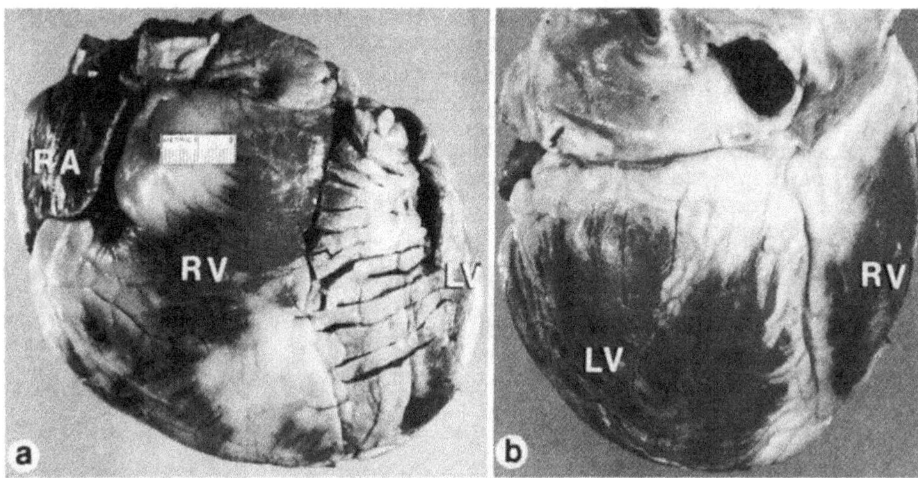

FIGURE 3. Patient 5 (age 40 years) (Table I). Exterior of heart: anterior view (a) and posterior view (b). The amount of epicardial fat does not appear to be increased. LV = left ventricle; RA = right atrium; RV = right ventricle.

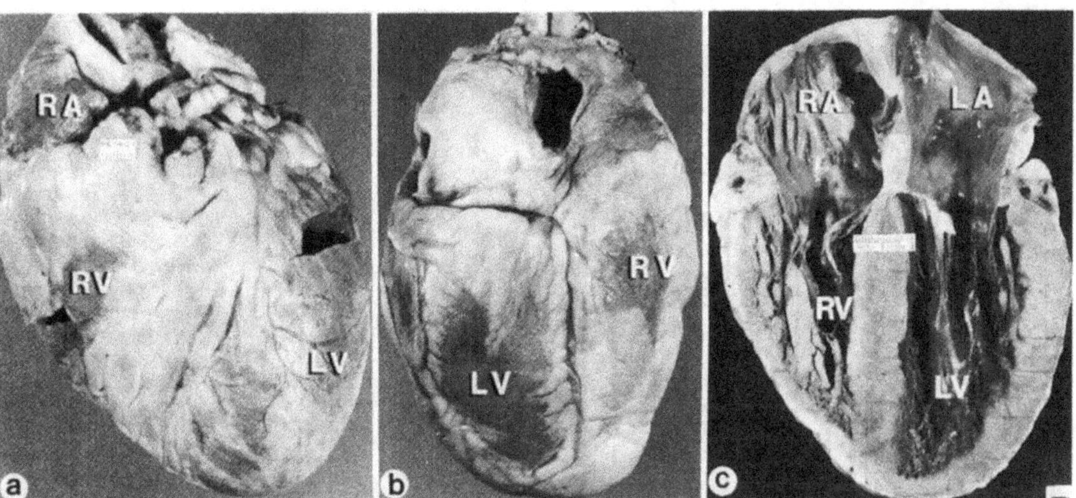

FIGURE 4. Patient 10 (age 48 years) (Table I). Exterior of heart (a and b) and after longitudinal cut (c). a, anterior view; b, posterior view. The subepicardial fat is moderately increased. c, all 4 chambers are dilated (heart weight 560 g). LA = left atrium; LV = left ventricle; RA = right atrium; RV = right ventricle.

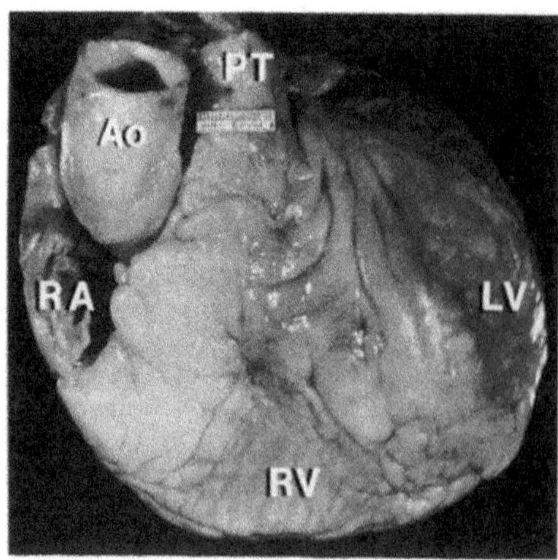

FIGURE 5. Patient 12 (age 59 years) (Table I). Exterior of heart as seen anteriorly, showing severe increase in amount of subepicardial adipose tissue. Ao = aorta; LV = left ventricle; PT = pulmonary trunk; RA = right atrium; RV = right ventricle.

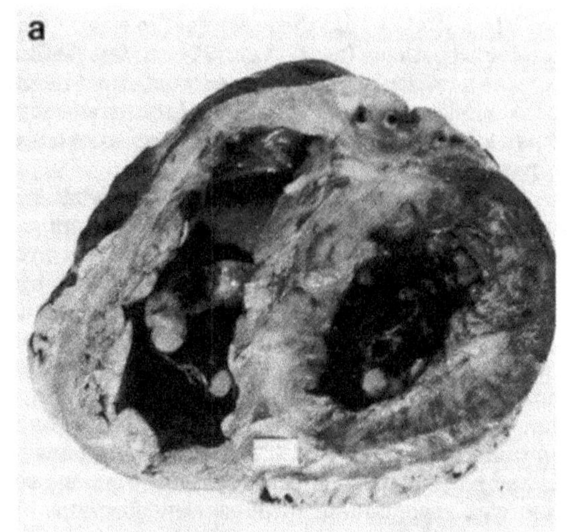

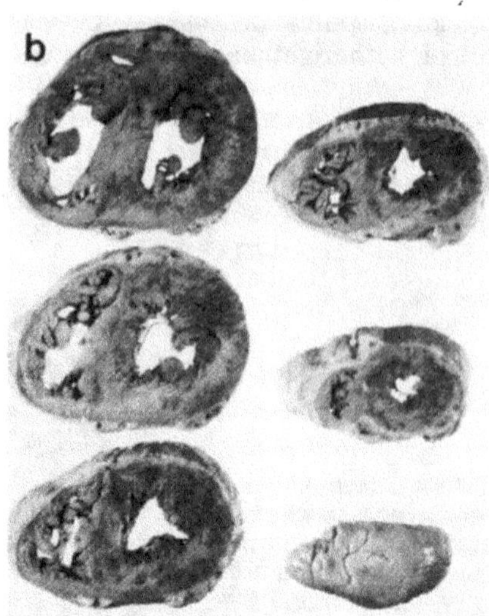

FIGURE 6. Patient 7 (age 34 years) (Table I). Base of the heart (a) and transverse slices of ventricles (b). Both ventricular walls are hypertrophied and both cavities are dilated.

in the 11 patients is shown in Figure 7. Only 2 patients (nos. 9 and 12) had any segments narrowed 76 to 100% in XSA. Of the 664 five-millimeter coronary segments, 431 (65%) were narrowed 0 to 25% in XSA; 143 (21%) were narrowed 26 to 50%; 73 (11%) were narrowed 51 to 75%; and 17 (3%) were narrowed 76 to 100%. No patient had any 5-mm segments narrowed 96 to 100%, although patient 12, with an acute myocardial infarction, had an occlusive thrombus in the proximal portion of the left anterior descending coronary artery at a site that was already narrowed 76 to 95% by atherosclerotic plaque.

Discussion

Examination of the 12 hearts described above disclosed that each was heavier than normal, that 9 contained increased amounts of subepicardial adipose

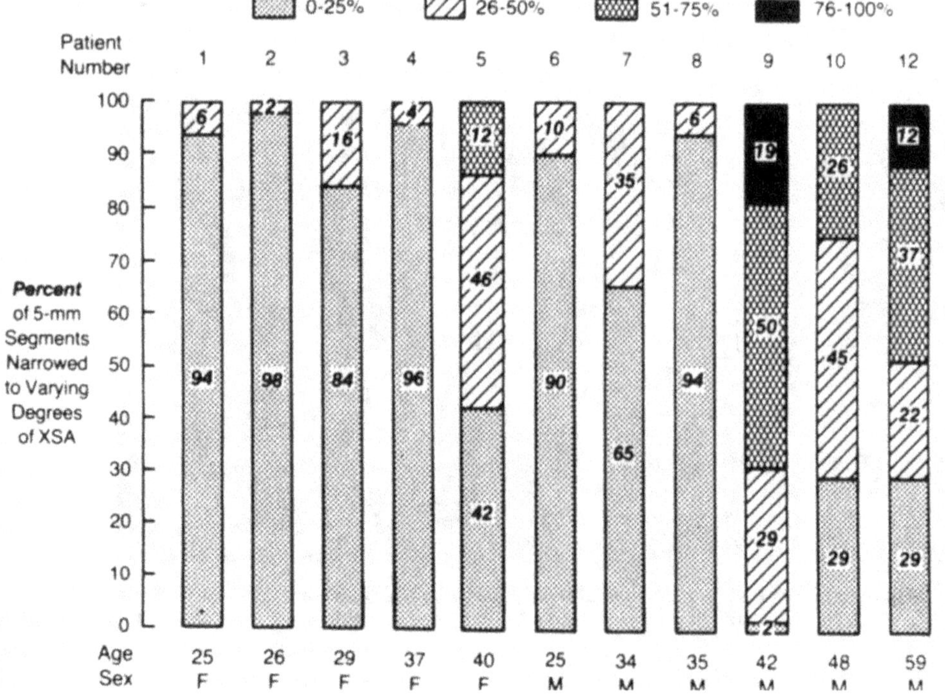

FIGURE 7. The percents of 5-mm segments of the 4 major epicardial coronary arteries narrowed to varying degrees in 11 patients with massive (>300 pounds) obesity. (Because the coronary arteries in patient 11 had been opened previously in longitudinal fashion, quantitation of them was not possible.) XSA = cross-sectional area.

tissue (none to the extent that the heart floated in water[2]), that all but 1 patient had dilated right and left ventricular cavities, and that only 2 patients had any significant coronary arterial luminal narrowing by atherosclerotic plaque.

The only other reported study describing cardiac necropsy findings in patients with extreme obesity was that of Amad et al.[5] Their 12 patients were 33 to 75 years old (mean 51). The 6 women, who were 155 to 171 cm tall (mean 163) (61 to 67 inches [mean 64]), weighed 108 to 159 kg (mean 136) (238 to 250 lb [mean 300]); the 6 men, who were 167 to 179 cm tall (mean 174) (66 to 71 inches [mean 69]), weighed 99 to 225 kg (mean 150) (218 to 496 lb [mean 331]). The amounts of excess body weight ranged from 25 to 159 kg, representing increments of 34 to 240% above predicted ideal weights. Amad et al excluded patients with indirect systemic arterial pressures ≥150/90 mm Hg, and patients with either clinical or morphologic evidence of coronary or valvular heart disease or hypothyroidism. Death in 3 of their 12 patients, however, was attributed to chronic congestive heart failure, each patient "... having had symptoms and signs of myocardial insufficiency for several months prior to death." The hearts in their 12 patients weighed 400 to 1,100 g (mean 575). (Their weights, in contrast to those in our study, were obtained from autopsy protocols, not by the weighing of each heart by the same investigator.) The mean body weight of their 12 patients was 143 kg (315 lb), giving them a 0.40 mean cardiac weight to body weight ratio, expressed as a percent (normal 0.43 for men [range 0.42 to 0.46] and 0.40 for women [range 0.38 to 0.46][6]). By gross examination, none of their 12 patients had fatty infiltration in myocardium, or grossly visible foci of myocardial necrosis or fibrosis, or "isolated" or "predominant" right ventricular hypertrophy.

Acknowledgment: We thank Dr. James L. Luke, formerly Chief Medical Examiner, Washington, D.C., for permission to use 9 cases studied by him and his associates.

References

1. **Bray GA, ed.** Obesity in Perspective. Fogarty International Center Series on Preventive Medicine. DHEW Publications, 1973, Vol 2, Part 1:7.
2. **Roberts WC, Roberts JD.** The floating heart or the heart too fat to sink: analysis of 55 necropsy patients. Am J Cardiol 1983;52:1286–1289.
3. **Movat HZ.** Demonstration of all connective tissue elements in a single section. Pentrachrome stains. Arch Pathol 1955;60:289–295.
4. **Isner JM, Wu M, Virmani R, Jones AA, Roberts WC.** Comparison of degrees of coronary arterial luminal narrowing determined by visual inspection of histologic sections under magnification among three independent observers and comparison to that obtained by videoplanimetry. An analysis of 559 five-millimeter segments of 61 coronary arteries from eleven patients. Lab Invest 1980;42:566–570.
5. **Amad KH, Brennan JC, Alexander JK.** The cardiac pathology of chronic exogenous obesity. Circulation 1965;32:740–745.
6. **Smith HL.** Relation of the weight of the heart to the weight of the body and of the weight of the heart to age. Am Heart J 1928;4:79–93.

Electrocardiographic Observations in Clinically Isolated, Pure, Chronic, Severe Aortic Regurgitation: Analysis of 30 Necropsy Patients Aged 19 to 65 Years

WILLIAM C. ROBERTS, MD, and PAUL J. DAY*

Certain electrocardiographic findings are described in 30 necropsy patients with clinically isolated pure, chronic, severe aortic regurgitation. They were 19 to 65 years old (mean 45). The hearts of the 22 men ranged in weight from 430 to 1,110 g (mean 717) and of the 8 women, from 375 to 950 g (mean 638). Four had grossly visible left ventricular (LV) scars. All but 1 patient was in sinus rhythm. The PR interval was >0.20 second in 8 patients (28%) and the QRS duration was ≥0.12 second in 6 patients (20%). Only 5 patients (17%) had 1 or more ventricular premature complexes recorded on the resting electrocardiogram analyzed. The mean QRS amplitude for each of the 12 leads averaged 23 mm. The highest mean QRS voltage occurred in leads V_2 and V_3 (each 38 mm), and the lowest in lead aVR (11 mm). The mean QRS voltage in V_5 was higher than in V_6 (33 vs 28 mm) and in 22 patients (73%) the QRS voltage in V_5 was higher than in V_6. The sum of the S wave in V_1 plus the larger of the R wave in V_5 or V_6 (Sokolow-Lyon index) averaged 51 mm and in only 22 patients (73%) was it >35 mm. The Romhilt-Estes voltage criteria for LV hypertrophy was fulfilled even less frequently, despite the severe degrees of LV hypertrophy in the patients studied. The total 12-lead QRS amplitude in the 30 patients ranged from 109 to 428 mm (mean 272) (10 mm = 1 mV) and in 27 patients (90%) it was >175 mm. The ratio of total 12-lead QRS voltage to heart weight in the 30 patients with aortic regurgitation was 0.42, only slightly higher than that in previously studied adults with severe aortic stenosis (0.39), an observation indicating that cavity dilatation does not magnify the QRS voltage generated by a given mass of myocardium.

(Am J Cardiol 1985;55:431–438)

Although many studies are available on electrocardiographic findings in patients with aortic valve stenosis, few studies have described electrocardiographic findings in patients with chronic aortic regurgitation (AR). Electrocardiographic QRS voltage observations[1-7] in patients with chronic AR usually have been limited to analysis of the presence of left ventricular (LV) hypertrophy as determined by criteria proposed by Sokolow and Lyon[8] or Romhilt and Estes.[9] No studies of patients with fatal, pure, isolated AR have compared electrocardiographic findings during life to necropsy cardiac findings. Such a correlation is the purpose of this report. The amplitude of the QRS complexes in all 12 leads, in addition to that of certain R and S waves, was measured in all patients.

Definitions

The terms describing AR in the patients were defined as follows: *Clinically isolated*—valvular dysfunction limited to the aortic valve. Function of the mitral, tricuspid and pulmonic valves was normal. *Pure*—no peak systolic pressure gradient present between left ventricle and systemic artery. *Chronic*—evidence of severe AR for more than 6 months.

Severe—AR graded 3+ or 4+/4+ by aortic root angiogram or symptoms of cardiac functional class III or IV (New York Heart Association criteria) and the symptoms attributable only to AR.

Patients

Inclusion criteria for this study were (1) presence of chronic, isolated, pure, severe AR; (2) age at death older than 15 years; (3) interval between aortic valve replacement and death within 2 months; (4) availability of 12-lead electrocardiogram (ECG) recorded either preoperatively or within 1 month of death; and (5) heart weight >350 g in women and >400 g in men. The ECG analyzed was always that obtained just before aortic valve replacement (19 patients) or in the patients who did not undergo aortic valve operation,[10] the one recorded in the last month of life. The amplitude of the QRS complexes was measured from the peak of the R wave to the maximal dip of the S or Q wave, whichever was greater (Fig. 1). The cardiac catheterization data were obtained just before aortic valve replacement (16 patients) or within 6 months of death in the patients who did not undergo aortic valve operation (6 patients).

Thirty patients fulfilled the inclusion criteria. Certain clinical and morphologic findings for these patients are summarized in Table I. In all 30 patients the clinical records were examined, the heart in each was examined initially and the hearts in 25 patients were reexamined. The amounts of coronary arterial narrowing present was determined by examination of 5-mm transverse sections of the 4 major coronary arteries by a method delineated elsewhere.[11] Of the 30 patients, the cause of the AR was infective endocarditis that had healed in 8,[10] cardiovascular syphilis in 6,[12] ankylosing spondylitis in 5,[13] Marfan's syndrome in 5,[14] uncertain cause

From the Pathology Branch, National Heart, Lung, and Blood Institute, National Institutes of Health, Bethesda, Maryland. Manuscript received September 12, 1984, accepted October 2, 1984.

* Student, Saint Mary's College, Saint Mary's City, Maryland 20686.

Address for reprints: William C. Roberts, MD, Building 10A, Room 3E-30, National Institutes of Health, Bethesda, Maryland 20205.

in 4, trauma in 1[15] and systemic hypertension in 1.[16] The patients were 19 to 65 years old (mean 45); 22 (73%) were men and 8 (27%) were women. Of the 30 patients, 29 had evidence of congestive heart failure (New York Heart Association functional class III or IV); patient 2 (Table I) was asymptomatic but had aortic valve replacement because of a LV end-systolic dimension >55 mm by echocardiogram. Of the 30 patients, 22 had left-sided cardiac catheterization and aortic root angiograms. LV peak systolic pressures ranged from 88 to 190 mm Hg (mean 133), LV end-diastolic pressures from 8 to 80 mm Hg (mean 32) and systemic arterial end-diastolic pressures from 20 to 65 mm Hg (mean 42). Nineteen patients died of complications of aortic valve replacement; the other 11 died from chronic congestive heart failure secondary to the AR.

At necropsy, the hearts in the 22 men weighed 430 to 1,100 g (mean 717) (normal ≤400 g) and the hearts in the 8 women weighed 375 to 950 g (mean 638) (normal ≤350 g). These weights were total heart weights, not just LV weights. A grossly visible, transmural (involving all the inner half and a portion or all of the outer half of the wall) LV scar (healed myocardial infarct) was present in 4 patients, but none during life had a clinical event diagnosed as, or compatible with, acute myocardial infarction.

The comparison of means was done using an unpaired Student t test, the comparison of ratios was done using a chi-square test, and the correlation coefficients were calculated using a Pearson's product moment test. Significance was judged if the test yielded a p valve <0.05.

Results

General electrocardiographic observations: Electrocardiographic findings are summarized in Tables I and II. The total 12-lead QRS amplitude in the 30 patients ranged from 109 to 428 mm (mean 272) (10 mm = 1 mV), and in 27 patients (90%) it was >175 mm (Table II). The relation of the total 12-lead QRS voltage to heart weight in the 30 patients is illustrated in Figure 2. The method of measuring various QRS complexes for this measurement is illustrated in Figure 1. The mean QRS voltage for each of the 12 leads in each patient was 23 mm. The individual and mean QRS amplitudes in each of the 12 leads is displayed in Table II. The highest mean QRS voltage occurred in leads V_2 and V_3 (each 38 mm), and the lowest mean voltage in lead aVR, 11 mm. The QRS mean voltage in V_5 was higher than that in V_6 (33 mm vs 28 mm); in 22 patients (73%), the QRS voltage in V_5 was higher than that in V_6.

Various previously recommended electrocardiographic QRS voltage criteria (summarized by Murphy et al[17]) for LV hypertrophy and the frequency of their occurrence in our 30 patients with chronic AR are summarized in Table III. A few criteria have been slightly modified to allow the number designating the upper limit of normal to end in a 0 or a 5, and to allow the elevated value to always be greater than a certain number rather than equal to or greater than a certain number. Of the 18 criteria analyzed, only 1 upper-limit number was evaluated in 3, two values were analyzed in 14, and 4 values in 1. Thus, a total of 35 values were analyzed for the 18 criteria: 34 were measurements in millimeters of QRS voltage and 1 was a ratio. The 2 criteria that had the highest positive frequency were the sum of the tallest limb-lead R wave plus the deepest limb-lead S wave >15 mm (90%, 27 of 30 patients) and the sum of the voltage of the QRS complex in all 12 leads, >175 mm (90%). The sum of the S wave in lead V_1 plus the larger of the R wave in V_5 or V_6 was >35 mm in 22 patients (73%). The sum of the larger S wave of leads V_1 or V_2 plus the larger of the R wave of V_5 or V_6 was >35 mm in 26 patients (87%) and >40 mm in 22 patients (73%). The sum of the deepest S wave in leads V_1, V_2 and V_3 plus the tallest R waves in leads V_4, V_5 and V_6 was >35 mm in 26 patients (87%), >40 mm in 25 patients (83%), >45 mm in 22 patients (73%) and >50 mm in 21 patients (70%). The tallest R wave plus the deepest S wave in any single V lead was >35 mm in 19 patients (63%).

The S-wave amplitude in lead V_1 ranged from 9 to 60 mm (mean 23); the R-wave amplitude in lead V_5 ranged from 9 to 64 mm (mean 25) and in V_6, from 11 to 47 mm (mean 25). The sum of the S wave in V_1 and the larger of the R waves in either V_5 or V_6 (Sokolow-Lyon index) ranged from 22 to 110 mm (mean 51). The deepest S wave in leads V_1, V_2 and V_3 ranged from 12 to 70 mm (mean 38) and in 23 patients (77%) it was >25 mm. The largest precordial S wave was in lead V_1 in 3 patients (10%), in lead V_2 in 12 patients (40%), in lead V_3 in 13 patients (43%) and in V_4 in 2 patients (7%). The average S-wave amplitude was higher in lead V_2 than V_1 (40 vs 24 mm).

The largest R wave in leads V_4, V_5 and V_6 ranged from 12 to 64 mm (mean 30) and in 19 patients (63%) it was >25 mm; the largest precordial R wave was in lead V_4 in 2 patients (7%), in V_5 in 19 (63%) and in V_6 in 9 (30%). The mean height of the R wave in both leads V_5 and V_6 averaged 25 mm. The R wave in V_6 was larger than the R wave in V_5 in 9 patients (30%).

Of the 30 patients, 29 (97%) were in sinus rhythm. The PR interval in them ranged from 0.16 to 0.36 second (mean 0.21) and it was >0.20 second in 8 (28%) patients. The width of the QRS complex ranged from 0.06 to 0.14 second (mean 0.10); in 6 (20%) patients it was ≥0.12 second. The QRS axes are listed in Table II. Of the 30

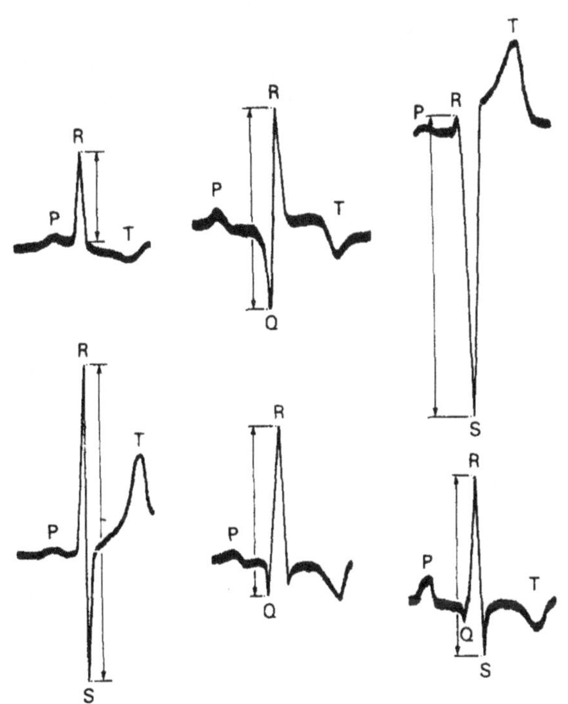

FIGURE 1. Method of measurement for various QRS complexes.

TABLE I Certain Clinical Morphologic and Electrocardiographic Features in 30 Necropsy Patients with Chronic, Severe, Pure Aortic Regurgitation

| | | | | | Pressures (mm Hg) | | | | | | | | | Electrocardiogram | | | | |
| | | | | | LV | | SA | | AR | | | | No. of | | | | Intervals (sec) | | |
Pt	Autopsy No.	Age (yr) & Sex	Cause of AR	AP	S	D	S	D	by Cine (1+–4+)	AVR	HW (g)	LV F	4 Major CA >75%	VR (bpm)	QRS axis (Degrees)	PR	QRS	VPC
1	A57-251	33M	IE	0	...	...	130	70	...	0	430	0	0	84	−40	0.27	0.14	0
2	A80-139	37M	IE	0	115	23	120	60	4+	+	610	0	0	90	−20	0.16	0.10	0
3	A69-254	39M	IE	0	140	20	140	38	4+	0	1010	0	0	68	0	0.20	0.12	0
4	71A-21	40M	IE	0	190	31	190	60	4+	+	575	+	0	72	+30	0.18	0.09	0
5	A70-117	45M	IE	0	120	50	120	50	4+	+	610	0	0	72	−15	0.20	0.11	0
6	71A-407	49M	IE	0	...	...	160	40	...	+	640	0	0	100	+30	0.18	0.11	+
7	A71-149	52F	IE	0	130	44	150	40	4+	+	500	0	0	75	0	0.15	0.10	0
8	A72-42	59M	IE	0	118	38	123	52	3+	+	840	0	0	70	+60	0.24	0.12	0
9	A58-280	19M	Syphilis	0	148	33	148	33	4+	0	750	0	0	100	+45	0.16	0.10	0
10	A61-192	37M	Syphilis	+	152	20	152	55	4+	0	600	0	0	66	+30	0.20	0.07	+
11	70A369	50M	Syphilis	+	...	...	160	60	...	0	720	+	2	90	−50	0.17	0.10	0
12	A65-106	55M	Syphilis	0	138	37	160	51	4+	+	940	0	3	75	−20	0.20	0.10	0
13	A64-223	56F	Syphilis	0	106	25	108	27	4+	+	800	+	3	72	+60	0.20	0.11	0
14	A77-241	65F	Syphilis	0	170	8	184	50	4+	+	710	0	1	81	+50	0.16	0.08	0
15	A61-274	34M	Anky Sp	0	100	22	120	25	4+	+	700	0	0	64	−30	0.26	0.10	0
16	A68-142	38M	Anky Sp	0	180	16	180	50	4+	+	1100	0	0	75	0	0.28	0.11	0
17	A61-99	52M	Anky Sp	0	160	18	168	30	4+	+	850	0	0	60	−15	0.36	0.14	0
18	A61-262	55M	Anky Sp	0	114	40	120	38	4+	0	680	0	0	82	−30	0.22	0.06	0
19	A66-127	57M	Anky Sp	0	...	...	200	80	...	0	500	0	0	110	0	0.17	0.09	0
20	A77-11	35F	Marfan	+	120	24	120	50	4+	+	375	0	0	66	−30	0.17	0.12	0
21	A58-206	36F	Marfan	0	...	...	130	40	...	0	700	0	0	95	−45	0.19	0.10	0
22	A65-64	41M	Marfan	0	100	30	100	40	3+	+	750	0	0	72	−10	0.20	0.10	+
23	A69-278	48F	Marfan	+	150	12	150	40	3+	+	520	0	0	72	+110	0.16	0.11	0
24	A59-169	59M	Marfan	0	190	25	200	80	3+	0	865	0	0	100	+20	...	0.08	+
25	71A27	34M	Uncertain	0	105	36	122	65	3+	+	460	0	0	84	−10	0.20	0.08	0
26	70A309	40F	Uncertain	0	...	...	180	60	...	0	950	0	0	70	+60	0.20	0.10	0
27	A64-102	41M	Uncertain	0	88	19	96	20	4+	+	920	0	0	75	+50	0.28	0.13	+
28	69A-135	59M	Uncertain	0	...	...	140	60	...	+	630	0	2	70	−20	0.167	0.08	0
29	A60-261	35M	Trauma	0	100	50	110	50	4+	0	550	+	0	85	+50	0.31	0.10	0
30	A68-325	51F	SH	+	...	...	210	80	...	+	600	0	0	76	−30	0.20	0.10	0
Mean or total	45	22M		5	132	28	139*	50*	22	19	696	4	5	79	+9	0.21	0.10	5

* Includes only the 23 patients in whom the systemic arterial pressure was measured directly at catheterization.

Anky Sp = ankylosing spondylitis; AP = angina pectrois; AR = aortic regurgitation; AVR = aortic valve replacement; CA = coronary artery; Cine-cineangiogram; D = end-diastole; F = grossly visible fibrosis; HW = heart weight; LV = left ventricle or left ventricular; S = peak systole; SA = systemic artery; SH = systemic hypertension; VPC = ventricular premature complex; VR = ventricular rate.

TABLE II Electrocardiographic QRS Amplitudes (in mm [10 mm = 1 mV]) in 30 Necropsy Patients with Chronic, Pure, Isolated Aortic Regurgitation

Pt	I	II	III	aVR	aVL	aVF	V_1	V_2	V_3	V_4	V_5	V_6	Total 12 Lead	S V_1	S V_2	R V_5	R V_6
1	7	7	12	5	9	9	11	33	42	42	29	34	240	10	33	22	32
2	13	20	23	14	19	19	11	14	11	12	15	11	182	10	12	12	11
3	12	8	15	9	12	10	30	56	52	37	24	50	315	27	54	23	47
4	15	15	12	15	11	10	31	33	20	48	35	28	273	29	28	35	28
5	8	30	28	18	15	26	32	72	44	58	50	29	410	25	62	48	28
6	9	12	8	7	9	7	33	37	40	41	32	28	263	27	32	31	28
7	7	8	7	7	7	7	26	48	47	28	30	20	242	24	48	27	20
8	8	9	5	7	6	7	24	25	12	17	17	16	153	23	24	16	14
9	5	18	17	11	6	17	25	53	49	55	36	19	311	17	36	21	17
10	9	7	4	8	5	4	18	29	35	14	31	29	193	20	31	32	30
11	16	5	14	8	16	11	16	31	38	34	30	15	234	16	30	23	15
12	20	7	24	10	21	15	27	58	46	17	23	31	299	28	49	29	31
13	13	18	21	10	15	19	21	28	32	29	39	36	281	20	24	27	34
14	11	14	9	11	8	9	10	12	15	20	30	20	169	9	16	18	17
15	19	17	28	13	23	19	31	64	74	24	68	48	428	30	59	64	44
16	29	13	21	22	27	9	50	58	72	42	21	50	414	50	59	9	42
17	21	11	12	14	17	4	21	18	16	8	27	27	196	15	15	26	24
18	9	4	11	6	10	8	14	18	31	31	27	24	193	13	16	15	21
19	19	21	8	21	11	12	50	54	37	70	45	26	374	39	38	37	25
20	11	8	6	8	8	5	14	34	46	40	42	24	246	7	13	15	12
21	21	18	35	12	28	26	39	44	37	39	45	37	381	31	39	37	30
22	21	14	19	18	16	10	64	74	62	20	46	27	391	60	72	50	27
23	9	32	42	13	30	37	8	23	28	38	62	62	384	9	21	12	16
24	9	9	13	5	12	12	15	29	34	16	26	22	202	17	35	16	14
25	5	5	6	5	5	4	9	22	18	6	15	9	109	8	18	14	8
26	12	9	10	9	12	5	32	39	40	27	20	35	250	29	37	10	31
27	8	11	6	8	8	9	31	52	76	52	25	29	367	22	52	11	27
28	11	15	8	11	6	11	14	19	26	33	29	19	202	13	19	20	15
29	10	8	11	6	10	9	22	22	30	24	30	25	207	21	21	29	24
30	18	20	15	18	13	17	35	25	16	15	29	28	249	33	22	28	26
Mean	13	14	15	11	13	13	25	38	38	32	33	28	272	23	34	25	25

Pt	Largest S V_1-V_3 (mm)	(Lead)	Largest R V_4-V_6 (mm)	(Lead)	Largest R 6 Limb Leads (mm)	(Lead)	Largest S 6 Limb Leads (mm)	(Lead)	R	S
1	33	V_3	32	V_6	8	aVL	11	III	5	11
2	12	V_2	12	V_5	16	aVL	17	III	12	17
3	54	V_2	47	V_6	12	I	10	III	12	10
4	29	V_1	35	V_5	15	I	15	aVR	15	7
5	62	V_2	48	V_5	18	II	17	III	9	17
6	39	V_4	31	V_5	12	II	3	aVL	7	0
7	48	V_2	27	V_5	8	I	8	aVR	8	5
8	24	V_2	16	V_5	9	I	9	aVR	9	2
9	40	V_4	21	V_5	11	II	7	AVF	3	6
10	35	V_3	32	V_5	10	I	8	AVR	10	4
11	35	V_3	23	V_5	15	I	13	III	15	13
12	49	V_2	31	V_6	23	aVL	22	III	18	22
13	29	V_3	34	V_6	19	aVF	11	aVR	11	0
14	16	V_2	18	V_5	14	II	12	aVR	10	0
15	68	V_3	64	V_5	20	aVL	22	III	18	22
16	68	V_3	42	V_6	30	I	23	aVR	30	20
17	15	V_1	26	V_5	19	I	16	aVR	19	12
18	27	V_3	21	V_6	9	I	11	III	9	11
19	38	V_2	46	V_4	20	I	19	aVR	20	7
20	16	V_3	15	V_5	11	I	8	aVR	11	5
21	39	V_2	37	V_5	29	aVL	32	III	19	32
22	72	V_2	50	V_5	23	I	18	aVR	23	15
23	27	V_3	16	V_6	37	aVF	29	aVL	2	41
24	40	V_3	16	V_5	11	aVL	11	III	10	11
25	18	V_2	14	V_5	3	I	3	aVR	3	3
26	39	V_3	31	V_6	9	I	10	aVR	9	4
27	72	V_3	27	V_6	7	I	7	aVR	7	2
28	19	V_2	25	V_4	11	I	9	aVR	11	8
29	32	V_3	29	V_5	10	I	10	III	10	10
30	34	V_1	28	V_5	20	II	17	aVR	17	0
Mean	38		30		15		14		12	10

single rest ECGs analyzed, 1 or more premature ventricular complexes were present in 5 patients (17%) (nos. 6, 10, 22, 24 and 27, Table I and II) and 1 or more premature atrial complexes in 1 patient (no. 2).

Comparison of men to women: No significant (p >0.05) differences were observed between the 22 men and 8 women in mean age; percent with significant coronary arterial narrowing, LV scarring, angina pectoris or widened ($\geq$0.12 second) QRS complexes; mean heart weight (717 vs 638 g); average total 12-lead QRS voltage (269 vs 275 mm); average Sokolow-Lyon index (52 vs 46 mm), or mean LV peak systolic pressure (134 vs 130 mm Hg).

TABLE III **Recommended or Modified Electrocardiographic Criteria for Determining Left Ventricular Hypertrophy as Applied to 30 Necropsy Patients with Severe Cardiomegaly from Chronic, Pure, Severe Aortic Regurgitation**

No.	QRS Complex Measured	Value Considered Upper Limit of Normal (mm)	No. (%) of 30 Patients Above Normal Limit
1a	$SV_1 + RV_5$ or V_6 (larger)	35	22 (73)
b	$SV_1 + RV_5$ or V_6 (larger)	40	18 (60)
2a	SV_1 or V_2 (larger) + RV_5 or V_6 (larger)	35	26 (87)
b	SV_1 or V_2 (larger) + RV_5 or V_6 (larger)	40	22 (73)
3a	SV_1 or V_2 (larger) + RV_6	35	25 (83)
b	SV_1 or V_2 (larger) + RV_6	40	21 (70)
4a	$SV_2 + RV_5$	35	24 (80)
b	$SV_2 + RV_5$	40	22 (73)
5a	Deepest $SV_1 - V_3$ + tallest $RV_4 - V_6$	35	26 (87)
b	Deepest $SV_1 - V_3$ + tallest $RV_4 - V_6$	40	25 (83)
c	Deepest $SV_1 - V_3$ + tallest $rV_4 - V_6$	45	22 (73)
d	Deepest $SV_1 - V_3$ + tallest $V_4 - V_6$	50	21 (70)
6a	Tallest R + deepest S in any V lead	35	19 (63)
b	Tallest R + deepest S in any V lead	40	16 (53)
7a	Deepest $SV_1 - V_3$	25	23 (77)
b	Deepest $SV_1 - V_3$	30	19 (63)
8a	Tallest $RV_4 - V_6$	25	19 (63)
b	Tallest $RV_4 - V_6$	30	14 (47)
9a	Deeper SV_1 or V_2	25	19 (63)
b	Deeper SV_1 or V_2	30	17 (57)
10a	Tallest RV_5 or V_6	25	26 (87)
b	Tallest RV_5 or V_6	30	14 (47)
11	$RV_6 > RV_5$	<1	9 (30)
12a	Tallest limb-lead R + deepest limb-lead S	15	27 (90)
b	Tallest limb-lead R + deepest limb-lead S	20	17 (57)
13a	$R_1 + S_3$	15	20 (67)
b	$R_1 + S_3$	20	14 (47)
14a	Tallest limb-lead R	10	21 (70)
b	Tallest limb-lead R	15	13 (43)
15a	Deepest limb-lead S	10	18 (60)
b	Deepest limb-lead S	15	11 (37)
16	R_1	10	15 (50)
17	S_3	10	13 (43)
18a	Total 12-lead QRS voltage	175	27 (90)
b	Total 12-lead QRS voltage	200	23 (77)

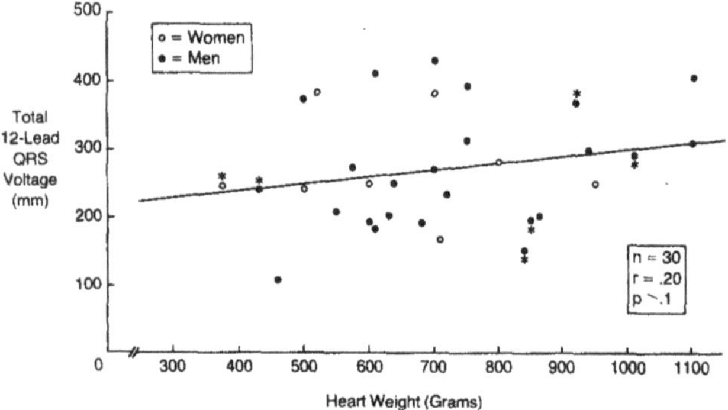

FIGURE 2. Relation of the total 12-lead QRS voltage (mm) to heart weight (grams) in the 30 patients with severe, pure aortic regurgitation. **Asterisks** designate the patients in whom the widths of the QRS complexes were at least 0.12 second.

Comparison of patients younger than 40 years and older than 40 years: No significant differences were observed between the 13 younger and the 17 older (older than 40 years) patients in sex ratio; percent with angina pectoris, widened QRS complexes or LV scarring; mean heart weight (677 vs 710 g); average Sokolow-Lyon index (50 vs 50 mm), or mean LV peak-systolic pressure (137 vs 129 mm Hg). The percent with significant (>75% cross-sectional area) coronary arterial narrowing was different (0 of 13 vs 5 of 17) (p <0.05).

Comparison of patients with and without angina pectoris: No significant differences were observed between the 6 patients with and the 24 patients without angina in mean age; sex ratio; frequency of coronary arterial narrowing or LV scarring; average total 12-lead QRS voltage (287 vs 267 mm); mean Sokolow-Lyon index (55 vs 49 mm); or LV peak systolic pressure (117 vs 138 mm Hg). The frequency of widened QRS complexes was different (3 of 6 vs 3 of 24) (p <0.05).

Comparison of patients with total 12-lead QRS voltage 250 mm or less to those with total voltage more than 250 mm: No significant differences were observed between the 17 patients with total 12-lead QRS voltage ≤250 mm and the 13 patients with larger total voltage in mean age, sex ratio, percent with significant coronary arterial narrowing, LV scarring, angina pectoris or widened QRS complexes; mean LV peak systolic pressure (135 vs 133 mm Hg), or mean heart weight (648 vs 760 g). The average Sokolow-Lyon index was different (39 vs 65 mm) (p <0.001).

Comparison of patients with normal and abnormal Sokolow-Lyon indexes: No significant differences were observed between the 8 patients with normal and the 22 patients with abnormal (>35 mm) indexes in mean age; sex ratio; percent with narrowed coronary arteries, LV scar, angina pectoris or widened QRS complexes, or mean LV peak systolic pressure (131 vs 136 mm Hg). The average total 12-lead QRS voltage was different (210 vs 296 mm) (p <0.05). The Sokolow-Lyon index in the 22 patients in whom this index was >35 mm ranged from 38 to 110 mm (mean 61) and their hearts weighed 430 to 1,100 g (mean 729); in the 8 patients in whom the Sokolow-Lyon index was <35 mm, the index ranged from 22 to 34 mm (mean 27) and their hearts weighed 375 to 865 g (mean 606).

Comparison of patients with normal and widened (more than 0.12 second) QRS complexes: No significant differences were observed between the 24 patients with QRS widths <0.12 second compared to the 6 with longer widths in mean age; sex ratio; percent with narrowed coronary arteries, LV scar or angina pectoris; mean heart weight (686 vs 738 g); average total 12-lead QRS voltage (276 vs 249 mm); mean Sokolow-Lyon index (51 vs 44 mm), or mean LV peak systolic pressure (138 vs 117 mm Hg). The frequency of angina pectoris was different (p <0.05): angina was present in 3 of 24 patients with normal-width QRS complexes and in 3 of 6 patients with widened complexes (p <0.05).

Comparison of patients with left ventricular peak systolic pressure less than 140 mm Hg to those with pressures greater than 140 mm Hg: No significant differences were observed between the 14 patients with the lower compared to the 8 patients with the higher (>140 mm) pressures in age; sex ratio; percent with angina, coronary arterial narrowing, LV scar, or widened QRS complexes; mean heart weight (696 vs 746 g), average total 12-lead QRS voltage (271 vs 267 mm), or mean Sokolow-Lyon index (52 vs 44 mm).

Comparison of patients with hearts weighing 600 g or less to those with hearts weighing more than 600 g: No significant differences were observed between the 10 patients with hearts ≤600 g compared to the 20 patients with larger hearts in mean age; sex ratio; percent with angina pectoris, coronary arterial narrowing, LV scar or widened QRS complexes; average total 12-lead QRS voltage (252 vs 280 mm); mean Sokolow-Lyon index (45 vs 53 mm), or mean LV peak-systolic pressure (130 vs 135 mm Hg).

Comparison of patients with and without coronary arterial narrowing: The mean age was older among the 5 patients with narrowing >75% in cross-sectional area of 1 or more major coronary arteries compared to that among the 25 patients without (57 vs 42 years), and the percent with LV scarring was higher (2 of 5 vs 2 of 25) (p <0.05). No significant differences were observed between the 2 groups in sex ratio; percent with angina or widened QRS complexes; mean heart weights (729 vs 688 g); average total 12-lead QRS voltage (243 vs 277 mm); mean Sokolow-Lyon index (47 vs 51 mm), or mean LV peak-systolic pressure (138 vs 140 mm Hg).

Comparison of patients with and without left ventricular scarring: Except for a higher frequency of coronary arterial narrowing in the patients with LV scars (2 of 4 vs 2 of 26) (p <0.05), no significant differences between these groups occurred in age; sex ratio; percent with angina or widened QRS complexes; mean heart weight (661 vs 701 g); average total 12-lead QRS voltage (249 vs 274 mm); mean Sokolow-Lyon index (50 vs 50 mm) or mean LV peak-systolic pressure (132 vs 135 mm Hg).

Discussion

Patients with chronic severe AR generally have hearts of greater weight than that observed in other conditions.[18] Thus, these patients should have larger QRS voltages than observed in other conditions. In addition to measuring R and S waves in 1 or more leads for LV hypertrophy as suggested by many investigators and summarized by Murphy et al[17] and in Table III, we measured the total QRS voltage in all 12 leads in each patient and compared its usefulness to that of other voltage criteria for LV hypertrophy.

Because patients with chronic, severe AR generally have the largest human hearts, these persons would appear to be the ideal group to examine the usefulness of the various QRS voltage criteria for LV hypertrophy. Many studies, of course, have compared LV mass determined at necropsy[9,19] or by angiography[20] or echocardiography[21–23] to QRS voltage, but few of the previous studies have included patients with chronic, severe, pure AR. All previous studies have demonstrated that all QRS voltage criteria for LV hypertrophy are unreliable. The present study demonstrates the same finding, but in a group of patients with larger hearts than those studied previously. Our patients as a group had hearts that weighed roughly 2 times normal.

The Sokolow-Lyon index[8] (sum of the S wave in V_1 plus the larger of the R wave in either V_5 or V_6), the most widely used QRS voltage criterion for LV hypertrophy, was >35 mm, i.e., abnormal, in only 22 of our 30 patients (73%) whose mean heart weight was 696 g. The QRS voltage for LV hypertrophy advocated by Romhilt and Estes[9] fared even worse, although these 2 investigators also incorporated non-QRS-voltage criteria for LV hypertrophy. Only 8 of our 30 patients (27%) had an R wave in the 6 limb leads ≥20 mm and only 5 (17%) had an S wave in these leads ≥20 mm (In our Table III, we use the criteria >20 mm rather than ≥20 mm to aid in comparisons to other criteria.); 23 patients (77%) had an S wave in leads V_1, V_2 and V_3 ≥25 mm and 20 (67%) had an R wave in leads V_4, V_5 and V_6 ≥25 mm. (Again, in the table we modified these voltage criteria to >25 mm rather than ≥25 mm.) A total of 25 patients (83%), however, satisfied the Romhilt-Estes QRS voltage criteria in 1 or more of the 4 lead sites (R in limb leads ≥20; S in limb leads ≥20; S in V_1, V_2 and V_3 ≥25 and R in V_4, V_5 and V_6 ≥25 mm).

A better criterion of LV hypertrophy was the sum of the tallest R wave and deepest S wave in the 6 limb leads. This sum was >15 mm in 27 (90%) of 30 patients.

In contrast to the disappointing frequency of fulfillment of the Sokolow-Lyon, Romhilt-Estes and most other criteria (Table III) for LV hypertrophy in our 30 patients with chronic, severe AR, measurement of the sum of the height and depth of the QRS complexes in all 12 leads did appear useful. Although the upper limit of normal QRS voltage in each of the 12 electrocardiographic leads in adults without evidence of cardiac disease has been well established,[17,24–27] the upper limit of total 12-lead QRS voltage has not been established in human adults whose LV mass has been determined by necropsy or by an angiographic or echocardiographic means. It is likely, however, that the total 12-lead QRS voltage in adults over 30 or so years of age with normal sized hearts is <175 mm. Indeed, Richard B. Devereux (AJC Editorial Board Member), in his review of the present manuscript, stated that 12-lead QRS voltage was <175 mm in 87 of 92 clinically normal patients (95%) studied by him, P.N. Casale and P. Kligfield (unpublished observations), indicating that this criterion has good specificity (100 times number of normal subjects with negative test divided by total number of normal subjects tested). Using 175 mm as the upper limit of normal, 27 of our 30 patients (90%) had LV hypertrophy by this criterion.

In the present study we also examined 10 other variables, further analyzing each to compare patients with to those without 1 or more variables or to compare patients with greater than to those with less than a certain figure. A total of 90 comparisons were examined among the 10 variables. Of the 90, only 8 (9%) showed a significant (p <0.05) difference in the variable analyzed. The 4 patients with transmural LV scars had a higher frequency of coronary narrowing (2 of 4 patients) than the 26 patients without LV scars (2 of 26 patients) (p <0.05) and vice versa. Patients older than 40 years had a significantly higher frequency of coronary narrowing than did the younger patients (p <0.05) and vice versa. Angina was significantly more frequent in pa-

TABLE IV Comparison of Total 12-Lead QRS Amplitude in Necropsy Patients with Chronic Aortic Regurgitation to Necropsy Patients with Aortic Valve Stenosis and Cardiac Amyloidosis

	Aortic Stenosis	p Value	Aortic Regurgitation	p Value	Cardiac Amyloidosis
No. of patients	50		30		30
Age (yr), range (mean)	16–65 (48)	NS	19–65 (45)	<0.001	21–93 (58)
Men (n)	36 (72%)	NS	22 (73%)	NS	15 (50%)
Women (n)	14 (28%)	NS	8 (27%)	NS	15 (50%)
Substernal pain (n)	34 (68%)	<0.01	11 (37%)	<0.05	4 (13%)
SA peak systole (mm Hg), range (average)	63–180 (112)	<0.001	96–200 (139)	<0.001	90–110 (104)
SA end-diastole (mm Hg), range (average)	34–88 (62)	<0.001	20–65 (42)	<0.001	60–80 (67)
Heart weight (g), range (mean)	380–880 (606)	<0.05	375–1110 (696)	<0.001	370–900 (532)
Narrowed coronary artery (n)	16 (32%)	NS	5 (17%)	NS	5 (17%)
Left ventricular scar (n)	7 (14%)	NS	4 (13%)	NS	4 (13%)
Total 12-lead QRS voltage (mm), range (average)	144–417 (257)	NS	109–428 (270)	<0.0001	58–199 (104)
Total 12-lead QRS voltage >175 mm, (n)	47 (94%)	NS	27 (90%)	<0.0001	2 (7%)

tients with QRS widths $\geq$0.12 second than in those with shorter QRS widths (3 of 6 vs 3 of 24) (p <0.05) and, conversely, the patients with the normal Sokolow-Lyon indices had significantly lower average total 12-lead QRS voltage than did the 21 patients with an abnormal (>35 mm) Sokolow-Lyon index (210 vs 296 mm); conversely, the 17 patients with total 12-lead QRS voltages $\leq$250 mm had lower mean Sokolow-Lyon indexes than did the 13 patients with total 12-lead QRS voltages >250 mm (39 vs 65 mm) (p <0.001).

Two other studies from this laboratory have used total 12-lead QRS voltage. One examined electrocardiograms in 50 necropsy patients with severe (LV systemic arterial peak systolic pressure gradients >50 mm Hg) aortic valve stenosis[28] and the other examined electrocardiograms in 30 necropsy patients with cardiac amyloidosis[29] (Table IV). Findings in these 2 groups of patients are summarized in Table IV and the findings are compared with those in the 30 patients with pure, chronic AR. The mean total QRS voltage was highest among patients with AR and lowest for those with amyloid. The percent of patients with AR or aortic stenosis having total 12-lead QRS voltage >175 mm was similar (90% and 94%), and 13 times higher than that in the amyloid group. The ratio of 12-lead QRS voltage to heart weight was slightly lower in the patients with aortic stenosis compared to those with pure AR (0.39 vs 0.42), indicating that cavity dilatation does not magnify the QRS voltage generated by a given mass of myocardium.

References

1. **Spagnuolo M, Kloth H, Taranta A, Doyle E, Pasternack B.** Natural history of rheumatic aortic regurgitation: criteria predictive of death, congestive heart failure, and angina in young patients. Circulation 1971;44:368–380.
2. **Angioff E.** Aortic incompetence: clinical haemodynamic and angiographic evaluation. IV. Physical signs and electrocardiographic findings. Acta Med Scand 1972;193:suppl 538:35–39.
3. **Goldschlager N, Pfeifer J, Cohn K, Popper R, Selzer A.** The natural history of aortic regurgitation: a clinical and hemodynamic study. Am J Med 1973;54:577–588.
4. **Hirshfeld JW, Jr, Epstein SE, Roberts AJ, Glancy DL, Morrow AG.** Indices predicting long-term survival after valve replacement in patients with aortic regurgitation and patients with aortic stenosis. Circulation 1974;50:1190–1199.
5. **Henry WL, Bonow RO, Borer JS, Ware JH, Kent KM, Redwood DR, McIntosh CL, Morrow AG, Epstein SE.** Observations on the optimum time for operative intervention for aortic regurgitation. I. Evaluation of the results of aortic valve replacement in symptomatic patients. Circulation 1980;61:471–483.
6. **Henry WL, Bonow RO, Rosing DR, Epstein SE.** Observations on the optimum time for operative intervention for aortic regurgitation. II. Serial echocardiographic evaluation of asymptomatic patients. Circulation 1980;61:484–492.
7. **Carroll JD, Gaasch WH, Naimi S, Levine HJ.** Regression of myocardial hypertrophy: electrocardiographic-echocardiographic correlations after aortic valve replacement in patients with chronic aortic regurgitation. Circulation 1982;65:980–987.
8. **Sokolow M, Lyon TP.** The ventricular complex in left ventricular hypertrophy as obtained by unipolar precordial and limb leads. Am Heart J 1949;37:161–186.
9. **Romhilt DW, Estes EH.** A point-score system for the ECG diagnosis of left ventricular hypertrophy. Am Heart J 1968;75:752–758.
10. **Roberts WC, Buchbinder NA.** Healed left-sided infective endocarditis: clinicopathologic study of 59 patients. Am J Cardiol 1977;40:876–888.
11. **Day PJ, McManus BM, Roberts WC.** Amounts of coronary arterial narrowing by atherosclerotic plaques in clinically isolated, chronic, pure aortic regurgitation: analysis of 37 necropsy patients older than 30 years. Am J Cardiol 1984;53:173–177.
12. **Roberts WC, Dangel JC, Bulkley BH.** Non-rheumatic valvular cardiac disease: a clinicopathologic survey of 27 different conditions causing valvular dysfunction. Cardiovasc Clin 1973;5:333–446.
13. **Bulkley BH, Roberts WC.** Ankylosing spondylitis and aortic regurgitation: description of the characteristic cardiovascular lesion from study of eight necropsy patients. Circulation 1973;48:1014–1027.
14. **Roberts WC, Honig HS.** The spectrum of cardiovascular disease in the Marfan syndrome: a clinico-morphologic study of 18 necropsy patients and comparison to 151 previously reported necropsy patients. Am Heart J 1982;104:115–135.
15. **Levine RJ, Roberts WC, Morrow AG.** Traumatic aortic regurgitation. Am J Cardiol 1962;10:752–763.
16. **Waller BF, Zoltick JM, Rosen JH, Katz NM, Gomes MN, Fletcher RD, Wallace RB, Roberts WC.** Severe aortic regurgitation from systemic hypertension (without aortic dissection) requiring aortic valve replacement. Analysis of four patients. Am J Cardiol 1982;49:473–477.
17. **Murphy ML, Thenabadu PN, Blue LR, Meade J, de Soyza N, Doherty JE, Baker BJ.** Descriptive characteristics of the electrocardiogram from autopsied men free of cardiopulmonary disease—a basis for evaluating criteria for ventricular hypertrophy. Am J Cardiol 1983;52:1275–1280.
18. **Roberts WC, Podolak MJ.** The king of hearts: analysis of 23 patients with hearts weighing 1000 grams or more. Am J Cardiol 1985; 55:485–494.
19. **Scott RC.** The correlation between the electrocardiographic patterns of ventricular hypertrophy and the anatomic findings. Circulation 1960;21:256–291.
20. **Baxley WA, Dodge HT, Sandler H.** A quantitative angiocardiographic study of left ventricular hypertrophy and the electrocardiogram. Circulation 1968;37:509–517.
21. **Bennett DH, Evans DW.** Correlation of left ventricular mass determined by echocardiography with vectorcardiographic and electrocardiographic voltage measurements. Br Heart J 1974;36:981–987.
22. **Reichek N, Devereux RB.** Left ventricular hypertrophy: relationship of anatomic, echocardiographic and electrocardiographic findings. Circulation 1981;63:1391–1398.
23. **Devereux RB, Phillips MC, Casale PN, Eisenberg RR, Kligfield P.** Geometric determinants of electrocardiographic left ventricular hypertrophy. Circulation 1983;67:907–911.
24. **Winsor T, ed.** Electrocardiographic Textbook. Vol. 1. New York: American Heart Association, 1956: appendix pages 144–160.
25. **Simonson E.** Differentiation Between Normal and Abnormal in Electrocardiography. St. Louis: CV Mosby, 1961;51,132.
26. Criteria Committee of the New York Heart Association. Diseases of the Heart and Blood Vessels. Nomenclature and Criteria for Diagnosis. 6th ed. Boston: Little, Brown, 1964;437.
27. **Cooksey JD, Dunn M, Massie E.** Clinical Vectocardiography and Electrocardiography. 2nd ed. Chicago: Year Book Medical, 1977:81.
28. **Siegel RJ, Roberts WC.** Electrocardiographic observations in severe aortic valve stenosis: correlative necropsy study to clinical, hemodynamic, and ECG variables demonstrating relation of 12-lead QRS amplitude to peak systolic transaortic pressure gradient. Am Heart J 1982;103:210–221.
29. **Roberts WC, Waller BF.** Cardiac amyloidosis causing cardiac dysfunction: analysis of 54 necropsy patients. Am J Cardiol 1983;52:137–147.

The King of Hearts: Analysis of 23 Patients with Hearts Weighing 1,000 Grams or More

WILLIAM C. ROBERTS, MD, and MICHAEL J. PODOLAK, BSE*

Certain clinical and morphologic features are described in 23 patients in whom the heart at necropsy weighed at least 1,000 g (mean 1,106). The heart weight to body weight ratio ranged from 1.2 to 2.7 (normal 0.40). The 23 patients were derived from examination of the hearts of 7,671 patients with various cardiovascular disorders over a 25-year period. The massive cardiomegaly was the result of aortic regurgitation in 14 patients (61%): isolated in 8, associated with mitral regurgitation in 4, and with ventricular septal defect in 2. Three others (13%) had combined aortic valve stenosis and aortic regurgitation and 1 patient (4%) had mitral stenosis and regurgitation and mild aortic stenosis. Four patients (17%) had hypertrophic cardiomyopathy, and 1 patient (4%) had ventricular septal defect with mitral stenosis. They were 20 to 64 years old (mean 42) and 21 (91%) were men. Four patients at necropsy had 1 or more major coronary arteries narrowed more than 75% in cross-sectional area by atherosclerotic plaques, and only 4 patients had grossly visible left ventricular (LV) scars, 2 of whom had insignificant coronary narrowing. Examination of electrocardiograms in 17 of the 23 patients disclosed that Sokolow-Lyon criteria for LV hypertrophy was achieved in only 12 patients (71%) and Romhilt-Holt QRS voltage criteria faired even worse. Total 12-lead QRS voltage was more than 175 mm (10 mm = 1 mV) in 16 patients (94%) and it was more than 250 mm in 13 patients (76%). Total 12-lead QRS voltage in 17 patients ranged from 140 to 601 mm (mean 323). Measurement of the sum of the 12-lead QRS voltage may be quite useful in diagnosing LV hypertrophy by electrocardiogram.

(Am J Cardiol 1985;55:485–494)

The upper limit of the normal heart weight in women is about 350 g and for men, about 400 g. Hearts that weigh 1,000 g or more* in human beings are rare. During the past 25 years one of us (WCR) has examined at necropsy the hearts of 23 patients in whom the heart weighed at least 1,000 g (>2.5 times normal weight). Certain clinical and morphologic findings in these 23 patients are described in this report.

Methods

From July 1, 1959, to July 30, 1984, the hearts of 7,671 patients with cardiovascular disease were examined at the National Institutes of Health by 1 of us (WCR). The file of each was reexamined and the records of those in whom the heart weight was recorded as at least 1,000 g were pulled. Thirty-two patients had hearts that weighed more than 1,000 g recorded in the necropsy protocol. Upon review of the records and on reexamination of most of the hearts it was apparent that the weights in 9 of the 32 patients were inaccurately recorded because ascending aorta or parietal pericardium or other tissues were still attached to the heart, and although the hearts weighed more than 900 g, they weighed less than 1,000 g. Thus, 23 patients remained in whom the heart itself weighed at least 1,000 g. In 21 of the 23 patients the weights were those recorded by 1 of us (WCR). In each, the weight was that obtained after the heart had been fixed in 10% formalin for about 48 hours, after the main right and left pulmonary arteries, ascending aorta (2 cm cephalad to the sinotubular junction), all parietal pericardium and all intracardiac clot or thrombus had been removed from the heart itself. The scale used to weigh most of the hearts was a Mettler P1210, a scale with a range from 10 mg to 1,200 g. A different scale was used for the 4 hearts that weighed more than 1,200 g.

The clinical and morphologic records in all 23 patients were then examined. The hearts in 15 of the 23 patients were reexamined.

Results

The data obtained in the 23 patients are recorded in Tables I, II and III. The patients were 29 to 64 years old

From the Pathology Branch, National Heart, Lung, and Blood Institute, National Institutes of Health, Bethesda, Maryland. Manuscript received September 7, 1984; revised manuscript received and accepted October 5, 1984.

* Freshman Student, Duke University Medical School, Durham, North Carolina.

Address for reprints: William C. Roberts, MD, Building 10A, Room 3E-30, National Institutes of Health, Bethesda, Maryland 20205.

* To better sense the feeling of 1,000 g, the June 1, 1984, issue of *The American Journal of Cardiology* weighed 967 g. It included 459 pages (279 editorial and 180 advertising).

TABLE I Clinical and Morphologic Observations in the 23 Patients with Hearts Weighing 1,000 Grams or More

Pt	Age (yr), Race & Sex	Cardiac Disorder	LV (s/d) (mm Hg)	SA (s/d) (mm Hg)	LV-SA psg (mm Hg)	RV (s/d)	AR by AA cine (0–4+)	MR by LV cine (0–4+)	CI	AVR	MVR	Interval Op to Death	Ht. (cm)	HW (kg)	BW (g)	HW/BW (%)	No. AV Cusps	LV F	No. CAs >75%
1	30WM	AR	140/33	140/38	0	50/9	4+	0	2.5	+	0	37 mo	167	1,200	79	1.5	3	0	0
2	32BM	AR	...	215/45	...	...	...	...	...	0	0	...	165	1,030	68	1.5	3	0	0
3	39WM	AR	170/16	175/50	0	34/6	4+	1+	4.5	+	0	25 days	170	1,100	63	1.7	3	0	0
4	39WM	AR	140/20	140/38	0	32/5	4+	1+	2.8	0	0	...	183	1,010	85	1.2	2	0	1
5	41BM	AR	120/12	120/75	0	24/8	3+	0	2.6	+	0	21 mo	190	1,270	109	1.2	3	0	0
6	43WM	AR	...	180/80	...	...	...	...	...	+	0	60 mo	183	1,020	87	1.2	3	0	0
7	44WM	AR	140/10	145/40	0	...	4+	...	...	+	0	2 days	...	1,050	...	...	2	0	0
8	51WM	AR	152/38	158/46	0	56/12	3+	1+	2.0	+	0	0	178	1,010	80	1.3	3	0	2
9	29WM	AR + MR	130/14	140/40	0	45/10	4+	2+	1.9	+	+	3 days	165	1,040	52	2.0	3	0	0
10	45WM	AR + MR	144/18	152/45	0	35/7	4+	2+	1.8	+	+	10 days	175	1,040	74	1.4	3	0	0
11	50WM	AR + MR	118/18	140/63	0	46/15	2+	4+	...	+	+	0	185	1,005	91	1.1	3	+	0
12	62BM	AR + MR	195/18	210/40	0	45/6	4+	2+	2.0	+	0*	52 mo	183	1,230	71	1.7	3	+	1
13	29WM	AR + VSD	155/20	170/70	0	70/4	4+	...	...	+†	0	12 mo	185	1,360	93	1.5	3	0	0
14	34WM	AR + VSD	168/22	145/48	23	68/6	4+	...	...	+†	0	1 day	178	1,150	58	2.0	3	0	0
15	53WM	AR + AS	120/36	100/40	20	60/10	4+	0	...	+	0	12 mo	183	1,100	70	1.6	2	0	0
16	56WM	AR + AS	190/14	130/75	60	24/8	2+	...	...	+	0	53 mo	186	1,100	57	1.9	2	0	0
17	60WM	AR + AS‡	...	100/60	...	...	...	...	...	0	0	...	173	1,050	55	1.9	2	+	1
18	64WM	MS§ + MR + AS	120/12	110/60	10	50/9	...	3+	3.9	0	+	76 days	176	1,055	73	1.4	3	0	0
19	20WF	HC	158/10	108/57	50	40/7	...	3+	3.9	0	0	...	161	1,250	47	2.7	3	+	0
20	32WM	HC	...	95/60	...	...	...	...	...	0	0	...	...	1,200	...	...	3	0	0
21	33WM	HC	105/25	117/70	0	33/7	0	0	2.7	0	0	...	179	1,020	82	1.2	3	0	0
22	45WF	HC	...	...	...||	...	...	...	...	0||	0||	144 mo	...	1,150	...	...	3	0	0
23	30BM	VSD + MS¶	...	160/110	...	...	...	...	...	0	0	...	...	1,005	78	1.3	3	0	0

* Aortic valve replacement 53 months before death; mitral valve replacement 2 days before death.
† Closure of ventricular septal defect at same time.
‡ Although the mitral valve was neither stenotic nor incompetent, its anulus contained heavy (4+/4+) calcific deposits.
§ Left atrial to left ventricular mean diastolic gradient = 13 mm Hg.
|| This patient also had obstruction to left ventricular outflow and partial ventricular septotomy-septectomy was performed 144 months before death.
¶ Parachute mitral valve (single papillary muscle syndrome).

AA = ascending aorta; AR = aortic regurgitation; AS = aortic valve stenosis: AV = aortic valve; AVR = aortic valve replacement; BW = body weight; CAs = coronary arteries; cine = cineangiogram; CI = cardiac index; F = grossly visible fibrosis; HC = hypertrophic cardiomyopathy; Ht = height; HW = heart weight; LV = left ventricle or ventricular; MR = mitral regurgitation; MS = mitral stenosis; MVR = mitral valve replacement; RV = right ventricle; SA = systemic artery; s/d = peak systole/end-diastole; VSD = ventricular septal defect.

TABLE II Electrocardiographic Findings in 17 Necropsy Patients with Hearts Weighing 1,000 Grams or More

Pt	Interval ECG to Death	Cardiac Disease	VR (bpm)	Intervals QRS (sec)	Intervals P-R (sec)	QRS Voltage I	II	III	aVR	aVL	aVF	V$_1$	V$_2$	V$_3$	V$_4$	V$_5$	V$_6$
1	37 mo	AR	54	0.12	0.24	10	9	15	6	13	11	50	50	52	37	10	16
2	1 day	AR	125	0.16	0.08	18	11	6	10	4	7	27	32	27	21	7	9
3	40 days	AR	75	0.12	0.28	29	13	21	22	27	9	50	58	72	42	21	50
4	75 days	AR	64	0.12	0.20	12	8	15	9	12	10	30	56	52	37	24	50
8	3 days	AR	73	0.10	0.20	15	12	19	10	16	14	27	52	39	37	38	32
9	8 days	AR-MR	112	0.12	0.22	16	10	20	11	18	12	42	86	82	46	43	28
10	11 days	AR-MR	90	0.12	. . .*	3	8	9	4	5	8	6	38	48	46	23	16
11	2 days	AR-MR	115	0.11	. . .*	3	14	14	7	7	13	13	38	40	44	40	20
12	52 mo	AR-MR	105	0.16	. . .*	16	20	32	10	21	26	30	60	68	60	18	41
13	12 mo	AR-VSD	102	0.08	0.18	12	15	25	12	18	18	31	68	72	68	28	30
14	9 days	AR-VSD	74	0.12	0.28	5	16	17	9	10	16	12	46	70	70	70	24
15	12 mo	AR-AS	73	0.12	0.20	13	10	16	10	13	7	39	50	40	28	26	35
16	53 mo	AR-AS	64	0.12	0.19	24	17	11	20	17	7	21	23	14	20	20	15
18	79 days	AR-MR-MS	55[†]	0.08	. . .[†]	4	6	5	5	3	5	6	12	25	34	20	15
19	41 mo	HC	56	0.12	0.08	34	37	23	30	33	74	70	40	52	64	74	70
21	4 mo	HC	76	0.10	0.16	21	23	27	16	22	20	30	60	54	40	56	36
23	6 mo	VSD-MS	71	0.12	0.32	31	14	35	17	31	22	17	13	22	29	44	33
	Mean			0.12	0.20	16	14	18	12	16	16	30	46	49	43	32	31

Pt	Total 12-Lead QRS Voltage	S V$_1$	S V$_2$	R V$_5$	R V$_6$	Largest S V$_1$–V$_3$ (mm)	(Lead)	Largest R V$_4$–V$_6$ (mm)	(Lead)	Largest R in 6 Limb Leads (mm)	Lead	Largest S in 6 Limb Leads (mm)	Lead	R I	S III
1	279	50	50	3	16	50	V$_1$	16	V$_6$	10	aVL	10	III	8	10
2	179	23	28	2	9	27	V$_3$	9	V$_6$	11	II	10	aVR	15	2
3	414	50	56	8	42	68	V$_3$	42	V$_6$	30	I	23	aVR	30	21
4	315	27	54	23	47	54	V$_2$	47	V$_6$	12	I	10	III	12	10
8	311	26	46	33	34	46	V$_2$	34	V$_6$	14	I	11	III	14	11
9	414	34	82	14	25	82	V$_2$	25	V$_6$	15	I	13	III	15	13
10	214	5	36	11	14	42	V$_3$	14	V$_6$	8	III	5	aVL	2	0
11	253	14	34	34	38	34	V$_2$	34	V$_5$	13	III	7	aVR	3	0
12	402	30	56	8	39	62	V$_3$	39	V$_6$	20	aVL	28	III	16	28
13	397	30	64	10	30	66	V$_3$	30	V$_6$	15	II	13	III	11	13
14	365	9	45	12	21	70	V$_3$	21	V$_6$	11	III	8	III	3	8
15	287	30	46	24	35	46	V$_2$	35	V$_6$	13	I	14	III	13	14
16	209	20	22	20	15	20	V$_1$	20	V$_5$	23	I	19	aVR	23	9
18	140	6	11	14	15	20	V$_3$	15	V$_6$	6	II	2	aVL	3	0
19	601	26	0	60	60	26	V$_1$	60	V$_5$,V$_6$	50	aVF	24	aVF	30	23
21	405	29	54	52	36	56	V$_2$	54	V$_5$	22	II	16	aVR	21	10
23	308	6	3	21	15	6	V$_1$	21	V$_5$	32	III	26	aVL	9	0
	323	24	40	21	28	45		30		18		14		13	10

* Atrial fibrillation: [†] atrioventricular junctional rhythm.
AR = aortic regurgitation; bpm = beats per minute; HC = hypertrophic cardiomyopathy; MR = mitral regurgitation; MS = mitral stenosis; VR = ventricular rate; VSD = ventricular septal defect.

(mean 42); 21 (91%) were men and 2 (9%) were women. Cardiac conditions producing the massive cardiomegaly were: (1) pure *aortic regurgitation* (AR) in 14 patients (isolated in 8, associated with mitral regurgitation [MR] in 4 and with ventricular septal defect [VSD] in 2); (2) *combined aortic stenosis (AS) and AR* in 3; (3) *hypertrophic cardiomyopathy* in 4; (4) *combined mitral stenosis (with MR) and AS* in 1 patient; and (5) *VSD with mitral stenosis* (parachute mitral valve) in 1. Of the 8 patients with isolated pure AR, the origin of the valve disease was infective endocarditis that healed in 2[1] (patients 4 and 6, Table I) (Fig. 1), congenitally bicuspid aortic valve that never was the site of infection in 1 (patient 6),[2] uncertain in 2 (patients 1 and 5), rheumatic in 1 patient (patient 2), ankylosing spondylitis in 1 (patient 3),[3] and syphilis in 1 (patient 8) (Fig. 2).[4] Of the 4 patients with combined AR and MR, the cause was rheumatic in 3 (patients 9, 11 and 12) and infective endocarditis that healed in 1 (patient 10) (Fig.

3). The AR in the 2 patients with VSD (nos. 13 and 14) resulted from prolapse of 1 of the 3 aortic valve cusps, with superimposed infective endocarditis that healed in 1 of the patients (no. 14) (Fig. 4 and 5). One patient (no. 14) with AR plus VSD also had a small (20-mm Hg) peak systolic pressure gradient between left ventricle and systemic artery (Fig. 5). Two patients (nos. 15 and 16) had congenitally bicuspid aortic valves causing combined aortic valve stenosis and regurgitation (Fig. 6);[5] the stenosis was the dominant hemodynamic lesion in 1 (patient 17) and he had a bicuspid aortic valve (Fig. 7). The cause of the combined mitral and aortic valve stenosis in patient 18 was rheumatic. The hypertrophic cardiomyopathy in patients 19 to 22 was congenital in origin (Fig. 8). Patient 23 obviously had congenital heart disease (Fig. 9).

Electrocardiograms were available for examination in 17 patients (Table II, Fig. 1, 3, 5 and 6). Twelve had had valve replacement operations; the electrocardio-

TABLE III Recommended or Modified Electrocardiographic Criteria for Determining Left Ventricular Hypertrophy as Applied to 17 Patients with Hearts at Necropsy Weighing More than 1,000 Grams

No.	QRS Complex Measured	Value Considered Upper Limit of Normal (mm)	No. (%) of 17 Patients Above Normal Limit
1a	$SV_1 + RV_5$ or V_6 (larger)	35	12 (71)
b	$SV_1 + RV_5$ or V_6 (larger)	40	11 (65)
2a	SV_1 or V_2 (larger) + RV_5 or V_6 (larger)	35	15 (88)
b	SV_1 or V_2 (larger) + RV_5 or V_6 (larger)	40	14 (82)
3a	SV_1 or V_2 (larger) + RV_6	35	15 (88)
b	SV_1 or V_2 (larger) + RV_6	40	13 (76)
4a	$SV_2 + RV_5$	35	14 (82)
b	$SV_2 + RV_5$	40	14 (82)
5a	Deepest $SV_1 - V_3$ + tallest $RV_4 - V_6$	35	14 (82)
b	Deepest $SV_1 - V_3$ + tallest $RV_4 - V_6$	40	13 (76)
c	Deepest $SV_1 - V_3$ + tallest $RV_4 - V_6$	45	13 (76)
d	Deepest $SV_1 - V_3$ + tallest $RV_4 - V_6$	50	13 (76)
6a	Tallest R + deepest S in any V lead	35	14 (82)
b	Tallest R + deepest S in any V lead	40	14 (82)
7a	Deepest $SV_1 - V_3$	25	14 (82)
b	Deepest $SV_1 - V_3$	30	12 (71)
8a	Tallest $RV_4 - V_6$	25	9 (53)
b	Tallest $RV_4 - V_6$	30	8 (27)
9a	Deeper SV_1 or V_2	25	14 (82)
b	Deeper SV_1 or V_2	30	12 (71)
10a	Tallest RV_5 or V_6	25	9 (53)
b	Tallest RV_5 or V_6	30	8 (47)
11	$RV_6 > RV_5$	≤ 1	13 (76)
12a	Tallest limb-lead R + deepest limb-lead S	15	15 (88)
b	Tallest limb-lead R + deepest limb-lead S	20	12 (71)
13a	$R_1 + S_3$	15	12 (71)
b	$R_1 + S_3$	20	10 (59)
14a	Tallest limb-lead R	10	14 (82)
b	Tallest limb-lead R	15	6 (35)
15a	Deepest limb-lead S	10	10 (59)
b	Deepest limb-lead S	15	6 (35)
16	R_1	10	11 (65)
17	S_3	10	7 (41)
18a	Total 12-lead QRS voltage	175	16 (94)
b	Total 12-lead QRS voltage	200	15 (88)
c	Total 12-lead QRS voltage	225	13 (76)
d	Total 12-lead QRS voltage	250	13 (76)

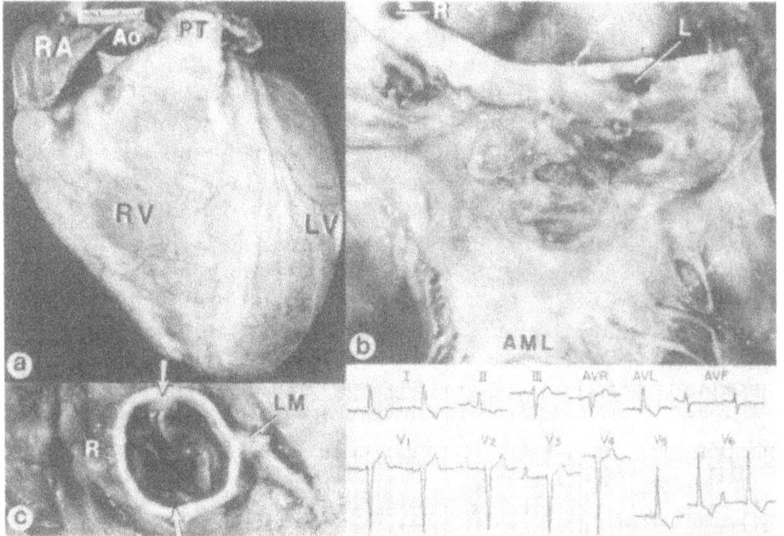

FIGURE 1. Patient 4 in Table I. Heart, weighing 1,010 g, and electrocardiogram from a 39-year-old man (A69-254) who had active infective endocarditis on a bicuspid aortic valve at age 24 years and aortic regurgitation thereafter. He refused operative treatment. He died suddenly while playing golf. **a,** exterior of heart. Ao = ascending aorta; LV = left ventricle; PT = pulmonary trunk; RA = right atrium; RV = right ventricle. **b,** opened aortic valve. Each cusp is perforated and the margins of the perforations contain small calcific deposits. AML = anterior mitral leaflet; L and R = left and right coronary ostia. **c,** congenitally bicuspid aortic valve from above. The **arrows** designate the 2 commissures. LM = left main and R = right coronary artery. The QRS voltage in the precordial leads is enormous. A strain pattern is present.

gram analyzed was recorded within the month preceding operation. Seven of these 12 patients died within 76 days (median 3) of operation; the other 5 patients died 12, 12, 37, 52 and 53 months (mean 33) after operation. In the latter 5 patients electrocardiograms were available for examination 12, 7, 22, 52 and 31 months (mean 25), respectively, after valve replacement.

A single QRS complex was measured in each lead in the 17 patients (Fig. 10). The total 12-lead QRS voltage ranged from 140 to 601 mm (mean 323) (10 mm = 1 mV); in 16 patients (94%) this voltage was more than 175 mm and in 13 (17%), more than 250 mm. In 5 patients with isolated severe AR, the total 12-lead QRS voltage ranged from 179 to 414 mm (mean 300); in 4 patients with combined AR and MR, it was 214 to 414 (mean 321); in 2 patients with AR plus VSD, it was 365 and 397 mm; in 2 patients (nos. 15 and 16) with AR plus AS, it was 209 and 287 mm, and in 2 patients with hypertrophic cardiomyopathy, it was 405 and 601 mm. The mean QRS voltage in each of the 12 leads in each of the 17 patients was 27 mm. The individual and mean QRS amplitudes in each of the 12 leads in the 17 patients are

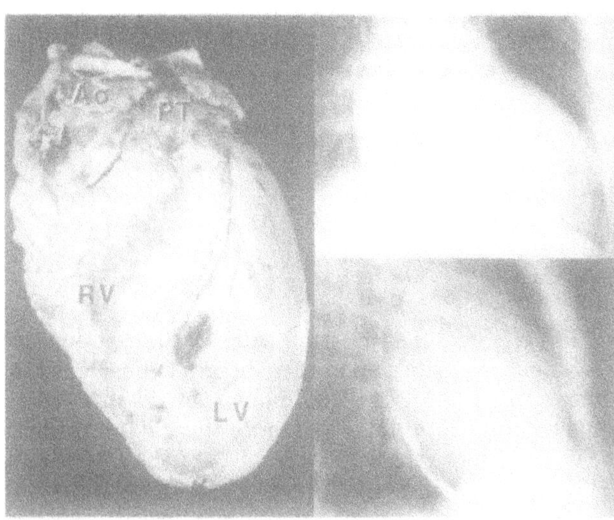

FIGURE 2. Patient 8. **left,** exterior view of heart weighing 1,010 g from a 51-year-old man (A68-8) with chronic aortic regurgitation from syphilis. The enormousness of the heart is apparent from the posteroanterior (**upper right**) and lateral (**lower right**) radiographs. Abbreviations as in Figure 1.

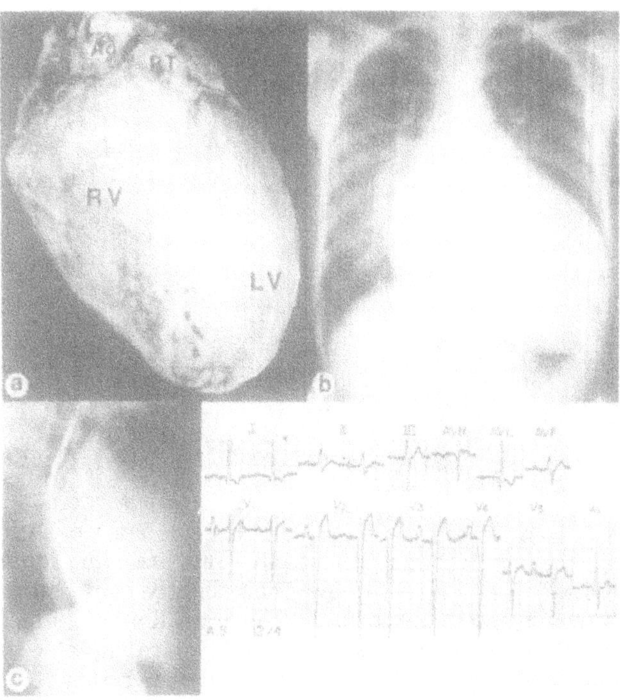

FIGURE 3. Patient 9. Heart weighing 1,040 g (**a**), chest radiographs (**b** and **c**) and electrocardiogram from a 29-year-old man (A68-3) with combined pure aortic and mitral regurgitation of rheumatic origin. Leads V_1 to V_5 are at one-half standard. Abbreviations as in Figure 1.

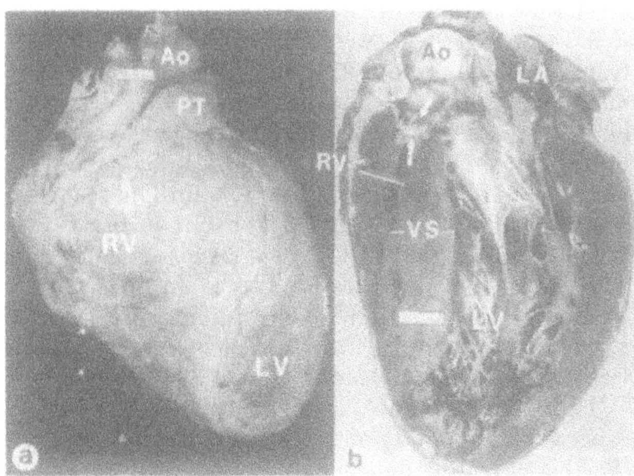

FIGURE 4. Patient 13. Heart from a 29-year-old man (A71-197) with ventricular septal defect (VSD) complicated by aortic regurgitation. He died 1 year after closure of the VSD and replacement of the aortic valve. The aortic regurgitation resulted from prolapse of 1 of the 3 aortic valve cusps. **a,** exterior view of heart. The heart weight (1,360 g) was determined after most of the ascending aorta and pulmonary trunk had been excised. **b,** longitudinal cut of heart. The **arrows** point to the site of the previous VSD. The caged-ball prosthesis has been removed. A thrombus is present in the left ventricular apex. VS = ventricular septum; other abbreviations as in Figure 1.

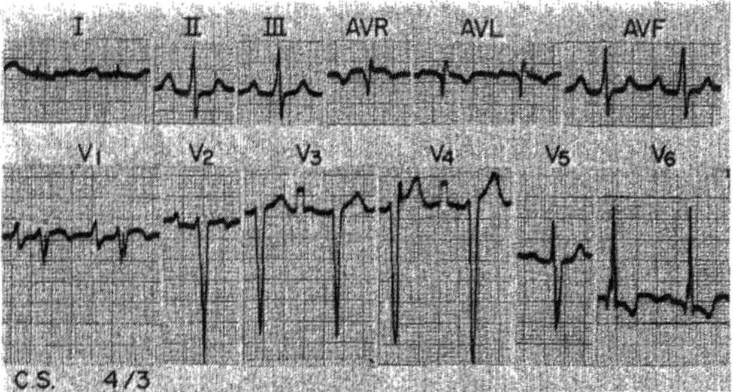

FIGURE 5. Patient 14. Electrocardiogram from a 34-year-old man (A64-92) with aortic regurgitation (AR) complicating ventricular septal defect (VSD). The heart weighed 1,150 g. He had active infective endocarditis at age 21 years and severe aortic regurgitation thereafter. A large perforation was present in the prolapsed aortic valve cusp at the time of closure of the ventricular septal defect and aortic valve replacement 1 year before death. The QRS voltage in the preoperative electrocardiogram is enormous. Leads V_3 and V_4 are at one-half standard.

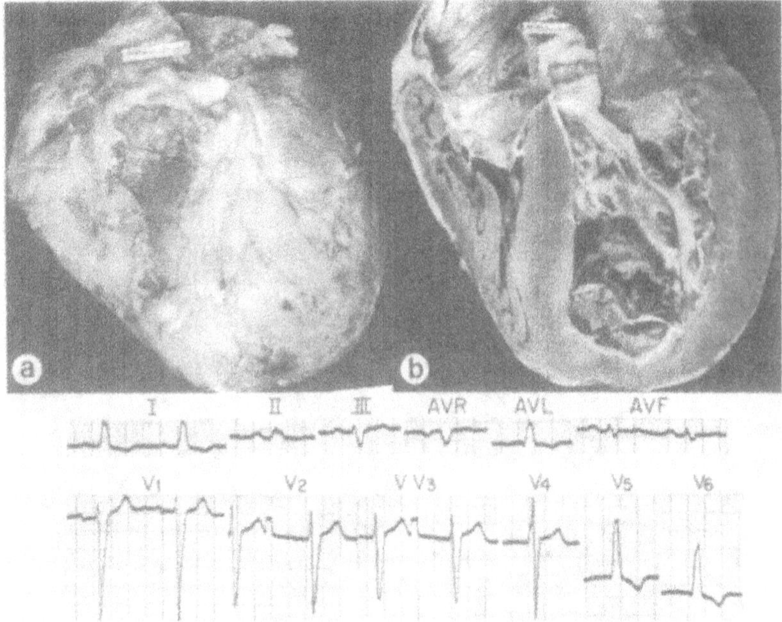

FIGURE 6. Patient 15. Heart and electrocardiogram in a 53-year-old man (A70-54) who developed active infective endocarditis on a congenitally bicuspid aortic valve with severe aortic regurgitation (AR) thereafter. At catheterization before aortic valve replacement, a 20-mm Hg peak systolic pressure gradient was present between left ventricle and aorta and aortic root cineangiogram disclosed 4+/4+ AR. He died 1 year after aortic valve replacement. **a,** exterior view of heart, which weighs 1,100 g. **b,** longitudinal view. The prosthetic aortic valve has been excised. A thrombus is present in the left ventricle. The electrocardiogram shows high QRS voltage in the precordial leads and a strain pattern. Leads V_2 and V_3 are at one-half standard.

listed in Table II. The highest mean 12-lead QRS voltage occurred in lead V_3 (49 mm), next in V_2 (46 mm), next in V_4 (43 mm), and it was lowest in lead aVR (12 mm). The QRS mean voltage in leads V_5 and V_6 were similar (32 and 31 mm).

Various electrocardiographic QRS voltage criteria for left ventricular hypertrophy and the frequency of their occurrence in the 17 patients are summarized in Table III.[6-10] A few criteria have been slightly modified to allow the number designating the upper limit of normal to end in a 0 or a 5 and to allow the elevated value to always be greater than a certain number rather than equal to or greater than a certain number. Of the 18 criteria analyzed, only 1 upper-limit number was evaluated in 3, two values were analyzed in 13, and 4 values in 2. Thus, a total of 37 values were analyzed for the 18 criteria: 36 were measurements in millimeters of QRS voltage and 1 was a ratio.

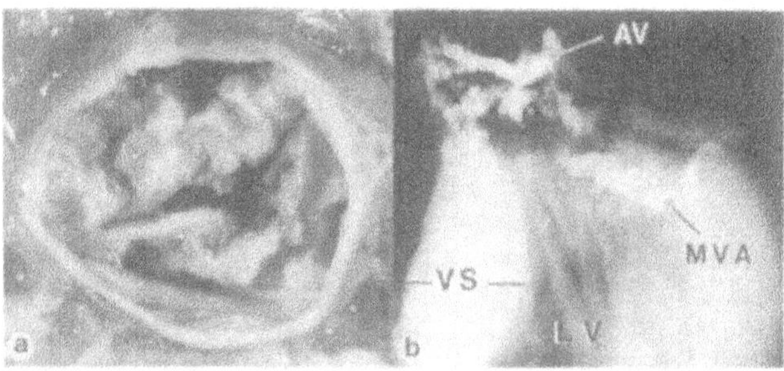

FIGURE 7. Patient 17. Stenotic and heavily calcified, bicuspid aortic valve and calcified mitral valve anulus in a 60-year-old man (A71-14). Congestive heart failure developed about a year before death. Electrocardiogram (not available for reexamination and therefore not included in the analysis of 17) disclosed atrial fibrillation, complete right bundle branch block and Q waves in leads II, III, aVF and V_4 to V_6. This patient had a large anterior wall transmural left ventricular scar. **a,** severely stenotic and mildly incompetent aortic valve from above. **b,** radiograph of heart showing calcium in both aortic valve (AV) and mitral valve anulus (MVA). The mitral valve functioned normally. LV = left ventricular cavity; VS = ventricular septum.

The QRS voltage criterion with the highest positive frequency was the sum of the voltage of the QRS complexes in all 12 leads being more than 175 mm (94%); this total QRS voltage was more than 200 mm in 15 (88%) and more than 250 mm in 13 of the 17 patients (17%).

Several recognized QRS voltage criteria for LV hypertrophy were met in 15 of the 17 patients (88%): (1) sum of the S wave in V_1 or V_2 (larger) plus the R wave in V_5 or V_6 (larger) being >35 mm; (2) sum of the S wave in V_1 or V_2 (larger) plus R in V_6 being >35 mm; and (3) sum of the tallest limb-lead R wave plus the deepest limb-lead S wave being >15 mm.

The S-wave amplitude in lead V_1 ranged from 5 to 50 mm (mean 24); the R-wave amplitude in lead V_5 ranged from 2 to 60 mm (mean 21) and in lead V_6, from 9 to 60 mm (mean 28). The sum of the S wave in lead V_1 and the larger of the R waves in either V_5 or V_6 (Sokolow-Lyon index) ranged from 19 to 92 mm (mean 55), and in 12 patients (71%) it was more than 35 mm. The deepest S wave in leads V_1 to V_3 ranged from 6 to 82 mm (mean 45) and in 14 patients (82%) it was more than 25 mm. The deepest S wave in leads V_1 to V_3 was in lead V_1 in 4 patients (24%), in lead V_2 in 6 patients (35%), and in V_3 in 7 patients (41%). The average S-wave amplitude was higher in lead V_2 than V_1 (40 vs 24 mm).

The largest R-wave amplitude in leads V_4 to V_6 ranged from 9 to 60 mm (mean 30), and in 9 patients (53%) it was more than 25 mm; the largest R wave in V_4 to V_6 was in lead V_5 in 5 patients (29%) and in lead V_6 in 12 patients (71%). The mean height of the R wave was higher in lead V_6 than in V_5 (28 vs 21 mm), and the R wave in V_6 was higher than the R wave in V_5 in 13 patients (76%).

Of the 17 patients with electrocardiograms available for analysis, 13 were in sinus rhythm, 3 had atrial fibrillation and 1 patient had atrioventricular junctional rhythm. The PR interval was prolonged (>0.20 second) in 5 of the 13 patients (38%) with sinus rhythm. The

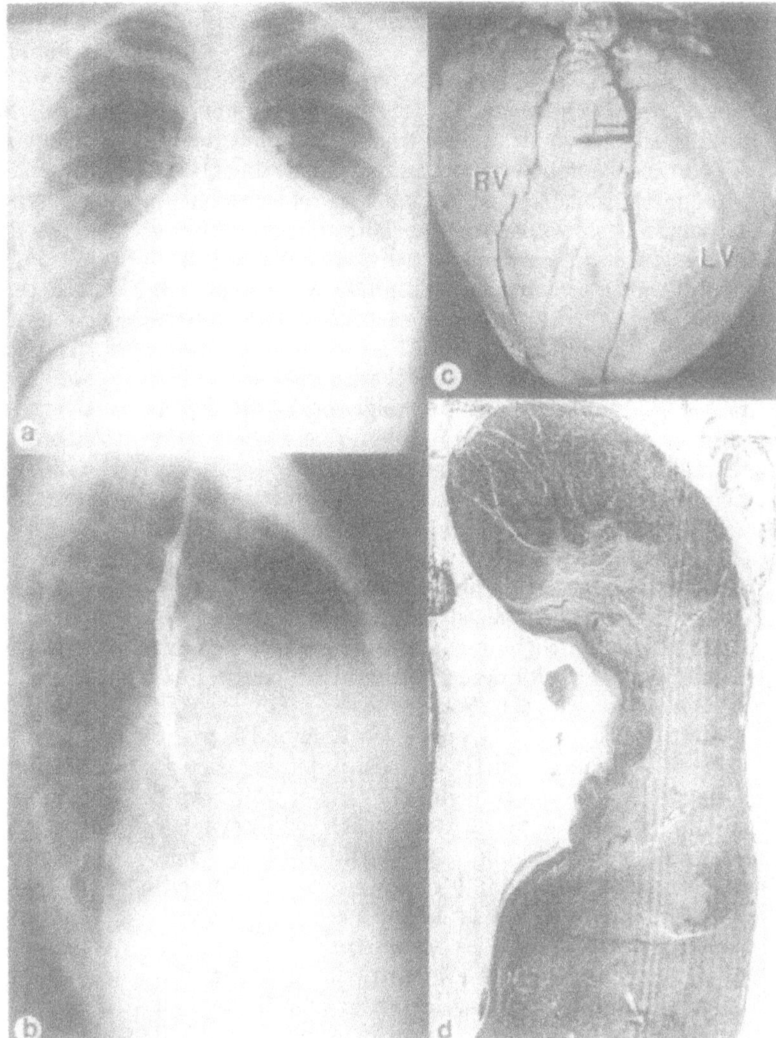

FIGURE 8. Patient 19. a and b, chest radiographs 4 years before death; c, heart weighing 1,250 g; and d, longitudinal section of left ventricular free wall showing a healed myocardial infarct in a 20-year-old woman (A72-197) with hypertrophic cardiomyopathy. She weighed 47 kg. The myocardial infarct likely was the result of inability of the normal epicardial coronary arteries to adequately supply the huge mass of myocardium. LV = left ventricle; RV = right ventricle.

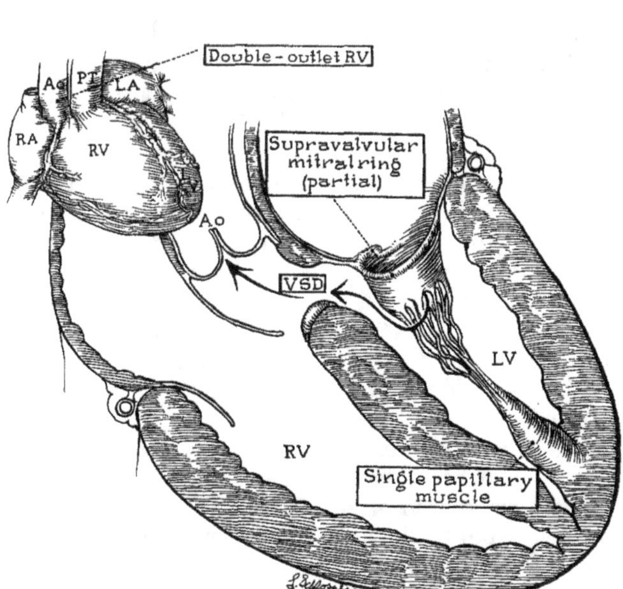

FIGURE 9. Patient 23. Diagram of heart from a 30-year-old man (83-02-106) with congenital mitral stenosis, ventricular septal defect (VSD) and double-outlet right ventricle (RV). The heart weight 1,005 g. Ao = aorta; LA = left atrium; LV = left ventricle; PT = pulmonary trunk; RA = right atrium.

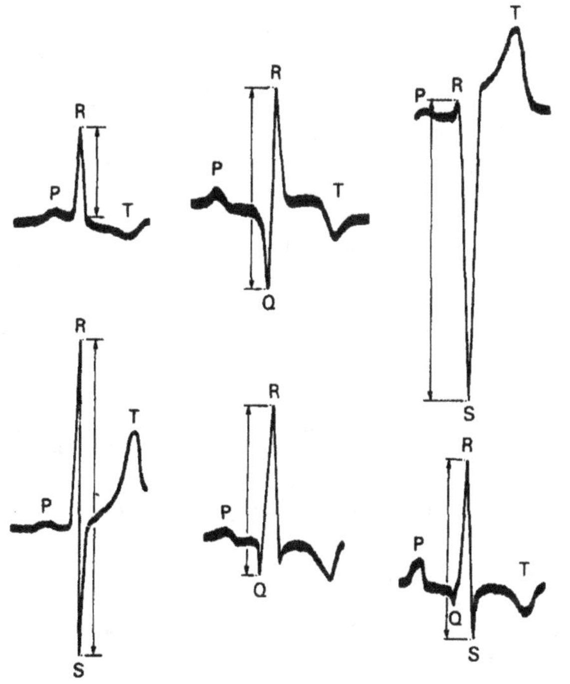

FIGURE 10. Various QRS complexes showing how each was measured.

QRS width was 0.12 second or longer in 12 patients (71%).

Cardiac valve operations were performed in 16 of the 23 patients (70%): isolated aortic valve replacement in 9, simultaneous aortic plus mitral valve replacements in 3, aortic valve replacement plus closure of ventricular septal defect in 2, isolated mitral valve replacement in 1 patient and partial ventricular septotomy-septectomy (for hypertrophic cardiomyopathy) in 1 (patient 22). Eight of the 16 patients died within 90 days (median 3) of operation and the other 8 died 12 to 144 months (mean 49) after operation.

At necropsy, the hearts weighed 1,005 to 1,360 g (mean 1,106); in 15 patients the range was 1,005 to 1,100 g and in 8 it was 1,150 to 1,360 g. The body weight (available in 20 patients) ranged from 47 to 109 kg (mean 74). The percent of body weight contributed by heart weight ranged from 1.1 to 2.7 (mean 1.6) (normal 0.38 to 0.46 [mean 0.40] for women and 0.42 to 0.46 [mean 0.43] for men). Four patients (17%) had congenitally bicuspid aortic valves.

One or more of the 4 major coronary arteries (right, left main, left anterior descending and left circumflex) were narrowed more than 75% in cross-sectional area in 4 of the 23 patients (17%), only 1 of whom had as many as 2 arteries so narrowed. Grossly visible left ventricular scars were found in 4 patients (17%), 2 of whom were among the 4 patients with severe (>75%) coronary narrowing. Two patients (nos. 11 and 12) had small, posterior wall, transmural (> inner one-half of the wall) left ventricular scars. Patient 17 had a large anterior wall scar and a narrowed single coronary artery. Patient 20 had extensive transmural left ventricular scarring with normal extramural coronary arteries; this 20-year-old woman had a 1,250-g heart and she weighed only 103 pounds. We believed that the myocardial ischemia was the result of the myocardial mass "outgrowing" the ability of the coronary bed to perfuse it.

Discussion

The present study includes the largest number of patients heretofore reported with hearts weighing 1,000 g or more. The present study differs from previous ones concerning massive cardiomegaly in that the weights of the hearts, with 2 exceptions, were those recorded by 1 person (WCR) and only after the attachments (great arteries, parietal pericardium, intracardiac clot, and so forth) to the heart had been removed. All previous studies including more than 1 patient with massive cardiomegaly have used heart weights recorded in necropsy protocols, an inaccurate method for obtaining accurate information.[11] Through the years one of us (WCR) has received many hearts originally stated to weigh more than 1,000 g, but after removing the noncardiac attachments the weight was usually less.

The present study demonstrates that there are relatively few conditions that cause the heart to weigh 1,000 g or more. Among our 23 patients, 14 (61%) had *pure "volume" lesions:* isolated AR in 8, AR plus MR in 4, and AR plus VSD in 2. Five patients (22%) had *combined "pressure" and "volume" lesions:* 3 had AS (2 of whom also had considerable AR and 1 [patient 17] of whom had mild AR); 1 patient had mitral stenosis with severe MR; and 1 had mitral stenosis with VSD. Four patients (17%) had *hypertrophic cardiomyopathy*, 2 of whom had peak systolic pressure gradients at rest between left ventricle and aorta. Thus, with the exception of hypertrophic cardiomyopathy and an occasional patient with combined valvular stenosis and regurgitation, it is usually the patient with AR with or without MR or VSD who has a heart that weighs 1,000 g or more.

Several other investigators have observed hearts weighing 1,000 g or more at necropsy. Cabot,[12] in 1926, described 7 men, aged 19 to 52 years (mean 33) whose hearts were recorded as weighing 1,000 to 1,328 g (mean 1150). Although he stated that "chronic pericarditis with mediastinitis produces the largest hearts . . ." all 6 of his patients with "chronic pericarditis and mediastinitis" had valvular heart disease (AR in 4 patients AS in 1 patient and probably both AR and MR in 1). His only patient without "chronic pericarditis and mediastinitis" had syphilitic AR. Golden and Brams[13] described 9 patients (8 men), aged 28 to 57 years (mean 46), with hearts recorded as weighing 1,000 to 1,475 (mean 1,131). The cause of the severe cardiomegaly was AR in 6 (isolated in 5 and associated with MR in 1), combined aortic and mitral valve stenosis in 1 patient and systemic hypertension in 2. Rosenow and Smith[14] reported 3 men, aged 40, 46 and 58 years, with hearts that weighed 1,017, 1,100 and 1,170 g, respectively. Two patients had AS (1 with associated MR) and 1 had systemic hypertension. Strong and Munroe[15] reported 8 patients (7 men), aged 28 to 62 years (mean 43), with hearts recorded as weighing 1,000 to 1,750 g (mean 1,108). The cause of the cardiomegaly was AR in 5 patients, (isolated in 4 and associated with MR in 1), AS in 1 patient and systemic hypertension in 1. Pena[16] reported 15 men, aged 25 to 65 years (mean 49), who had hearts that were recorded as weighing 1,000 to 2,000 g (mean 1,158). The cause of the cardiomegaly was AR in 6 patients (isolated in 4 and associated with MR in 2), isolated MR in 1 patient and systemic hypertension in 8. One of the latter patients also had acromegaly, and his heart weighed 1,525 g. The heart recorded as weighing 2,000 g was in a patient with MR; his blood pressure was 130/70 mm Hg. (We doubt the accuracy of this weight; it is unlikely that the heart can enlarge more than 5 times normal size.) Several investigators in this century have described a single patient in whom the heart weighed 1,000 g or more.[17–24] The cause of the enlargement was AS in 2,[19,22] AR or MR or both in 2,[18,23] cardiac amyloidosis in 1,[24] acromegaly in 1[17] and uncertain cause in 2.[20,21]

Thus, the reports of others cited herein also indicate that valvular heart disease, primarily AR, is the most frequent cause of massive ($\geq$1,000 g) cardiomegaly. In contrast to our study, however, systemic hypertension was mentioned as a cause of massive cardiomegaly. We suspect this cause is unlikely and that more likely the heart was not weighed accurately. Examination by 1 of us (WCR) of hearts of 756 patients with systemic hy-

TABLE IV Frequency of Hearts Weighing 1,000 Grams or More Among Necropsy Patients with Cardiac Disease Studied in the Pathology Branch, National Heart, Lung, and Blood Institute*

	No. of Patients	Number Heart Weight $\geq$ 1,000 g
Valvular heart disease		
Aortic stenosis (AS)	355	3 (1%)
Mitral stenosis (MS)	216	0
AS + MS	167	1
Aortic regurgitation (AR)	138	8 (6%)
Mitral regurgitation (MR)	122	0
MS + AR	70	0
MR + AR	49	4 (8%)
AS + MR	23	0
Tricuspid stenosis + MS $\pm$ AS	29	0
Hypertrophic cardiomyopathy	171	4 (2%)
Ventricular septal defect[†]	30	3[‡]
Idiopathic dilated cardiomyopathy	165	0
Amyloid heart disease	57	0
Systemic hypertension	756	0
Acromegaly	9	0
Massive obesity (body weight > 176 kg)	12	0
Totals	2369	23

* Excludes coronary heart disease.
† Without associated right ventricular outflow obstruction and age older than 15 years.
‡ Two had associated severe aortic regurgitation and 1 had associated congenital mitral stenosis (parachute mitral valve).
Abbreviations as in Table I.

pertension during life disclosed none weighing 1,000 g or more (Table III). Likewise, among 57 hearts of patients with cardiac amyloidosis extensive enough to cause cardiac dysfunction, none weighed 1,000 g or more (Table IV).[25] Although acromegaly has been reported as causing a human heart to weigh 1,000 g or more,[16,17,26] 1 of us (WCR) has not observed such an occurrence among 9 patients with acromegaly studied at necropsy (Table III).[27] Although in persons of normal weight and without heart disease, heart size is proportional to body weight,[28] such is not the case in patients with massive obesity.[29] Warnes and Roberts[29] studied 12 patients at necropsy whose body weight was more than 176 g (>300 lbs) and their hearts weighed 380 to 990 g (mean 616). No one, to our knowledge, has reported a heart in a human being weighing 1,000 g or more on the basis of massive obesity alone.

Our report is the first to demonstrate hypertrophic cardiomyopathy to be a cause of massive ($\geq$1,000 g) cardiomegaly. Of our 4 patients, 2 were women, the only 2 women among our 23 patients. As a group, the largest hearts among our 23 patients were the 2 with AR plus VSD (mean 1,255 g) and the next largest were the 4 with hypertrophic cardiomyopathy (mean 1,155 g), a weight greater than that of the 8 patients with isolated AR (mean 1,086 g), the 4 patients with AR plus MR (mean 1,079 g), or the 4 with AS (mean 1,100 g). It is not surprising that hypertrophic cardiomyopathy has not been described previously as a cause of massive ($\geq$1000 g) cardiomegaly because the last article on causes of massive cardiomegaly was in 1962 (by Pena[16]) and hypertrophic cardiomyopathy was described only 4 years earlier (1958).[30] Our study also is the first to demonstrate massive cardiomegaly in a patient with VSD. Two of our 3 patients with VSD, however, had AR and the third also had congenital mitral stenosis. It is doubtful that VSD as an isolated anomaly can cause cardiomegaly to the extent that the heart could weigh 1,000 g or more.

The frequency of massive ($\geq$1,000 g) cardiomegaly among certain groups of cardiac patients studied at necropsy by one of us (WCR) is summarized in Table IV. Of the 138 patients with clinically isolated pure AR, 8 (6%) had hearts weighing at least 1,000 g; of the 49 patients with combined pure AR plus MR, 4 (8%) had massive cardiomegaly. Of the 355 patients with AS with or without AR, only 3 (1%) had hearts weighing 1,000 g or more. Of the 171 patients with hypertrophic cardiomyopathy studied at necropsy, 4 (2%) had massive cardiomegaly. None of the 152 patients with idiopathic dilated cardiomyopathy had massive cardiomegaly.[31] Of the hundreds of patients with atherosclerotic coronary heart disease unassociated with another condition and studied at necropsy by one of us (WCR), none had hearts weighing 1,000 g or more.

All but 1 previous study on patients with hearts weighing 1,000 g or more referred to herein were published before 1950 or before 12-lead electrocardiograms became routine (rather than 3 or 6-lead electrocardiograms). The 1 study on huge hearts since 1950 did not describe electrocardiographic findings.[16] Thus, our study is the first to examine 12-lead electrocardiograms in patients in whom the heart weighed 1,000 g or more. Total 12-lead QRS voltage in adults with hearts of normal weight has not been determined but 175 mm (10 mm = 1 mV) would probably be a reasonable upper limit. Of our 17 patients in whom electrocardiograms were available, 16 (94%) had total 12-lead QRS voltage more than 175 mm and in them it ranged from 179 to 601 mm (mean 335); 13 of the 16 patients had total 12-lead QRS voltage more than 250 mm. The largest voltage occurred in 2 patients with hypertrophic cardiomyopathy (405 and 601 mm), and next in the 2 patients with AR plus VSD (365 and 397 mm). In the 1 patient (no. 18) in whom the total 12-lead QRS voltage was less than 175 mm, the total voltage was 140 mm. This patient had diffuse LV hypokinesia on angiography with an ejection fraction of 23%, insignificant aortic valve disease, severe mitral stenosis and MR, and a large thrombus in the body of the left ventricle (not included in the cardiac weight). Thus, the amount of left ventricle hypertrophy in this patient was much less than in the other 16 patients.

The Sokolow-Lyon index[6] was not a sensitive indicator of left ventricular hypertrophy. The sum of S_{V_1} and R_{V_5} or $_{V_6}$ (larger) was more than 35 mm in only 12 (71%) of the 17 patients, and in these 12 it ranged from 40 to 92 (mean 67); in the 5 patients in whom this index was normal ($\leq$35 mm), it ranged from 19 to 32 (mean 26). The Romhilt-Estes[7] QRS voltage criteria for left ventricular hypertrophy faired worse although it is recognized that non-voltage criteria also were used by these 2 investigators. The patients fulfilling their QRS voltage criteria were as follows: (1) largest R wave in any of the 6 limb leads of 20 mm or more, 6 patients (35%); (2) largest S wave in any of the 6 limb leads of 20 mm or more, 6 patients (35%); (3) largest S wave in leads V_1 to V_3 of 25 mm or more, 14 patients (82%); (4) largest R wave in V_4 to V_6 of 25 mm or more, 10 patients (59%). The criteria for left ventricular hypertrophy examined by Scott et al[8] yielded the following: (1) R wave in lead I and S wave in lead III of more than 25 mm, 7 patients (41%); (2) R wave in V_5 or V_6 of more than 26 mm, 9 patients (53%). (3) R wave plus S wave in any precordial lead of more than 45 mm, 13 patients (76%). Griep[9] and, later, Holt and Spodick[10] used the R_{V_6}:R_{V_5} voltage ratio for diagnosing left ventricular hypertrophy. They found that when the R-wave voltage in lead V_6 was larger than that in lead V_5 that left ventricular hypertrophy was usually present. In 13 of our 17 patients (76%), the R_{V_6}:R_{V_5} ratio was >1. Thus, despite using several ECG criteria for diagnosis of hypertrophy in hearts known to be enormous ($\geq$1,000 g), voltage criteria for left ventricular hypertrophy was present only 35 to 88% of the time (Table III). Measuring total 12-lead QRS voltage appears to be useful in diagnosing left ventricular hypertrophy by electrocardiogram.

References

1. **Roberts WC, Buchbinder NA.** Healed left-sided infective endocarditis. A clinicopathologic study of 59 patients. Am J Cardiol 1977;40:876–888.
2. **Roberts WC, Morrow AG, McIntosh CL, Jones M, Epstein SE.** Congenitally bicuspid aortic valve causing severe, pure aortic regurgitation without superimposed infective endocarditis. Analysis of 13 patients requiring aortic valve replacement. Am J Cardiol 1981;47:206–209.
3. **Bulkley BH, Roberts WC.** Ankylosing spondylitis and aortic regurgitation. Description of the characteristic cardiovascular lesion from study of eight necropsy patients. Circulation 1973;48:1014–1027.
4. **Roberts WC, Dangel JC, Bulkley BH.** Non-rheumatic valvular cardiac disease: a clinicopathologic survey of 27 different conditions causing valvular dysfunction. Cardiovasc Clin 1973;5:333–446.
5. **Roberts WC.** The congenitally bicuspid aortic valve. A study of 85 autopsy cases. Am J Cardiol 1970;49:151–159.
6. **Sokolow M, Lyon TP.** The ventricular complex in left ventricular hypertrophy as obtained by unipolar precordial and limb leads. Am Heart J 1949;37:161–186.
7. **Romhilt DW, Estes EH.** A point-score system for the ECG diagnosis of left ventricular hypertrophy. Am Heart J 1968;75:752–758.
8. **Scott RC, Seiwert VJ, Simon DL, McGuire J.** Left ventricular hypertrophy. A study of the accuracy of current electrocardiographic criteria when compared with autopsy findings in one hundred cases. Circulation 1955;11:89–96.
9. **Griep AH.** Pitfalls in the electrocardiographic diagnosis of left ventricular hypertrophy. A correlative study of 200 autopsied patients. Circulation 1959;20:30–34.
10. **Holt DH, Spodick DH.** The R_{V_6}:R_{V_5} voltage ratio in left ventricular hypertrophy. Am Heart J 1962;63:65–66.
11. **Roberts WC.** The autopsy: its decline and a suggestion for its revival. N Engl J Med 1978;299:332–338.
12. **Cabot RC.** Facts on the Heart. Philadelphia: WB Saunders, 1926:429–432.
13. **Golden JS, Brams WA.** Extreme cardiac enlargement. Am Heart J 1937;13:207–216.
14. **Rosenow EC Jr, Smith HL.** Extreme cardiac hypertrophy. A report of forty-four cases in which the heart weighed 800 grams or more. Minn Med 1939;22:739–743.
15. **Strong GF, Munroe DS.** Cardiac hypertrophy; forty-two hearts weighing 750 grams or more. Ann Intern Med 1940;13:2253–2264.
16. **Pena C.** Massive cardiac hypertrophy. Report of 15 hearts weighing 1000 gm or more. Am J Cardiol 1963;11:18–23.
17. **Humphry L, Dixon WE.** A case of acromegaly with hypertrophied heart: pressor substances in the urine. Br Med J 1910;2:1047–1050.
18. **Clawson BJ, Bell ET, Hartzell TB.** Valvular diseases of the heart with special reference to the pathogenesis of old valvular defects. Am J Pathol 1926;2:193–234.
19. **Christian HA.** Aortic stenosis with calcification of the cusps. A distinct clinical entity. JAMA 1931;97:158–161.
20. **Cooke WT, Cloake PCP.** Extreme cardiac hypertrophy. Report of two cases with aortic hypoplasia and endocrine disorders. Br Heart J 1943;5:139–146.
21. **Doane JC, Skversky NJ.** Massive cardiac hypertrophy. A case report. Am Heart J 1944;28:816–818.
22. **Karsner HT, Koletsky S.** Calcific Disease of the Aortic Valve. Philadelphia: JB Lippincott, 1947:25.
23. **Evans LR, White PD.** Massive hypertrophy of the heart with special reference to Bernheim's syndrome. Am J Med Sci 1948;216:485–491.
24. **Eliot RS, McGee HJ, Blount SG.** Cardiac amyloidosis. Circulation 1961;23:613–622.
25. **Roberts WC, Waller BF.** Cardiac amyloidosis causing cardiac dysfunction: analysis of 54 necropsy patients. Am J Cardiol 1983;52:137–147.
26. **Courville C, Mason VR.** The heart in acromegaly. Arch Intern Med 1936;61:704–713.
27. **McGuffin WL Jr, Sherman BM, Roth J, Gordon P, Kahn CR, Roberts WC, Frommer PL.** Acromegaly and cardiovascular disorders. A prospective study. Ann Intern Med 1974;81:11–18.
28. **Grande F, Taylor HL.** Adaptive changes in the heart, vessels, and patterns of control under chronically high loads. In: Hamilton WF, Dow P, eds. Handbook of Physiology. A Critical, Comprehensive Presentation of Physiological Knowledge and Concepts. Section 2. Circulation Vol III. Washington, DC: Am Physiol 1965:2615–2677.
29. **Warnes CA, Roberts WC.** The heart in massive (more than 300 pounds or more than 136 Kilograms) obesity: Analysis of 12 patients studied at necropsy. Am J Cardiol 1984;54:1087–1091.
30. **Teare D.** Asymmetrical hypertrophy of the heart in young adults. Br Heart J 1958;20:1–18.
31. **Roberts WC, Siegel RJ, McManus BM.** Idiopathic dilated cardiomyopathy. Analysis of 152 necropsy patients. Am J Cardiol 1985;56, in press.

The Carcinoid Syndrome: Comparison of 21 Necropsy Subjects with Carcinoid Heart Disease to 15 Necropsy Subjects without Carcinoid Heart Disease

ELIZABETH M. ROSS, M.D.
WILLIAM C. ROBERTS, M.D.

Bethesda, Maryland

Carcinoid heart disease is a morphologically specific type of cardiac disorder that involves the mural and valvular endocardium on the right side of the heart. Twenty-one subjects (57 percent) (Group I) with carcinoid heart disease and 15 subjects (43 percent) (Group II) without carcinoid heart disease were studied at necropsy. The two groups were similar in mean age (54 years versus 55 years), duration of clinical illness (4.7 years versus 6.3 years), body weight (50 kg versus 52 kg), systemic blood pressure (117/77 mm Hg versus 128/77 mm Hg), blood hematocrit levels (37 percent versus 36 percent), total serum protein levels (6.0 g/dl), and serum albumin levels (2.2 g/dl versus 2.6 g/dl). The two groups were different in the frequency of the presence of precordial murmurs consistent with tricuspid regurgitation and/or pulmonic stenosis (95 percent versus 13 percent), cardiomegaly by chest radiography (38 percent versus 0), low voltage on electrocardiography (47 percent versus 0), and location of the primary site of the carcinoid tumor. Total electrocardiographic 12-lead QRS voltage was similar in each group (105 mm versus 132 mm) (10 mm = 1 mV). Of Group I subjects, 43 percent died of cardiac causes; none of the Group II subjects died of cardiac causes. Of the 21 subjects with carcinoid heart disease, seven had left-sided cardiac involvement, but in none was it of functional significance. Thus, although carcinoid heart disease frequently is the cause of death in patients with the carcinoid syndrome, the development of carcinoid heart disease is not related to the duration of symptoms of the carcinoid syndrome.

In 1964, Roberts and Sjoerdsma [1] reported clinical and necrospy findings in 17 subjects with the carcinoid syndrome, nine with and eight without carcinoid heart disease. Since that date, we have studied both clinically and at necropsy an additional 19 subjects with this syndrome. This report summarizes findings in the entire group of 36 subjects, specifically seeking clues to distinguish clinically those subjects with carcinoid heart disease from those without carcinoid heart disease, and it evaluates the effect of carcinoid heart disease on prognosis.

SUBJECTS AND METHODS

Definitions.   *Carcinoid syndrome*—the presence of histologically proved carcinoid tumor in a site other than the appendix with metastases to both local lymph nodes and to one or more other sites, and the presence of diarrhea, wheezing, and/or cutaneous flushing. *Carcinoid heart disease*—the presence of grossly visible, focal, uniform fibrous lesions on the mural endocardium of the right atrium, right ventricle, or left ventricle and the presence of diffuse or focal thickening of the cusps of tricuspid and/or pulmonic valves with or without involvement of the mitral and/or aortic valves; histologic examination

From the Pathology Branch, National Heart, Lung and Blood Institute, National Institutes of Health, Bethesda, Maryland. Requests for reprints should be addressed either to Dr. Elizabeth M. Ross, Washington Hospital Center, 110 Irving Street, NW, Room 3B-44B, Washington, D.C. 20010, or to Dr. William C. Roberts, Building 10A, Room 3E-30, National Institutes of Health, Bethesda, Maryland 20205. Manuscript accepted December 28, 1984.

TABLE I   Clinical and Morphologic Findings in 21 Subjects with Carcinoid Heart Disease

Subject	Necropsy Number	Age (years) and Sex	Length of Illness (years)	SAP (mm Hg)	Site of Primary Carcinoid	Precordial Murmur (grade 0–6)			CT Ratio >0.5	Hct (percent)	TP (g/dl)	Alb (mg/dl)
						TR	PS	Other				
1	A-63-222	28F	1.5	120/70	SI	0	+	PR	0	34	—	—
2	A-64-217	32F	9	95/70	Ileum	+	+	TS	0	39	5.0	1.4
3	A-63-96	39M	3	90/70	SI	+	0	PR	0	39	7.3	0.6
4	A-57-49	41M	3	110/70	Ileum	0	+	0	0	36	6.6	2.2
5	A-65-180	42M	5	125/80	Ileum	+	0	0	+	43	7.6	1.9
6	A-66-165	47M	13	100/70	Ileum	0	+	0	0	30	4.8	2.5
7	A-57-238	50F	12	100/70	Ileum	0	+	PR	0	37	4.7	2.6
8	A-62-9	52F	1.5	120/80	Jejunum	0	+	0	0	30	5.1	2.0
9	A-70-214	52M	4	—	Ileum	0	0	0	0	29	—	2.2
10	A-65-93	53M	3.5	100/65	Ileum	+	+	0	+	35	6.5	2.8
11	A-61-68	57F	4	140/90	Ileum	0	+	PR	+	37	6.6	3.3
12	A-61-266	57F	4	110/65	Ileum	+	+	0	0	35	5.7	2.5
13	A-68-49	57F	8	120/76	Ileum	+	0	TS	0	40	5.3	2.3
14	A-59-223	59M	6	100/60	Ileum	+	0	PR	+	43	6.5	2.2
15	A-72-96	61F	1	110/80	Ileum	+	0	0	0	45	6.9	3.0
16	A-61-193	64M	1.5	130/80	Jejunum	+	+	TS/PR	+	43	4.9	1.4
17	A-65-127	64F	1	110/75	Ileum	0	+	0	+	37	5.1	1.8
18	A-59-192	67M	7	110/70	Ileum	0	+	0	0	35	5.0	2.8
19	A-76-210	68M	9	130/80	—	+	0	0	0	38	7.2	3.8
20	A-62-34	69M	1	120/80	Ileum	+	+	0	+	33	6.7	3.3
21	83-A-94	72M	0.5	180/130	Ileum	+	0	0	+	—	—	2.3

* Zero indicates amount of pericardial fluid to be less than 50 ml.

† Zero indicates amount of pleural fluid to be less than 100 ml on either side.

‡ Zero indicates amount of peritoneal fluid to be less than 100 ml.

A = ascites; Alb = serum albumin; BW = body weight; CT = cardiothoracic; Hct = hematocrit; HIAA = hydroxyindole acetic acid; HW = heart weight; MV = mitral valve; Pe = pericardial; Pl = pleural; PR = pulmonic regurgitation; PS = pulmonic stenosis; PV = pulmonic valve; RA = right atrium; RV = right ventricle; SAP = systemic artery pressure; SE = subcutaneous pitting edema; SI = small intestine; TP = total protein; TR = tricuspid regurgitation; TS = tricuspid stenosis; TV = tricuspid valve; VC = vena cava.

of the thickened valvular cusps and thickened mural endocardium discloses uniform-appearing fibrous tissue devoid of elastic fibrils. These specific mural and valvular endocardial lesions will be referred to herein as *carcinoid plaques.*

Methods.   The medical records of cases coded as "carcinoid syndrome" in the files of the Pathology Branch, National Heart, Lung, and Blood Institute, were retrieved and examined, and pertinent clinical and morphologic data (to be summarized later) recorded. The 19 hearts studied since 1964 were re-examined by both of us. (The hearts in the first 17 cases had been examined earlier by one of us [W.C.R.].) The necropsy records of all 36 cases were examined. At least two histologic sections of one or more grossly visible carcinoid plaques were examined in each subject; the range was two to 37 sections (average 12) per subject. Data were analyzed using the Student t test. A p value of 0.05 was accepted as indicating a significant difference between the groups.

HW (g)	BW (kg)	Highest Urinary 5-HIAA (mg/24 hours)	Hepatic Weight (g)	Location of Carcinoid Plaque						Effusion (amount in ml)			
				RA	TV	RV	PV	MV	VC	Pe*	PI†	A‡	SE
250	—	263	—	+	+	0	+	+	+	—	—	—	+
250	37	288	1,950	+	+	+	+	0	0	0	+ (500)	+ (350)	+
280	48	432	2,900	+	+	0	+	+	0	0	0	+ (1,950)	+
220	42	890	7,400	+	+	0	+	0	0	0	0	+ (200)	0
420	55	450	2,130	+	+	+	+	+	0	0	0	+ (500)	+
250	67	§	4,000	+	0**	0	+	0	0	0	+ (200)	+ (1,500)	0
250	38	1,270	4,500	+	+	+	+	0	0	+ (100)	+ (2,500)	+ (20)	+
200	43	220	2,800	+	+	+	+	+	+	0	0	+ (4,600)	+
350	50	—	3,000	+	+	+	+	0	0	0	+ (600)	+ (3,000)	+
320	40	350	2,150	+	+	0	+	0	+	0	+ (250)	0	+
270	60	283	2,300	+	+	+	+	0	+	0	0	0	+
210	50	274	1,800	+	+	+	+	+	+	0	+ (750)	+ (525)	+
290	45	§	1,800	+	+	+	+	0	0	+ (50)	+ (1,100)	+ (500)	+
350	56	580	1,800	+	+	0	+	0	+	+ (150)	0	+	+
240	46	285	1,700	+	+	0	+	0	+	0	0	+ (750)	+
400	50	524	1,600	+	+	+	+††	+	0	0	0	0	+
250	47	135	2,150	+	+	0	+	0	+	0	0	+ (1,500)	+
280	62	—	2,500	+	+	+	+	0	0	+ (50)	+ (1,000)	+ (700)	+
480	67	500	5,700	0	+	+	+	+	0	0	0	+ (500)	+
475	52	120	2,600	0	+	0	+††	0	0	0	0	+	+
370	—	—	1,800	+	+	+	+	0	0	0	0	+	+

§ Markedly positive.
** Grossly normal; histologically abnormal.
†† Pulmonary trunk involved also.

RESULTS

Of the 36 subjects with the carcinoid syndrome, 21 (57 percent) at necropsy had carcinoid heart disease (Group I) and 15 (43 percent) did not (Group II). Certain findings in the subjects with carcinoid heart disease are summarized in **Table I,** and in those without in **Table II.**

Morphologic Findings. All 36 subjects had histologically proved carcinoid tumors with local lymph node involvement and metastases to one or more distant sites. Only one subject did not have hepatic metastases (Subject 15, Group II). Metastases to organs other than the liver occurred in 14 (67 percent) of 21 subjects in Group I and in 11 (73 percent) of 15 subjects in Group II. Pulmonary metastases occurred in five subjects in Group I and in eight in Group II. Bone metastases oc-

TABLE II Clinical and Morphologic Findings in 15 Subjects with Carcinoid Syndrome but without Carcinoid Heart Disease

Subject	Necropsy Number	Age (years) and Sex	Length of Illness (years)	SAP (mm Hg)	Site of Primary Carcinoid	Precordial Systolic Murmur	CT Ratio >0.5	Hct (percent)	TP (g/dl)	Alb (mg/dl)	HW (g)	BW (kg)	Highest Urinary 5-HIAA (mg/24 hours)	Hepatic Weight (g)	Pe*	Effusion (amount in ml) Pl†	A‡	SE
1	A-67-232	28F	1	130/80	Stomach	+	0	34	7.5	2.9	150	39	—	5,660	0	+ (1,450)	+ (2,000)	+
2	A-62-75	40F	4	90/50	Ileum	0	0	34	4.8	1.4	230	42	60	3,500	0	+ (130)	0	+
3	A-72-43	42M	25	170/110	Bronchus	+	—	29	5.9	3.8	570	75	119	6,400	0	0	+ (1,000)	+
4	A-70-29	43M	20	110/60	Ileum	0	0	36	6.1	2.1	335	59	153	4,700	0	+ (800)	0	+
5	A-59-44	45M	5	120/80	Bronchus	0	0	37	6.6	3.1	450	75	588	6,100	0	0	0	0
6	A-56-199	47M	3	135/90	Cecum	0	0	47	—	—	300	68	124	2,100	+ (70)	0	0	0
7	A-64-118	51F	3.5	125/60	Ileum	+	0	28	5.6	1.8	250	41	§	2,100	0	0	0	+
8	A-72-139	59M	8	130/85	Ileum	0	0	34	7.0	2.7	240	47	196	1,300	0	0	+	+
9	A-69-275	60M	2	160/80	Bronchus	+	0	39	6.5	3.8	430	60	14.3	3,600	0	0	0	+
10	A-63-67	65F	3	95/60	Ileum	0	0	28	5.6	1.8	250	28	23	510	0	+ (450)	0	+
11	A-60-46	67M	8	130/80	Ileum	0	0	38	7.4	3.3	300	55	43	2,100	0	0	+ (4,000)	+
12	A-60-68	67F	1	170/90	Ileum	0	0	33	6.6	2.3	270	48	§	1,650	0	0	0	0
13	A-57-219	69M	9	120/80	Meckel's	+	0	43	5.2	2.7	270	59	854	3,800	+ (50)	+ (700)	0	+
14	A-58-166	74M	1.5	100/80	SI	0	0	27	5.4	1.9	290	31	400	2,500	0	0	0	+
15	A-58-32	75M	1	130/75	Ileum	0	0	38	—	—	320	57	73	1,700	0	0	+ (2,000)	0

* Zero indicates amount of pericardial fluid to be less than 50 ml.
† Zero indicates amount of pleural fluid to be less than 100 ml on either side.
‡ Zero indicates amount of peritoneal fluid to be less than 100 ml.
§ Markedly positive.
Abbreviations as in Table I.

curred in nine Group I subjects and in six Group II subjects.

Carcinoid plaques were present on tricuspid and pulmonic cusps in all 21 Group I subjects (**Figures 1** to **6**). Carcinoid plaques also were present on one or both left-sided cardiac valves in seven subjects: mitral valve only in six and both mitral and aortic valves in one. The thickening of the tricuspid and pulmonic leaflets was diffuse and uniform in 19 of the 21 subjects (Figures 3, 5, and 6). In the other two patients (Subjects 6 and 8, Group I), the thickening on both right-sided valves was focal. In contrast, the thickening of the mitral leaflets, except for one subject (Subject 16, Group I), was focal and to far less degree than the involvement of either tricuspid or pulmonic cusps (Figure 2). The involvement of the aortic valve in the one subject consisted of a small fibrous plaque on one of the three aortic valve cusps. Carcinoid plaques were present on the mural endocardium of the right atrium in 19 subjects, on the mural endocardium of the right ventricle in 13, and on the mural endocardium of the left ventricle in seven. The mural endocardial plaques of the right atrium were always thicker and covered a larger area than those in the right ventricle; mural plaques in the left ventricle always were small. In several subjects, focal carcinoid plaques also were observed in the coronary sinus, inferior and superior caval veins, brachiocephalic vein, and pulmonary trunk. In one subject, a small carcinoid plaque was present in the ascending aorta.

Histologically, carcinoid plaques consisted of fibrous tissue, devoid of elastic fibrils, deposited on the endocardial surfaces of the valve cusps and the cardiac chambers and on the intima of the vessels (Figures 1 to 6). The underlying endocardium and intima were not involved and were delineated by an elastic membrane. The fibrotic process was located on the ventricular aspect of the posterior and septal tricuspid valve leaflets, usually causing them to adhere to the underlying ventricular wall. The fibrotic process involved both atrial and ventricular aspects of the anterior tricuspid valve leaflet. The fibrotic process involved the pulmonic valve cusps on their arterial or downstream aspects, causing infolding of the distal third or so of the cusps toward the sinuses. As with the tricuspid septal and posterior leaflets, the carcinoid involvement of the mitral leaflets was also entirely on their ventricular aspects.

The tricuspid valve was usually fixed in an open position, producing regurgitation with or without some degree of stenosis (Figure 3). The left side of the heart never had lesions severe enough to cause dysfunction. The carcinoid plaques on the pulmonic valve cusps caused relative rigidity of the cusps and relative constriction of the circumference of the pulmonary trunk at the level of the valve sinuses. (Figures 3, 5, and 6). The result was usually a pulmonic valve orifice that was

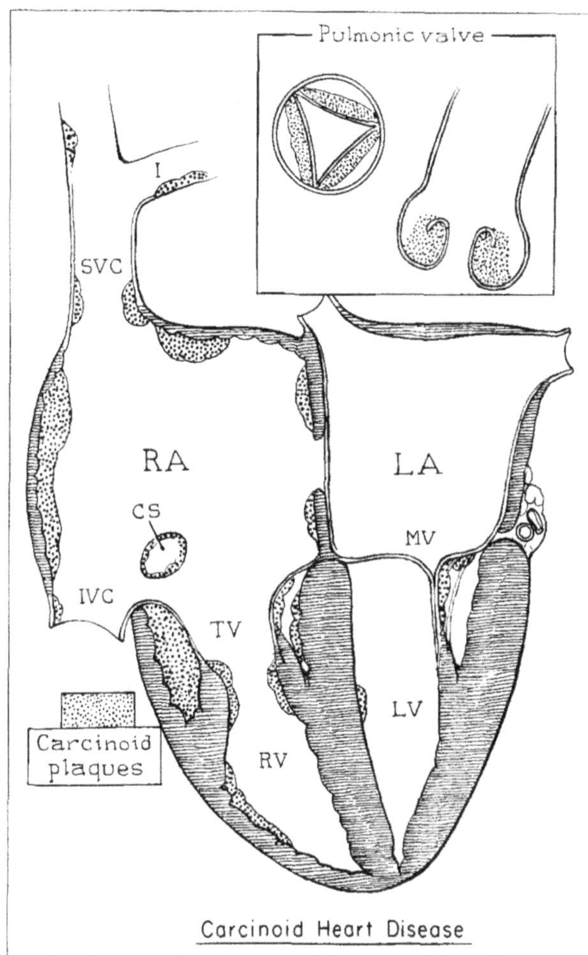

Figure 1. *Illustration of location and distribution of carcinoid plaques. CS = ostium of coronary sinus; I = innominate (brachiocephalic) vein; IVC = inferior vena cava; LA = left atrium; LV = left ventricle; MV = mitral valve; RA = right atrium; RV = right ventricle; SVC = superior vena cava; TV = tricuspid valve.*

smaller than normal, thus producing some degree of stenosis. Because the cusps were thickened and relatively immobile, they were not able to appose one another during ventricular diastole, and pulmonic regurgitation was the usual result.

Clinical Findings. No significant differences were observed between the subjects with carcinoid heart disease and those without carcinoid heart disease in sex (57 percent men versus 67 percent men); mean age (54 years versus 55 years); frequency of diarrhea (100 percent versus 93 percent); flushing (81 percent versus 93 percent); pericardial effusion (25 percent versus 13 percent); pleural effusions (40 percent versus 33 percent); and subcutaneous edema (90 percent versus 73 percent). Both groups had similar mean body weights (50 kg versus 52 kg) and mean heights (169 cm versus 168 cm); systemic blood pressures (117/77 mm Hg

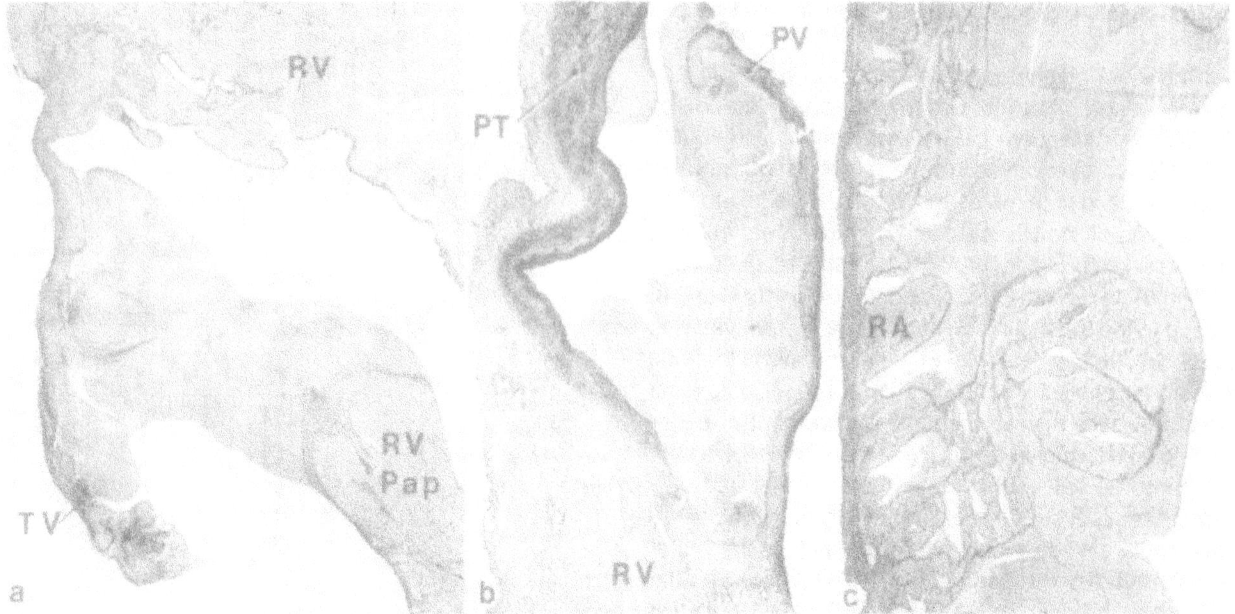

Figure 2. (Subject 2, Table I) **A,** photomicrograph of tricuspid valve (TV) cusp with underlying right ventricular (RV) wall and papillary (Pap) muscle. The cusp is adherent to the papillary muscle by carcinoid plaque. **B,** photomicrograph of pulmonic valve (PV) cusp, wall of pulmonary trunk (PT), and right ventricle. Carcinoid plaque is present in the pulmonic sinus and on the endothelium of the pulmonary trunk. The distal portion of the cusp is folded inward. **C,** photomicrograph of a portion of the wall of the right atrium (RA) showing deposit of carcinoid plaque on the endocardium. The plaque is thicker than the original atrial wall (Verhõeff-van Gieson elastic tissue stains; original magnification × 15 [**A** and **B**], × 19 [**C**], reduced by 35 percent).

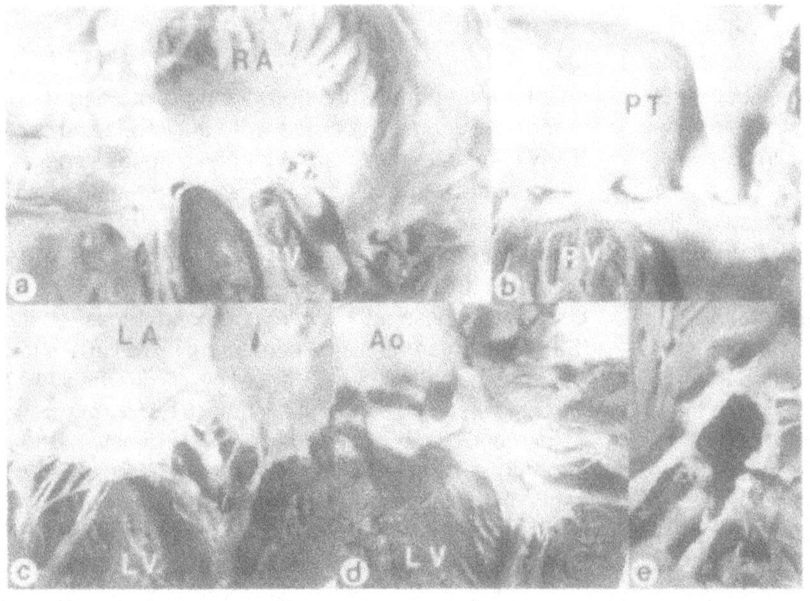

Figure 3. (Subject 5, Table I) **A,** opened right atrium (RA) and right ventricle (RV) showing carcinoid plaque; the tricuspid valve leaflets and attached chordae are thick and shortened. **B,** opened pulmonic valve showing diffuse involvement by carcinoid plaque resulting in marked shortening and retraction of the cusps. The wall of the pulmonary trunk (PT) is folded at the level of the valve. **C,** opened left atrium (LA), mitral valve, and left ventricle (LV) showing focal plaque deposits on the leaflets. **D,** opened aorta (Ao), aortic valve, and left ventricle showing focal plaque deposits. **E,** tricuspid valve seen from the right ventricle showing a fixed and incompetent orifice.

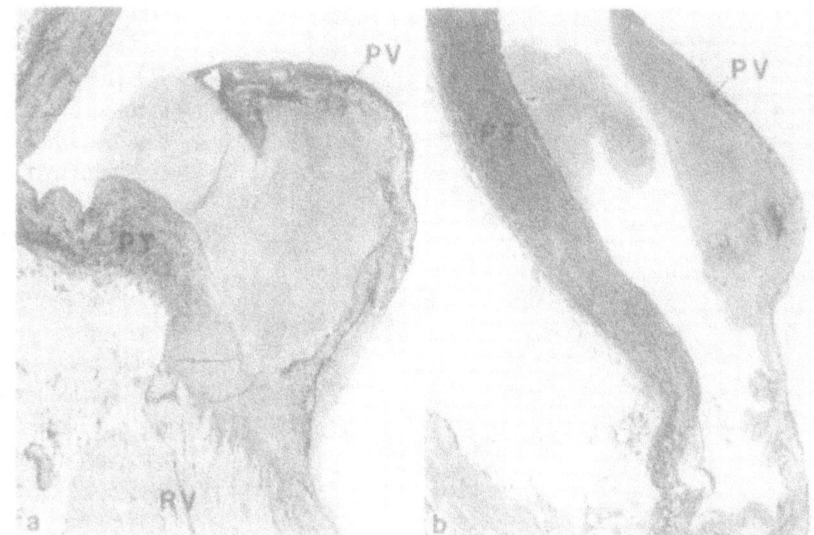

Figure 4. *(Subject 5, Table I)* **A,** *photomicrograph of a pulmonic valve (PV) cusp showing infolding of its distal portion and complete obliteration of the sinus by carcinoid plaque. PT = pulmonary trunk; RV = right ventricle.* **B,** *photomicrograph of another pulmonic valve cusp showing carcinoid plaque on one side of the cusp and on the pulmonary trunk but no fixation of the cusp (Verhoeff-van Gieson elastic tissue stain; original magnification each ✕ 11, reduced by 43 percent).*

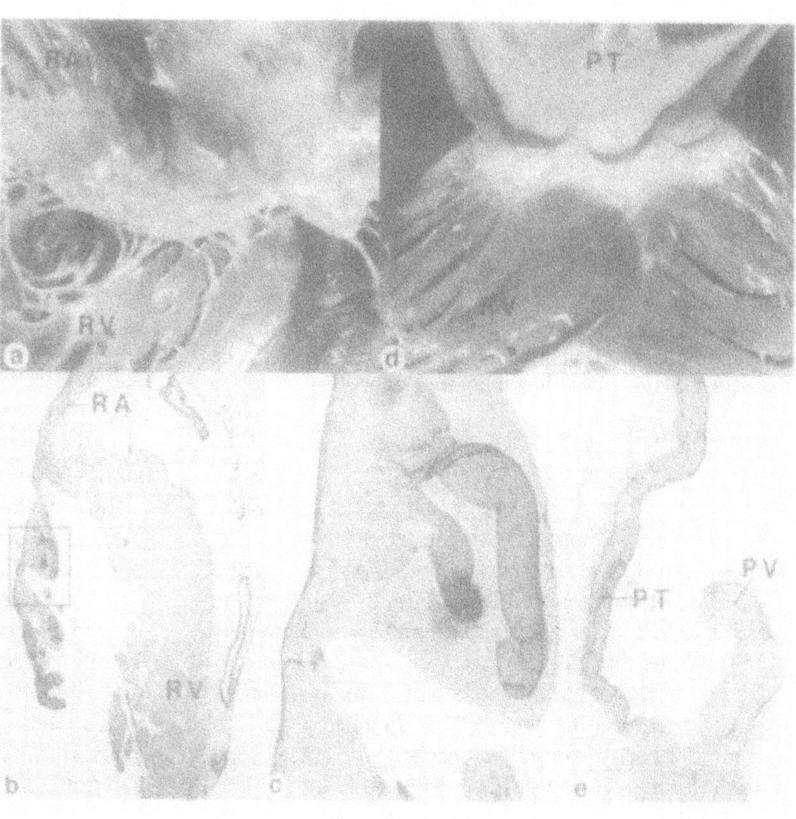

Figure 5. *(Subject 15, Table I)* **A,** *opened right atrium (RA), tricuspid valve, and right ventricle (RV) showing a thickened valve and atrial carcinoid plaques.* **B,** *photomicrograph of a portion of the right atrium, tricuspid valve, and right ventricle showing carcinoid plaque involving the leaflet and chordae.* **C,** *photomicrograph of the leaflet and chordae of the tricuspid valve indicated by a* **box** *in* **B.** **D,** *opened pulmonary trunk (PT), pulmonic valve, and right ventricle showing diffusely thickened and retracted valve cusps.* **E,** *photomicrograph of a pulmonic valve (PV) cusp and pulmonary trunk showing carcinoid plaque primarily on the "downstream" aspect of the cusp (Verhoeff-van Gieson elastic tissue stains; original magnification ✕ 6[* **B** *], ✕ 25 [* **C** *], ✕ 8 [* **E** *], reduced by 45 percent).*

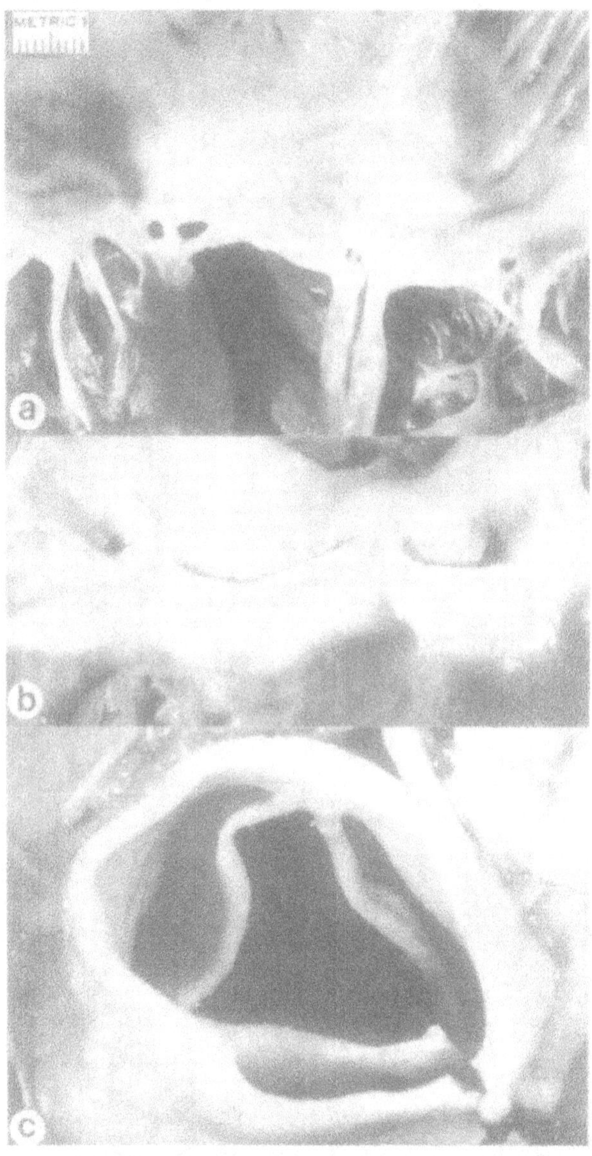

Figure 6. (*Subject 21, Table I*) *A, opened right atrium, tricuspid valve, and right ventricle showing thickened leaflets and chordae. B, opened pulmonic valve showing diffusely thickened cusps. C, nearly intact pulmonic valve showing thickened cusps and an incompetent orifice.*

versus 128/77 mm Hg); blood hematocrit levels (37 percent versus 35 percent); total serum protein (6.0 g/dl versus 6.0 g/dl) and albumin levels (2.3 g/dl versus 2.6 g/dl); cardiac weights (305 g versus 304 g); hepatic weights (2,830 g versus 3,180 g); and splenic weights (155 g versus 245 g).

The average length of illness was 1.6 years shorter (4.7 years versus 6.3 years) (NS) for the group with carcinoid heart disease compared with the group without carcinoid heart disease (**Figures 7** and **8**). Two subjects without carcinoid heart disease had extraor-

dinarily long survivals (20 years and 25 years) from onset of symptoms attributable to carcinoid syndrome. The range of survival from onset of symptoms to death in the group with heart disease was 0.5 to 13 years. Of the 21 subjects with carcinoid heart disease, seven lived less than two years from onset of symptoms and seven lived longer than five years. The range of survival from onset of symptoms to death in the group without heart disease was one to 25 years; of the 15 subjects, five survived less than two years and five lived longer than five years.

Of the 28 subjects that had urinary 5-hydroxyindole acetic acid levels measured, the average was insignificantly higher in the group with carcinoid heart disease compared with the group without carcinoid heart disease (429 mg/dl versus 221 mg/dl). The duration of symptoms did not correlate with the level of 5-hydroxyindole acetic acid.

The two groups differed from each other in the location of the primary tumor. In Group I, the small intestine was the site of the primary tumor in 20 (95 percent) subjects, whereas it was the site of the primary tumor in 10 (67 percent) of the 15 subjects in Group II (p < 0.05).

The two groups differed in the frequency of precordial murmurs. Systolic murmurs were recorded in 20 of 21 subjects with carcinoid heart disease and in five of 15 subjects without carcinoid heart disease. A murmur consistent with tricuspid regurgitation (systolic, over left sternal border with increase in intensity during inspiration) was heard in 12 (57 percent) of the 21 subjects in Group I and in two (13 percent) of 15 subjects in Group II. A murmur consistent with pulmonic valve stenosis was described in 13 (62 percent) of 21 subjects in Group I, and a flow murmur was noted in three (20 percent) of 15 subjects in Group II. A diastolic murmur consistent with pulmonic regurgitation was described in six of 21 subjects in Group I, and in no subject in Group II. A diastolic murmur consistent with tricuspid valve stenosis was heard in three (14 percent) of the 21 subjects in Group I and in none of the 15 subjects in Group II.

Other features also helped differentiate the two groups. Compared with the Group II subjects, the Group I subjects had a higher frequency of wheezing (48 percent versus 20 percent) and peritoneal effusions (75 percent versus 33 percent); a higher percent of cardiothoracic ratios of more than 0.5 (38 percent versus 0); and a higher frequency of low voltage (sum of QRS complexes in leads I to III 15 mm or less) (10 mm = 1 mV) (9 of 19 [47 percent] versus 0 of 15). Death appeared to be attributable at least in part to the cardiac involvement in nine (43 percent) of the 21 Group I subjects, but in none of the 15 Group II subjects.

Electrocardiographic Findings. Electrocardiograms

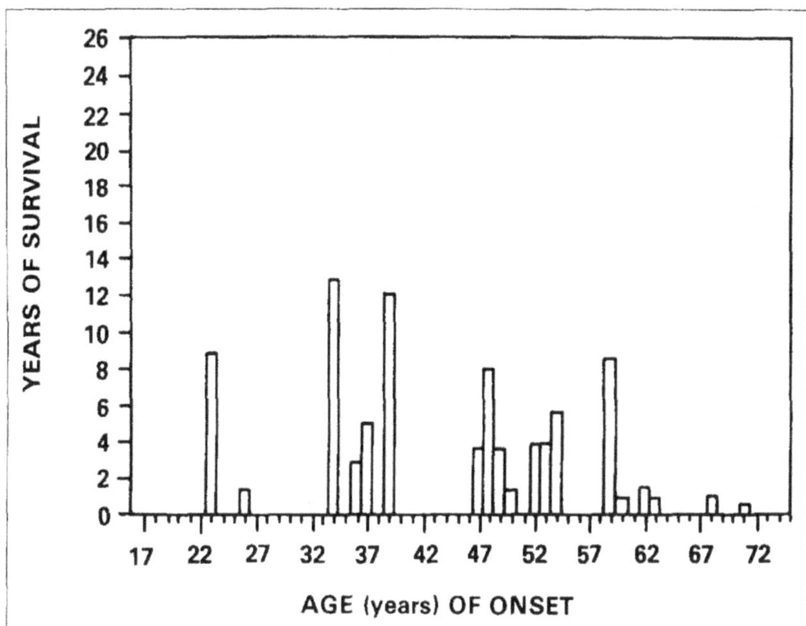

Figure 7. Graph showing years of survival from onset of symptoms of carcinoid syndrome for individual subjects with carcinoid heart disease (Table I).

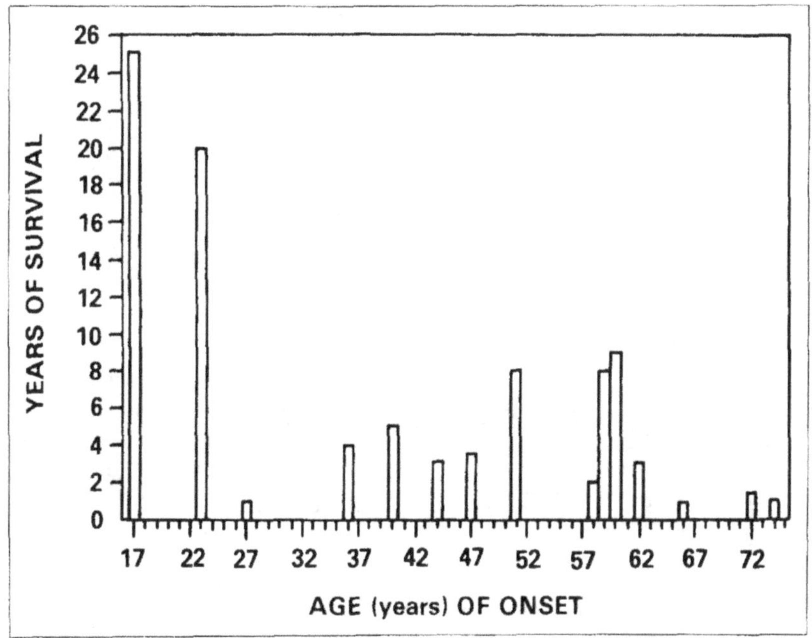

Figure 8. Graph showing years of survival from onset of symptoms of carcinoid syndrome for individual subjects without carcinoid heart disease (Table II).

were re-examined in 34 of the 36 subjects, and the findings are recorded in each subject in **Tables III** and **IV (Figures 9** and **10)**. The interval from the electrocardiographic recording to death ranged from seven to 186 days (mean 69) in the 19 Group I subjects with electrocardiograms and from 11 to 232 days (mean 73) in the 15 Group II subjects.

The ventricular rates were similar in Groups I and II (88 beats per minute versus 91 beats per minute). One

subject had premature atrial beats (Subject 19, Group I) on a resting electrocardiogram and two subjects had ventricular premature complexes (Subjects 8 and 13, Group II). The duration of the P-R, QRS, and Q-T intervals was similar in both groups.

The QRS voltage in each of the 12 leads was measured in 34 subjects. In the 19 Group I subjects, it ranged from 58 to 227 mm (mean 105), and in the 15 Group II subjects total 12-lead QRS voltage ranged from 89 to

TABLE III   Electrocardiographic Findings in 19 Subjects with Carcinoid Heart Disease

Subject	Interval ECG to Death (days)	VR (beats/minute)	Intervals (seconds)			Voltage (mm)												Total QRS 12-Lead Voltage (mm)	Axis
			P-R	QRS	Q-T	I	II	III	aVR	aVL	aVF	V_1	V_2	V_3	V_4	V_5	V_6		
2	34	85	0.16	0.08	0.28	3	6	5	3	3	5	6	9	7	6	5	4	59	120°
3	10	83	0.16	0.08	0.30	3	5	4	3	2	4	15	13	10	7	6	7	79	60°
4	104	120	0.16	0.06	0.32	4	7	4	5	3	5	21	37	23	28	17	13	167	0°
5	7	110	0.18	0.10	0.30	7	9	7	7	5	7	8	9	11	11	15	15	104	110°
6	115	52	0.20	0.08	0.42	6	7	6	7	6	5	4	13	15	16	20	14	119	30°
7	33	100	0.13	0.06	0.28	2	4	4	3	3	4	5	12	12	6	7	6	68	90°
8	186	110	0.14	0.08	0.32	7	5	2	5	3	3	10	15	13	13	11	7	94	0°
10	13	100	0.16	0.08	0.30	3	7	6	4	5	6	5	13	20	20	16	12	117	110°
11	28	65	0.20	0.08	0.48	5	7	5	5	3	6	6	19	17	14	10	7	104	30°
12	47	80	0.14	0.08	0.26	4	5	7	3	4	6	5	10	17	13	8	5	87	90°
13	107	100	0.18	0.08	0.30	4	10	8	8	5	9	9	23	20	11	10	11	128	0°
14	16	73	0.20	0.06	0.36	3	3	4	2	3	3	4	8	10	6	6	6	58	110°
15	42	85	0.16	0.08	0.36	4	4	4	4	2	4	3	8	6	7	6	6	58	60°
16	59	100	0.14	0.08	0.36	6	5	3	6	4	4	13	22	24	16	17	8	129	30°
17	39	80	0.12	0.08	0.36	7	5	7	4	6	5	5	12	6	4	8	7	76	30°
18	105	82	0.19	0.06	0.36	3	7	5	6	3	6	16	22	18	6	8	6	106	60°
19	160	75	0.16	0.08	0.36	3	3	2	3	2	2	2	16	18	18	18	9	96	60°
20	35	90	0.16	0.10	0.36	4	6	9	3	6	8	9	13	24	17	11	6	116	−60°
21	180	75	0.24	0.08	0.36	13	9	10	11	10	7	15	30	38	39	30	15	227	−30°
Mean	69	88	0.17	0.07	0.34	5	6	5	5	4	5	8	16	16	14	12	9	105	

ECG = electrocardiography; VR = ventricular rate.

TABLE IV   Electrocardiographic Observations in 15 Subjects with Carcinoid Syndrome but without Carcinoid Heart Disease

Subject	Interval ECG to Death (days)	VR (beats/minute)	Intervals (seconds)			Voltage (mm)												Total QRS 12-Lead Voltage (mm)	Axis
			P-R	QRS	Q-T	I	II	III	aVR	aVL	aVF	V_1	V_2	V_3	V_4	V_5	V_6		
1	134	90	0.16	0.08	0.38	4	8	8	6	2	7	5	8	9	19	24	16	116	60°
2	232	110	0.13	0.09	0.38	7	7	3	6	3	4	11	23	30	21	13	7	135	30°
3	65	75	0.18	0.08	0.36	8	8	3	7	5	5	5	22	14	24	17	14	132	45°
4	67	110	0.16	0.06	0.35	5	11	6	8	3	8	9	19	16	15	12	10	122	60°
5	31	92	0.15	0.07	0.36	6	9	5	6	3	7	10	11	13	21	18	10	119	30°
6	35	80	0.16	0.08	0.37	10	9	4	10	6	5	19	36	37	23	15	9	183	30°
7	71	80	0.20	0.08	0.36	8	8	5	7	6	6	8	15	11	8	12	8	102	30°
8	35	55	0.14	0.08	0.44	2	16	15	8	8	16	16	28	22	30	19	12	192	30°
9	106	133	0.16	0.06	0.36	5	12	9	6	3	10	8	20	13	25	23	18	152	60°
10	45	71	0.11	0.07	0.39	2	9	9	4	3	9	8	17	20	15	10	9	115	90°
11	102	75	0.16	0.08	0.32	6	7	5	6	3	6	6	14	17	15	8	6	99	30°
12	24	100	0.12	0.06	0.34	13	9	9	10	9	6	13	15	15	15	12	9	135	0°
13	35	78	0.14	0.09	0.36	3	9	8	5	3	9	6	6	9	13	11	7	89	60°
14	95	120	0.12	0.08	0.34	6	16	13	12	4	15	26	29	8	18	15	13	175	60°
15	11	98	0.16	0.10	0.36	4	12	16	5	9	13	5	6	11	9	9	8	107	−60°
Mean	73	91	0.15	0.08	0.36	6	10	8	7	5	8	10	18	16	18	14	10	132	

Abbreviations as in Table III.

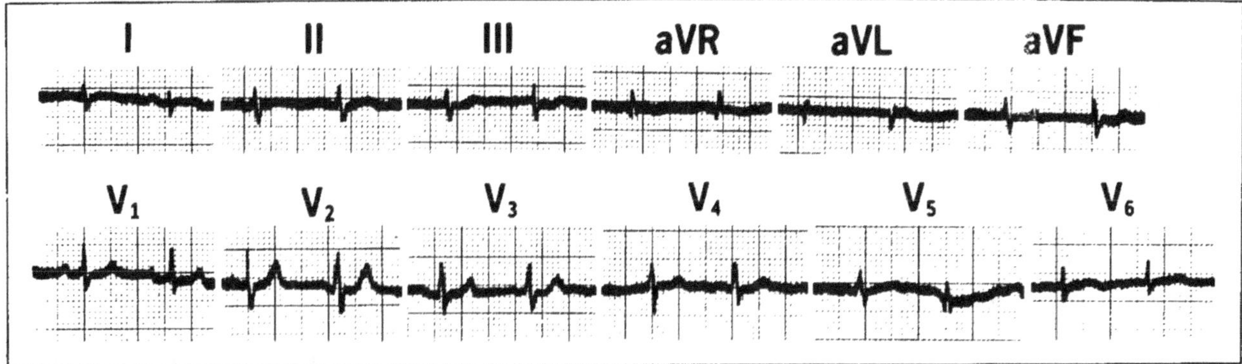

Figure 9. (Subject 2, Table I) Electrocardiogram showing low QRS voltage in limb leads and an R wave that is greater than the S wave in V_1 to V_6.

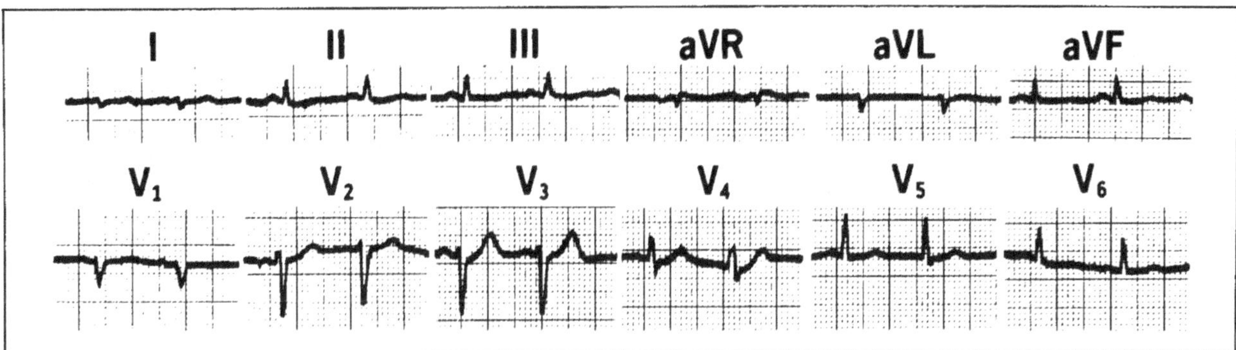

Figure 10. (Subject 7, Table I) Electrocardiogram showing low QRS voltage in limb leads, vertical axis, T wave changes, and delayed precordial transition.

192 mm (mean 132) (NS). Total 12-lead QRS voltage was 175 mm or less in 20 (95 percent) of 21 subjects with carcinoid heart disease and in 12 (80 percent) of 15 subjects without carcinoid heart disease. Of the 34 subjects with electrocardiograms, six (18 percent) had hearts weighing more than 400 g (clearly above normal). The total 12-lead QRS voltage in the six subjects with hearts of increased weight ranged from 96 to 152 mm (mean 120), and in the 28 subjects with normal-sized hearts it ranged from 58 to 227 mm (mean 116) (NS).

Of the 36 subjects, cardiac catheterization data are available in three. Right-sided pressure tracings in Subject 2, Group I, are shown in **Figures 11** and **12**.

COMMENTS

Examination of the hearts in our 36 subjects with the carcinoid syndrome disclosed that over half (58 percent) had carcinoid heart disease. Why carcinoid heart disease occurs in some patients with the carcinoid syndrome and not in others remains unexplained. Our data refute the earlier suggestions that patients with carcinoid heart disease have longer symptomatic illnesses compared with those without carcinoid heart disease [2–5]. The mean survival after onset of dermal flushing or diarrhea or wheezing (whichever symptom came first) was 4.7 years in our 21 subjects with carcinoid heart disease and 6.3 years in the 15 subjects without carcinoid heart disease (NS). Another proposal explaining the presence of carcinoid heart disease in some but not in other patients with the carcinoid syndrome is differing blood serotonin levels between the two groups. The mean urinary 5-hydroxyindole acetic acid levels in 16 subjects with carcinoid heart disease was 429 mg per 24 hours, and 221 mg per 24 hours (NS) in the 12 subjects without carcinoid heart disease.

Although its cause and mechanism of formation is unclear, carcinoid heart disease is a unique form of heart disease. It consists of the deposition of a peculiar type of fibrous tissue devoid of elastic fibrils within which are smooth muscle cells and mucopolysaccharide material on the mural and valvular endocardium, primarily on the right side of the heart [6]. A fascinating feature of the deposits (carcinoid plaques) is that by histologic and electron microscopic examination they all look alike. In other words, the deposits do not appear to go through various developmental stages—there are no early and late stages, only one stage. This morpho-

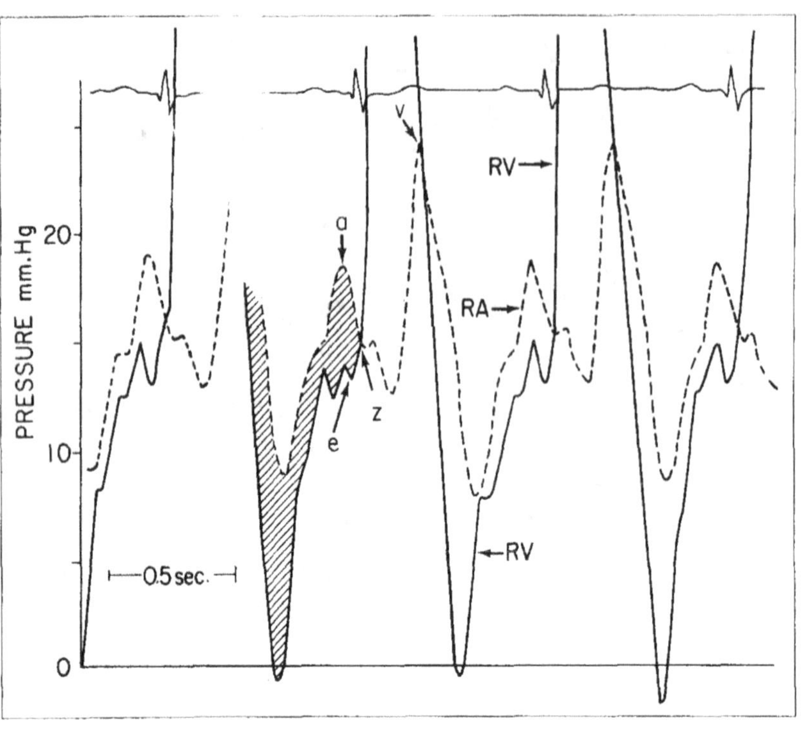

Figure 11. (Subject 2, Table I) Right-sided pressure tracing in a patient with tricuspid regurgitation and stenosis. The **hatched** area indicates the pressure gradient between right atrium (RA) and right ventricle (RV). a = A wave; e = E point; v = v wave; z = Z point. Lead II of the electrocardiogram is at the **top.** (Reproduced with permission from Roberts WC, Mason DT, Wright LD Jr: The non-distensible right atrium of carcinoid disease of the heart. Am J Clin Pathol 1965; 44: 627–631.)

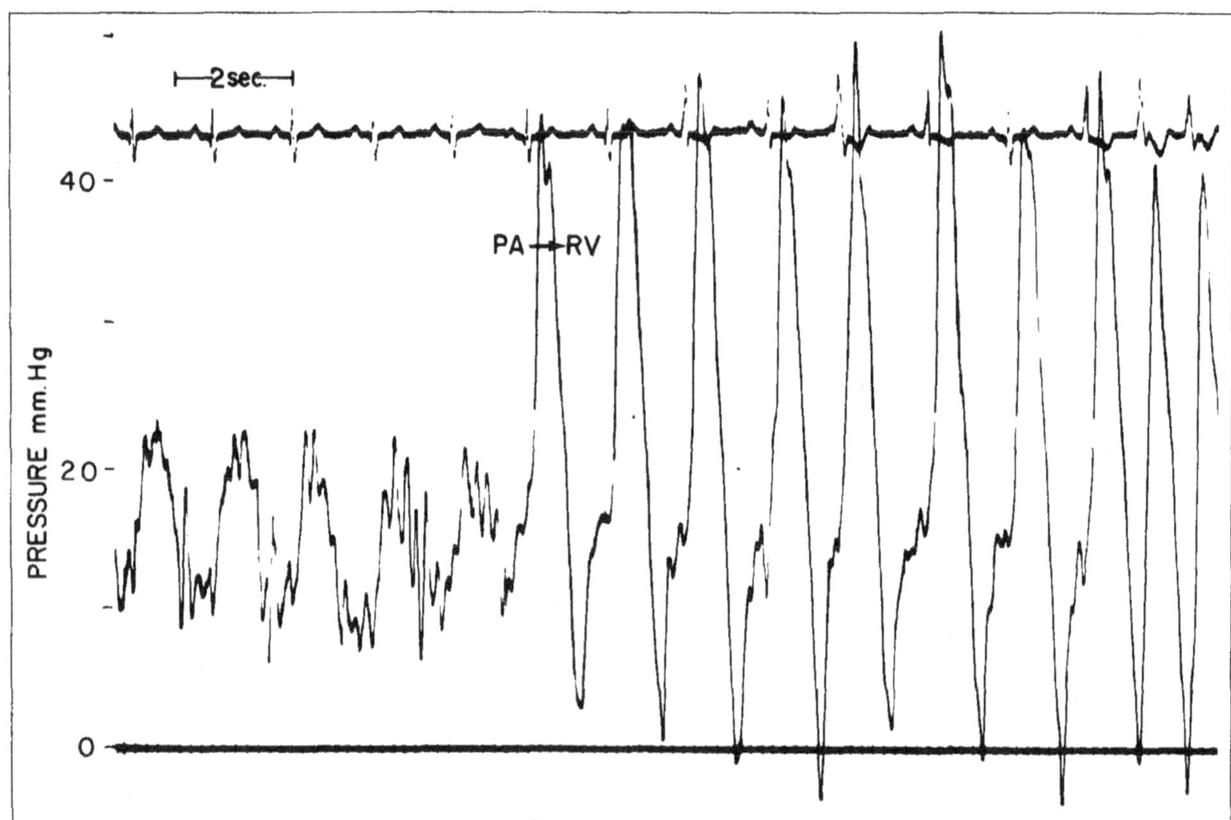

Figure 12. (Subject 2, Table I) Pullback pressure tracing from pulmonary trunk (PA) to right ventricle (RV) showing a 20 mm Hg peak systolic pressure gradient. The lead II electrocardiogram is shown at the **top.** (Reproduced with permission from Roberts WC, Mason DT, Wright LD Jr: The non-distensible right atrium of carcinoid disease of the heart. Am J Clin Pathol 1965; 44:

logic observation supports the view that the carcinoid endocardial plaque results from the deposit of a substance from the blood.

Not only is the composition of the carcinoid endocardial plaque unique [1,2], but the site of its occurrence in the heart is unique. The plaques are far more common on the right side of the heart than on the left, and even when present on the left, the right-sided plaques are always more extensive and larger. Among our 21 subjects with carcinoid heart disease, the carcinoid plaques were limited to the right side of the heart in 15 (71 percent).

All of our 21 subjects with carcinoid heart disease had involvement of both tricuspid and pulmonic valves by carcinoid plaques, and 19 of them also had carcinoid plaques on the mural endocardium of the right atrium and usually also on the mural endocardium of the right ventricle. The number of subjects with right-sided valvular dysfunction as a consequence of the carcinoid plaques on the valvular leaflets is less certain because of the relative difficulty in diagnosing by auscultation mild degrees of tricuspid and pulmonic valve dysfunction. In two of the 21 subjects with right-sided carcinoid heart disease, the degree of morphologic involvement of both valves was minimal and valvular function clearly was not affected. Of the remaining 19 subjects, 18 had precordial systolic and/or diastolic murmurs of grade 2/6 or greater intensity. The carcinoid deposits on the left-sided valve(s) in the six subjects did not appear extensive enough to cause valvular dysfunction.

Although the composition and location of the carcinoid plaques on both right-sided cardiac valves are similar, the functional consequences of the carcinoid plaques are different. The deposits occur nearly entirely on the downstream side of the valvular leaflets, i.e., on the ventricular aspects of the septal and posterior tricuspid leaflets and on the pulmonary arterial side of the pulmonic valve cusps. On the anterior tricuspid valve leaflet, the deposits can be on both sides. The consequences of the "downstream" deposition is an adherence of the leaflet to the underlying mural endocardium (tricuspid septal and posterior leaflets) or to the underlying pulmonary arterial endothelium (pulmonic valve) via the carcinoid plaques. The fibrous tissue of the carcinoid plaque acts as a constricting substance such that the "ring" of both right-sided cardiac valves is made smaller than normal and at the same time leaflet mobility is diminished. The consequence is tricuspid regurgitation with or without some degree of stenosis. Nearly all patients with pure tricuspid regurgitation (no element of stenosis) have dilated valve rings, but patients with some degree of stenosis in addition to regurgitation do not have dilated anuli. Patients with carcinoid heart disease follow this principle. Thus, patients with carcinoid heart disease have much more

tricuspid regurgitation than stenosis, but usually there is some degree of stenosis, albeit small.

In contrast to the tricuspid valve, the dominant functional pulmonic valve lesion is stenosis, although all patients with stenosis have some degree of pulmonic regurgitation. The reason for the difference—compared with the tricuspid valve—is that the orifice of the normal pulmonic valve is much smaller initially than the orifice of the tricuspid valve. Thus, the constriction by deposition of carcinoid plaques within the pulmonic sinuses causes constriction of the pulmonic root with the production of pulmonic stenosis. Because the distal portions of the pulmonic cusps are inverted toward the sinuses and the mobility of the cusps is lost, some degree of regurgitation is inevitable in all patients with carcinoid who have any degree of pulmonic stenosis.

Although combined lesions of both mitral and aortic valves are fairly common as a consequence of either rheumatic heart disease or infective endocarditis or both, combined lesions of both tricuspid and pulmonic valves are rare, and carcinoid is the only condition in which uniformly both—not just one—right-sided valves are involved together. The two dominant functional consequences of right-sided carcinoid heart disease are pulmonic stenosis and tricuspid regurgitation. These two lesions in the same patient are particularly unfavorable because the pulmonic stenosis increases the degree of tricuspid regurgitation. A commonly employed method of producing chronic congestive heart failure in experimental animals is by banding the pulmonary trunk to create pulmonic stenosis, and excising or destroying one or more tricuspid valve cusps to make the valve purely regurgitant. Thus, right-sided carcinoid heart disease in essence creates this experimental model. If a patient with carcinoid heart disease had only dysfunction of the pulmonic or the tricuspid valve, probably the functional consequence would be insignificant. It is the combination of both right-sided valvular lesions—namely pulmonic stenosis and tricuspid regurgitation—that has the potential of being devastating.

Clinical diagnosis of carcinoid heart disease can usually be established by noninvasive means. Auscultation, of course, is the first clue. In 20 (95 percent) of our 21 subjects with carcinoid heart disease and in five (33 percent) of our 15 subjects without carcinoid heart disease, one or more precordial murmurs were recorded (p <0.05). Of the 20 subjects with precordial murmurs and carcinoid heart disease, eight had both systolic and diastolic murmurs and 12 had only systolic murmurs; of the five subjects with precordial murmurs but without carcinoid heart disease, the murmurs in all were systolic only. Thus, nearly all patients with carcinoid heart disease have precordial murmurs, and when the murmur has a diastolic component, diagnosis

TABLE V Observations in 15 Previously Reported Patients with Carcinoid Heart Disease and Right-Sided Cardiac Operation

Reference	Age (years) at Time of Operation and Sex	Interval (years) First Carcinoid Symptom to Surgery	Operation (type) TV	Operation (type) PV	Interval (months) Cardiac Symptoms to Cardiac Operation	Interval (months) Cardiac Operation to Death	Preoperative Catheterization RA-RV MDG (mm Hg)	TR	RV-PA PSG (mm Hg)	PR	Murmurs TR	TS	PR	PS	Type (size) Prosthesis or Bioprosthesis
[2]	35F	19	+ (A)	+ (C)	5	Died postop	12	+	32	0	+	+	0	+	0
[9]	50M	15	+ (R)	+ (C)	60	72	24	+	48	0	+	+	+	+	Starr-Edwards (3 M)
[11]	31M	7	0	+ (E)	—	1	10	+	40	0	+	0	0	+	0
[10]	26F	9	+ (R)	+ (C)	5	132*	6	+	45	0	+	+	0	+	Kay-Shiley (6)
[3]	57M	3	+ (R)	0	18	4	0	+	3	0	+	0	+	+	Bjorck-Shiley (27)
[4]	46F	33	+ (R)	0	6	21*	4	—	10	0	0	+	0	+	Bjorck-Shiley (31)
[12]	24F	<0.5	+ (R)	+ (R)	4	24	4	+	32	0	+	0	0	+	Porcine(—)
[14]	64F	10	+ (R)	+ (R)	3	1	—	+	18	+	+	0	0	+	Bioprosthesis (—)
[16]	34M	5	+ (R)	+ (C)	12	96*	11	0	50	0	0	0	0	+	Starr-Edwards (3 M)
[13]	30F	18	+ (R)	+ (C)	12	4*	22	+	45	0	+	+	0	+	Porcine (27)
[15]	60F	<1	+ (R)	0	15	12*	5	+	—	0	+	0	0	0	Carpenter-Edwards (27)
[5]	53M	4.5	+ (R)	0	18	8	0	+	0	0	+	0	0	0	Porcine (27)
[17]	62M	25	+ (R)	+ (R)	—	24*	5	+	20	+	+	+	0	+	Porcine (—)
[18]	63F	1.5	+ (R)	+ (C)	18	2	4	+	8	0	+	0	0	+	Porcine (—)
[19]	56F	3	+ (R)	0	<8	23*	4	+	0	—	—	—	—	—	St. Jude (31)

* Alive.

A = annuloplasty; C = commissurotomy; E = excision; MDG = mean diastolic gradient; PA = pulmonary artery; postop = postoperatively; PR = pulmonic regurgitation; PS = pulmonic stenosis; PSG = peak systolic gradient; PV = pulmonic valve; R = replacement; RA = right atrium; RV = right ventricle; TR = tricuspid regurgitation; TS = tricuspid stenosis; TV = tricuspid valve; — = no information available.

of carcinoid heart disease can be made with confidence.

The systemic arterial blood pressure is not helpful in either diagnosing carcinoid syndrome or distinguishing those with carcinoid heart disease from those without carcinoid heart disease. Only three of our 36 subjects had indirect systolic systemic arterial pressures of more than 140 mm Hg and/or diastolic arterial pressures of more than 90 mm Hg: one of the 21 with carcinoid heart disease and two of the 15 without carcinoid heart disease. The average peak systolic pressure was 117 mm Hg in the 21 subjects with carcinoid heart disease, and 128 mm Hg in the 15 subjects without carcinoid heart disease; the average diastolic pressure in both groups was 77 mm Hg.

Chest radiography was helpful in diagnosing carcinoid heart disease. The cardiothoracic ratio was more than 0.50 in eight (38 percent) of 21 subjects with carcinoid heart disease and in none of 15 subjects without carcinoid heart disease. Thus, the cardiothoracic ratio is not a very sensitive test for carcinoid heart disease, but it is specific.

Resting electrocardiography was somewhat useful in distinguishing the subjects with carcinoid heart disease from those without carcinoid heart disease. The sum of the QRS voltage in leads I, II, and III was 15 mm or less in nine of the 21 subjects with carcinoid heart disease and in none of the 15 subjects without carcinoid heart disease (p <0.05). The sum of the total 12-lead QRS voltage ranged from 58 to 227 mm (10 mm = 1 mV) in 34 subjects, and the mean values were not significantly different between the two groups (105 mm versus 132 mm). In only three subjects (one with carcinoid heart disease) was this total 12-lead QRS voltage more than 175 mm. Evidence of right ventricular hypertrophy was rare. The R wave was greater than the S wave in either lead V_1 or V_2 in only four of the 19 subjects with carcinoid heart disease and in none of the 15 subjects without carcinoid heart disease. Right axis deviation (more than 90 degrees) was present in only 4 of the 19 subjects with carcinoid heart disease and in none of the 15 subjects without carcinoid heart disease. Despite right atrial dilatation in most of the subjects with carcinoid heart disease, all 19 with carcinoid heart disease and all 15 without carcinoid heart disease had sinus rhythm. The P-R interval was normal (0.20 second or less) in 18 of 19 subjects with carcinoid heart disease and in 14 of 15 subjects without carcinoid heart disease. The width of the QRS complex was normal (0.12 second or less) in all subjects, irrespective of whether or not they had carcinoid heart disease. Thus, other than the higher frequency of low voltage in the subjects with carcinoid heart disease, electrocardiography was not helpful in distinguishing those subjects with carcinoid heart disease from those without carcinoid heart disease.

Although not performed in any of our 36 subjects, echocardiography, particularly cross-sectional, is helpful in diagnosing carcinoid heart disease. Two reports have described echocardiographic features in relatively large groups of patients with carcinoid heart disease. Callahan and associates [7] described retrospectively echocardiographic features in 20 patients with the carcinoid syndrome. By physical examination, 15 patients had a diagnosis of carcinoid heart disease and the other five did not. Both M-mode and cross-sectional examinations in the latter five patients disclosed no abnormal findings. Of the 15 patients with auscultatory evidence of carcinoid heart disease, five had normal M-mode and cross-sectional echocardiographic findings. The other 10, all of whom had tricuspid regurgitation by physical examination, had dilated right ventricular cavities, abnormal motion of the ventricular septum, and of the nine in whom the tricuspid valve leaflets were visualized by cross-sectional echocardiography, strikingly abnormal tricuspid leaflets (thickened and retracted with fixed orifice). The pulmonic valve cusps were not visualized in any patient by M-mode echocardiography, but in the four in whom they were visualized by cross-sectional echocardiography, the pulmonic valve cusps were abnormal in each.

Howard and associates [8] prospectively examined by cross-sectional echocardiography 14 patients with the carcinoid syndrome, and eight had definite abnormalities of one or both right-sided cardiac valves. Clinically, five had auscultatory evidence of tricuspid regurgitation and all five had diffusely thickened and retracted tricuspid valve leaflets; the other nine patients had normal tricuspid valves by echocardiography. Four patients by auscultation had evidence of pulmonic stenosis with or without pulmonic regurgitation. The pulmonic valve cusps were visualized by echocardiography in seven patients: two had retracted pulmonic cusps with decreased systolic motion (one of whom had pulmonic stenosis by auscultation) and five had normal cusps (none of whom had auscultatory evidence of pulmonic stenosis).

Although none of our 21 subjects with carcinoid heart disease had an operative procedure performed on either the tricuspid or pulmonic valve or both, right-sided cardiac valve excision with or without valve replacement or valve commissurotomy or annuloplasty has been carried out in at least 15 patients [2–5,9–20]. The findings in these patients are summarized in **Table V.** At operation, the patients ranged in age from 26 to 64 years (mean 46); three were women and six were men. The interval from onset of symptoms and signs of congestive heart failure to cardiac valve operation ranged from three to 60 months (mean 14) and the interval from onset of symptoms of the carcinoid syndrome to cardiac valve operation ranged from 0.5 to 33 years (mean 10). Preoperatively, at least 12 of the 15 patients had hemodynamic evidence of tricuspid valve stenosis with mean diastolic pressure gradients between right atrium and right ventricle ranging from 4 to 24 mm Hg (mean 9). Of 15 patients, 14 had tricuspid regurgitation, which was graded as severe at angiography in at least seven patients. Pullback pressures between pulmonary artery and right ventricle were recorded in 14 patients, 12 of whom had peak systolic pressure gradients ranging from 3 to 50 mm Hg (average 29). The presence or absence of pulmonic regurgitation as determined by pulmonary angiography was noted in 12 patients, and only two apparently had regurgitation into the right ventricle during ventricular diastole. Of the 15 patients, 14 had tricuspid valve procedures: replacement in 13 and anuloplasty in one; 10 patients had pulmonic valve procedures: commissurotomy in six, replacement in three, and excision only in one. Of the 15 patients, eight had died at the time of the report: four within two months of operation, and one each four, eight, 24, and 72 months after operation. The other seven patients were alive 4 to 132 months (median 23) after operation.

REFERENCES

1. Roberts WC, Sjoerdsma A: The cardiac disease associated with the carcinoid syndrome (carcinoid heart disease). Am J Med 1964; 36: 5–34.

2. Wright PW, Mulder DG: Carcinoid heart disease. Report of a case treated by open heart surgery. Am J Cardiol 1963; 12: 864–868.

3. Lund HG, Cleveland RJ, Greenberg LH, Lippmann M, Dollinger MR: Tricuspid valve replacement in carcinoid heart disease. West J Med 1974; 120: 412–415.

4. Honey M, Paneth M. Carcinoid heart disease: successful tricuspid valve replacement. Thorax 1975; 30: 464–469.

5. Schoen FJ, Hausner RJ, Howell JF, Beazley HL, Titus JL: Porcine heterograft valve replacement in carcinoid heart disease. J Thorac Cardiovasc Surg 1981; 81: 100–105.

6. Ferrans VJ, Roberts WC: The carcinoid endocardial plaque. An ultrastructural study. Hum Pathol 1976; 7: 387–409.

7. Callahan JA, Wroblewski EM, Reeder GS, Edwards WD, Seward JB, Tajik AJ: Echocardiographic features of carcinoid heart disease. Am J Cardiol 1982; 50: 762–768.

8. Howard RJ, Drobac M, Rider WD, et al: Carcinoid heart disease: diagnosis by two-dimensional echocardiography, Circulation 1982; 66: 1059–1065.

9. Aroesty JM, DeWeese JA, Hoffman MJ, Yu PN: Carcinoid heart disease. Successful repair of the valvular lesions under cardiopulmonary bypass. Circulation 1966; 34: 105–110.

10. Carpena C, Kay JG, Mendex AM, Redington JV, Zubiate P, Zucker R: Carcinoid heart disease. Surgery for tricuspid and pulmonary valve lesions. Am J Cardiol 1973; 32: 229–233.

11. Garcia E, Taboada CF, Hall RJ, Cooley DA: Carcinoid heart disease: cardiac surgery for intractable heart failure. Cardiovasc Dis Bull Texas Heart Institute 1974; 1: 408–412.

12. McGuire MR, Pugh DM, Dunn MI: Carcinoid heart disease. Restrictive cardiomyopathy as a late complication. J Kans Med Soc 1978; 79: 661–665.

13. Okada RD, Ewy GA, Copeland JG: Echocardiography and surgery in tricuspid and pulmonary valve stenosis due to carcinoid syndrome. Cardiovasc Med 1979; 4: 871–881.

14. Nielsen MS, Manners JM: Valve replacement in carcinoid syndrome. Anaesthesia 1979; 34: 494–499.

15. Sworn MJ, Edlin GP, McGill GA, Mousley JS, Monro JL: Tricuspid valve replacement in carcinoid syndrome due to ovarian primary. Br Med J 1980; 280: 85–86.

16. Hendel N, Leckie B, Richards J: Carcinoid heart disease: eight-year survival following tricuspid valve replacement and pulmonary valvotomy. Ann Thorac Surg 1980; 30: 391–395.

17. Gutierrez FR, McKnight RC, Jaffe AS, Ludbrook PA, Biello D, Weldon CS: Double porcine valve replacement in carcinoid heart disease. Chest 1982; 81: 101–103.

18. Come PC, Come SE, Hawley CR, Gwon N, Riley MF: Echocardiographic manifestations of carcinoid heart disease. J Clin Ultrasound 1982; 10: 233–237.

19. Miller BR, Vohr FH, Christian FV, Singh AK: Cardiac valvular replacement in carcinoid heart disease. Am J Med 1983; 75: 896–898.

20. Kay JH: Eleven-year follow-up after tricuspid valve replacement and pulmonic valvulotomy in the carcinoid syndrome (letter). Am J Cardiol 1984; 53: 651.

QRS Voltage Measurements in Autopsied Men Free of Cardiopulmonary Disease: A Basis for Evaluating Total QRS Voltage as an Index of Left Ventricular Hypertrophy

HARRELL ODOM II, MD, J. LYNN DAVIS, MD, HA DINH, MD, BONNIE J. BAKER, MD, WILLIAM C. ROBERTS, MD, and MARVIN L. MURPHY, MD

Use of total 12-lead QRS electrocardiographic voltage as a criterion for left ventricular (LV) hypertrophy has been of recent interest. Although upper and lower limits of QRS voltage for individual electrocardiographic leads have been reported in clinically healthy men and women, the upper limit of total 12-lead QRS voltage has not been established in adults free of cardiopulmonary disease by clinical and necropsy criteria. Therefore, the total QRS voltage from all 12 electrocardiographic leads was determined in 30 autopsied men known to be free of cardiopulmonary disease by clinical assessment and by a special cardiac examination using postmortem coronary angiography and chamber partition determination of LV weight. Gross heart weight, LV weight and total QRS voltage are reported. Comparisons were made between disease-free patients and previously reported patients with aortic valve stenosis, aortic regurgitation and cardiac amyloidosis with respect to total QRS voltage and gross heart weight. Total QRS voltage and gross heart weight were significantly greater in patients with severe aortic stenosis (mean 245 mm) and severe aortic regurgitation (mean 274 mm) than in our patients (mean 127 mm). Total QRS voltage was significantly less, whereas gross heart weight was significantly greater in patients with cardiac amyloidosis (mean 101 mm) than in our normal subjects (mean 127 mm). These data provide a basis for evaluating the total 12-lead QRS voltage as a criterion for LV hypertrophy.

(Am J Cardiol 1986;58:801–804)

The total QRS voltage from all 12 electrocardiographic leads has been evaluated in several recent autopsy studies as a criterion for determining the presence of left ventricular (LV) hypertrophy in a variety of disease states.[1-3] The sum of the voltage from 1 limb lead (R wave in lead aVL) and 1 precordial lead (S wave in lead V_3) was found to be a useful predictor of LV hypertrophy in a study using echocardiographically determined LV mass.[4] Simonson[5] reported the upper and lower limits of QRS voltage for each of the 12 electrocardiographic leads in clinically healthy men and women aged 20 to 59 years. The upper limit of total QRS voltage has not been established in adults free of cardiopulmonary disease by clinical and necropsy criteria. This study describes the total QRS voltage from all 12 electrocardiographic leads in autopsied men free of cardiopulmonary disease. These normal values provide a basis for evaluating the use of the total QRS voltage as a criterion of LV hypertrophy.

From the Veterans Administration Medical Center and the Department of Medicine, University of Arkansas for Medical Sciences, Little Rock, Arkansas, and the Pathology Branch, National Heart, Lung, and Blood Institute, National Institutes of Health, Bethesda, Maryland. This study was supported in part by Little Rock Veterans Administration Medical Center Grant 4737-009. Manuscript received March 20, 1986; revised manuscript received April 24, 1986, accepted May 5, 1986.

Address for reprints: Marvin L. Murphy, MD, John L. McClellan Memorial Veterans Hospital (111B), 4300 West 7th Street, Little Rock, Arkansas 72205.

Methods

From 1966 through 1979, 3,202 autopsies were performed at the Little Rock Veterans' Administration Medical Center. Of these, 513 (16%) had a special cardiac examination including a postmortem coronary angiogram, chamber partition determination of LV

TABLE I Total Electrocardiographic QRS Voltage and Heart Weights in Autopsied Men Older Than 40 Years Free of Cardiopulmonary Disease

Pt	Age (yr)	QRS Voltage (mm)												Total QRS Voltage	R_{aVL} + S_{V3}*	LV Weight (g)	Heart Weight (g)
		I	II	III	aVR	aVL	aVF	V_1	V_2	V_3	V_4	V_5	V_6				
1	69	6	5	3	6	4	2	9	6	6	11	10	14	80	11	112	405
2	44	4	4	4	4	3	3	3	9	13	15	14	8	84	5	113	352
3	46	4	9	5	7	1	6	7	12	9	8	9	9	86	6	120	288
4	55	5	7	2	6	3	4	6	9	9	12	13	12	88	7	162	420
5	50	0	9	8	3	4	9	4	16	13	12	8	7	94	11	129	445
6	63	4	3	1	4	2	1	6	13	21	20	13	7	95	13	132	345
7	74	4	5	5	4	3	4	5	16	17	19	11	8	101	11	135	374
8	74	3	8	5	6	2	7	5	9	13	19	15	11	105	8	168	523
9	67	6	5	7	5	6	4	8	14	13	17	16	9	107	14	176	500
10	74	6	5	7	4	7	6	9	12	18	22	10	4	108	13	137	362
11	55	5	8	9	6	7	8	8	23	16	9	8	8	115	12	145	468
12	46	5	5	5	5	6	4	9	26	21	18	9	6	120	16	143	359
13	44	8	4	8	5	9	5	3	14	16	21	17	9	120	16	113	310
14	41	6	10	5	8	1	9	14	13	11	17	15	12	122	5	135	355
15	57	5	7	4	5	4	6	9	20	23	19	14	9	123	15	103	318
16	61	2	5	6	2	3	5	9	26	22	27	13	5	125	20	134	350
17	64	5	13	6	8	2	10	8	10	17	19	15	14	128	15	153	364
18	48	11	9	2	10	6	4	10	22	13	18	14	13	131	13	128	380
19	52	13	7	10	10	12	4	4	15	18	15	14	10	132	14	160	412
20	64	2	13	10	6	4	13	6	15	20	19	17	15	138	7	134	438
21	48	6	9	2	9	4	6	20	21	21	26	14	9	146	14	134	392
22	62	8	7	9	7	8	6	9	12	30	29	15	8	149	13	135	355
23	54	7	7	5	7	6	4	17	25	35	20	11	6	149	14	140	362
24	56	4	9	7	8	3	8	13	18	22	29	20	11	150	16	117	412
25	52	6	10	5	8	3	5	13	19	26	28	21	14	159	9	122	350
26	47	7	7	8	6	6	6	13	31	34	23	11	7	159	23	138	352
27	50	10	14	5	11	7	10	10	12	19	26	22	16	163	11	102	450
28	71	8	11	4	10	3	7	13	17	27	27	21	17	166	10	131	431
29	45	7	15	8	12	3	11	23	34	27	18	12	9	178	1	153	451
30	56	11	8	9	10	9	6	12	22	25	28	25	22	185	20	146	456
Mean	56	6	8	6	7	5	6	10	17	19	20	14	10	127	12	135	393
±SD	±10	±3	±3	±3	±2	±3	±3	±5	±7	±7	±6	±4	±4	±29	±5	±18	±57

* See reference 4.

LV = left ventricular; SD = standard deviation.

weight, and gross and microscopic examination as previously described.[6] Of the 513 patients, 48 (9%) were classified as being free of cardiopulmonary disease by previously described criteria.[6] Of these patients, 30 had electrocardiograms available for determining the total QRS voltage from all 12 leads. The last technically satisfactory electrocardiogram for each patient was selected for interpretation and was considered as the index tracing. The interval from the index tracing until death ranged from 0 to 11 weeks (average 2.8). Additional electrocardiograms obtained at least 12 months before the index tracing were evaluated in 8 patients and compared to the index tracing with respect to total QRS voltage.

The amplitude of the QRS complexes was measured from the peak of the R wave to the dip of the S or Q wave, whichever was greater, according to the method of Siegel and Roberts.[3] All patients were men aged 41 to 74 years (mean ± standard deviation 56 ± 10).

Comparisons of total QRS voltage measurements and gross heart weights were made between our patients free of cardiopulmonary disease and groups of men of comparable age with aortic valve stenosis, aortic regurgitation, and cardiac amyloidosis previously reported by Siegel and Roberts,[3] Roberts and Waller,[1] and Roberts and Day.[2] The sum of the R wave in lead aVL and the S wave in lead V_3 was determined to assess specificity as a criterion for LV hypertrophy.[4] Statistical analysis was performed using the 2-tailed Student t test. Significance was defined by a p value <0.05. The usual definitions of statistical terms were used.[7]

Results

Autopsy and electrocardiographic data: The values for each patient are presented in Table I. For these 30 normal patients, gross heart weight ranged from 288 to 523 g (mean 393 ± 57) and LV weight ranged from 102 to 176 g (mean 135 ± 18). Total QRS voltage averaged 127 ± 29 mm (range 80 to 185). The sum of the R wave in lead aVL and the S wave in lead V_3 averaged 12 ± 5 mm (range 1 to 23).

In 8 patients, additional electrocardiograms performed an average of 260 weeks (range 118 to 590) before the index tracing were available for comparison of total QRS voltage. In these 8 patients total QRS voltage averaged 116 ± 32 mm (range 88 to 185) in the index tracing and 120 ± 26 mm (range 70 to 146) in serial tracings (p >0.1).

TABLE II Comparison of 30 Male Patients Free of Cardiopulmonary Disease to Male Patients with Aortic Stenosis, Aortic Regurgitation and Cardiac Amyloidosis

	Present Study	Aortic Stenosis[3]	Aortic Regurgitation[2]	Cardiac Amyloidosis[1]
No. of pts	30	30	12	11
Age (yr)	56 ± 10	52 ± 5	52 ± 6	58 ± 9
Heart weight (g)	393 ± 57	630 ± 14*	745 ± 132*	563 ± 128*
Total QRS voltage (mm)	127 ± 29	245 ± 56*	274 ± 87*	101 ± 40†

* p < 0.001; † p < 0.05 compared with patients in present study.

Comparison: A comparison is summarized in Table II. There was no significant difference in age between the patients in our study and the men (older than 40 years) with aortic valve stenosis, pure aortic regurgitation and fatal cardiac amyloidosis studied by Siegel and Roberts,[3] Roberts and Day,[2] and Roberts and Waller.[1]

Gross heart weights were 630 ± 114 g for our 30 patients with severe aortic valve stenosis, 745 ± 132 g for 12 patients with severe aortic regurgitation, and 563 ± 128 g for 11 patients with cardiac amyloidosis. These are significantly greater (p <0.001) than the average gross heart weight of 393 ± 57 g in our disease-free patients.

Total QRS voltage from 12 electrocardiographic leads was significantly greater (p <0.001) in patients with aortic stenosis (245 ± 56 mm) and aortic regurgitation (274 ± 87 mm) than in our patients (127 ± 29 mm). A significantly lower total QRS voltage (p <0.05) was found in patients with cardiac amyloidosis (101 ± 40 mm) than in our patients.

Using 175 mm as the upper limit of normal for total QRS voltage as proposed by Roberts and Day,[2] 2 of our 30 patients would have been classified as having LV hypertrophy. This yields a specificity of 93%. LV weights in these 2 patients were 146 and 153 g. These values are clearly within the normal range for LV weight.[6] Casale et al[4] proposed that where the sum of the R wave in lead aVL and the S wave in lead V_3 exceeds 35 mm, LV hypertrophy is suggested. None of our 30 patients would have been designated as having LV hypertrophy by this criterion. This results in a specificity of 100%.

Discussion

Our study reports the total QRS voltage in all 12 electrocardiographic leads in autopsied men free of cardiopulmonary disease. These normal values provide a basis for evaluating the total QRS voltage as a criterion for LV hypertrophy. Several recent studies have examined the relation between QRS voltage and the presence of LV hypertrophy in a variety of disease states.[1-3] Siegel and Roberts[2] observed that total QRS voltage from all 12 electrocardiographic leads is predictive of the peak systolic transaortic pressure gradient and the degree of LV hypertrophy in patients with severe aortic valve stenosis who come to autopsy. Furthermore, Siegel and Roberts[3] found the total QRS voltage in 50 patients with severe aortic valve stenosis and in 30 patients with severe pure aortic regurgitation

to be comparable. Patients with aortic valve stenosis and those with pure aortic regurgitation had mean gross heart weights 60% and 90% greater than those in our patients, respectively. Total QRS voltage was 93% greater in patients with aortic valve stenosis and 116% greater in patients with pure aortic regurgitation than in our disease-free group. In patients with cardiac amyloidosis, low total QRS voltage is the usual finding despite an increased heart weight.[1,8] In the patients with cardiac amyloidosis studied by Roberts and Waller,[1] total QRS voltage was 20% less than the mean for our patients, whereas mean gross heart weight was 43% greater.

Factors other than cardiac muscle mass have been shown to affect the magnitude and orientation of QRS voltage. Geometric effects, cardiac volume (size and shape), lung conductivity, body habitus and surface muscle mass influence QRS voltage.[9-12] Murphy et al[13] showed that the sensitivity of traditional and modified voltage criteria for LV hypertrophy vary according to the nature of underlying cardiac disease. Among 13 of 14 voltage criteria for LV hypertrophy, sensitivity was greatest in patients with valvular and hypertensive heart diseases. These same voltage criteria failed to diagnose LV hypertrophy in 85 to 90% of patients with coronary artery disease. Significantly lower total QRS voltage has been reported in patients with aortic valve stenosis and concomitant significant coronary artery disease compared to patients with aortic valve stenosis alone.[3] In patients with severe pure aortic regurgitation, total QRS voltage is elevated to the same degree in the presence or absence of underlying coronary artery disease.[2] Because of these observations multiple-criteria methods for the diagnosis of LV hypertrophy have been recommended for application to populations with multiple cardiac diseases.[13] To our knowledge, total QRS voltage as a criterion for LV hypertrophy has not been systematically applied to other diagnostic categories of cardiac disease.

It has been suggested that QRS voltage measurements from electrocardiograms performed in the end stages of chronic disease or in acute illness may not be representative of the normal healthy state.[14-16] In comparing serial tracings up to an average of 260 weeks before the index tracing, no significant difference in total QRS voltage was noted in our patients. Therefore, we believe that the QRS voltage measurements in our patients are representative of patients free of cardiopulmonary disease. These results help to validate our data.

The data used to generate normal values for electrocardiographic measurements have routinely been acquired from a clinically healthy, free-living population.[17-20] Only recently have electrocardiograms from hospitalized patients, shown clinically and at autopsy to be free of cardiopulmonary disease, been evaluated to develop normal values.[6] With the reporting of new electrocardiographic criteria for LV hypertrophy that rely on voltage, a basis of normal values is needed. This study is the first to provide values for total QRS voltage from all 12 electrocardiographic leads in autopsied men free of cardiopulmonary disease.

References

1. Roberts WC, Waller BF. *Cardiac amyloidosis causing cardiac dysfunction: analysis of 54 necropsy patients. Am J Cardiol 1983;52:137-146.*
2. Roberts WC, Day PJ. *Electrocardiographic observations in clinically isolated, pure, chronic, severe aortic regurgitation: analysis of 30 necropsy patients aged 19 to 65 years. Am J Cardiol 1985;55:432-438.*
3. Siegel RJ, Roberts WC. *Electrocardiographic observations in severe aortic valve stenosis: correlative necropsy study to clinical, hemodynamic, and ECG variables demonstrating relation of 12-lead QRS amplitude to peak systolic transaortic pressure gradient. Am Heart J 1982;103:210-221.*
4. Casale PN, Devereux RB, Kligfield P, Eisenberg RR, Miller DH, Chaudhary BS, Phillips MC. *Electrocardiographic detection of left ventricular hypertrophy: development and prospective validation of improved criteria. JACC 1985;6:571-580.*
5. Simonson E. *Differentiation Between Normal and Abnormal in Electrocardiography. St. Louis: CV Mosby, 1961:136.*
6. Murphy ML, Thenabadu PN, Blue LR, Meade J, deSoyza N, Doherty JE. *Descriptive characteristics of the electrocardiogram from autopsied men free of cardiopulmonary disease—a basis for evaluating criteria for ventricular hypertrophy. Am J Cardiol 1983;52:1275-1280.*
7. Griner PF, Mayewski RJ, Mushlin AL, Greenland P. *Selection and interpretation of diagnostic tests and procedures. Ann Intern Med 1981;94:553-600.*
8. Carroll JD, Gaasch WH, McAdam KPWJ. *Amyloid cardiomyopathy characterization by a distinctive voltage/mass relation. Am J Cardiol 1982;49:9-13.*
9. Kossman CE, Burchell HB, Pruitt R, Scott RC. *The electrocardiogram in ventricular hypertrophy and bundle-branch block. Circulation 1962;26:1337-1351.*
10. Rudy Y, Wood R, Plonsey R, Liebman J. *The effect of high lung conductivity on electrocardiographic potentials: results from human subjects undergoing bronchopulmonary lavage. Circulation 1982;65:440-445.*
11. Rudy Y, Plonsey R. *A comparison of volume conductor and source geometry effects on body surface and epicardial potentials. Circ Res 1980;46:283-291.*
12. Rudy Y, Plonsey R. *Comments on the effect of variations in the size of the heart on magnitude of ECG potentials. J Electrocardiol 1980;13:79-82.*
13. Murphy ML, Thenabadu PN, de Soyza N, Meade J, Doherty JE, Baker BJ. *Sensitivity of electrocardiographic criteria for left ventricular hypertrophy according to type of cardiac disease. Am J Cardiol 1985;55:545-549.*
14. Simonson E, Henschel A, Keys A. *The electrocardiograms of men in semistarvation and subsequent rehabilitation. Am Heart J 1948;35:584-602.*
15. Lopes-Cardozo E, Eggink P. *Circulation failure in hunger oedema. Can Med Assoc J 1946;54:145-147.*
16. Bove KE, Rowlands DT, Scott RC. *Observations on the assessment of cardiac hypertrophy utilizing a chamber partition technique. Circulation 1966;33:558-568.*
17. Ferrer MI. *Electrocardiographic Notebook. New York: Futura Publishing, 1973:101.*
18. The Criteria Committee of the New York Heart Association. *Nomenclature and Criteria for Diagnosis of Diseases of the Heart and Great Vessels. 6th ed. Boston; Little, Brown, 1964:437.*
19. Cooksey JD, Dunn M, Massie E. *Clinical Vectorcardiography and Electrocardiography. 2nd ed, Chicago: Yearbook Medical Publishers, 1977:81.*
20. Winsor T, ed. *Electrocardiographic Text Book. Vol I. Dallas: American Heart Association, 1956: appendix pages 144-160.*

Idiopathic Dilated Cardiomyopathy: Analysis of 152 Necropsy Patients

WILLIAM C. ROBERTS, MD, ROBERT J. SIEGEL, MD,
and BRUCE M. McMANUS, MD, PhD

Certain clinical and cardiac necropsy findings are described in 152 patients aged 16 to 78 years (mean 45) with idiopathic dilated cardiomyopathy: 109 (72%) were men and 43 (28%) were women. Compared with the women, the men had a significantly (p <0.05) shorter mean duration of chronic congestive heart failure (CHF) (43 vs 69 months), a higher percentage of habitual alcoholism (40 vs 24%) and a higher mean heart weight (632 vs 551 g). The male to female ratio among the 58 known alcoholics was 7.3:1 and among the 70 known nonalcoholics, 1.5:1 (p <0.05). The mean duration of clinical evidence of CHF was similar among the known alcoholics and the known nonalcoholics (each 50 months). Of the 152 patients, 148 (97%) had clinical evidence of chronic CHF; in 114 patients it was the initial manifestation of idiopathic dilated cardiomyopathy, and in most it became intractable and caused death. The interval from onset of chronic CHF to death (known in 120 patients) ranged from 1 to 264 months (mean 54). Comparison of the 27 patients surviving >72 months after onset of chronic CHF to the 64 patients surviving ≤36 months disclosed a significantly higher frequency in the longer survival group of older patients, of women, of habitual alcoholics, of patients with chest pain syndromes, diabetes mellitus, pulmonary emboli, of patients treated with warfarin and of patients with larger hearts at necropsy. Each of the 4 patients without chronic CHF died suddenly and sudden death was the initial manifestation of idiopathic dilated cardiomyopathy in them.

An additional 33 patients also died suddenly, but each of them previously had had chronic CHF. Of the 79 patients (of the 131 for whom information was available) with either pulmonary or systemic emboli or both, 67 (85%) had either right- or left-sided thrombi or mural endocardial plaques or both, whereas of the 52 patients without emboli, 36 (69%) had intracardiac thrombi or plaques (p <0.05). Electrocardiograms in the last 6 months of life in 101 patients disclosed atrial fibrillation in 25; complete left (41 patients) or right (6 patients) bundle branch block or indeterminate intraventricular conduction delay (4 patients) in 51 patients; QRS voltage indicative of ventricular hypertrophy in 44 patients (left ventricular in 39 patients). The patients with left bundle branch block compared with those without had a significantly longer duration of CHF, (83 vs 43 months), larger mean heart weights (628 vs 590 g) and a higher frequency of grossly visible scars (44 vs 13%). The total 12-lead QRS amplitude in 35 men ranged from 74 to 250 mm (mean 147) (10 mm = 1 mV) and in the 14 women from 75 to 243 mm (mean 167). The hearts at necropsy in the women ranged from 360 to 860 g (mean 551) and in the men from 400 to 940 g (mean 632) (p <0.05). Grossly visible left ventricular scars were observed in 22 (14%) patients. Histologic examination (96 patients) of sections of the ventricular myocardium disclosed interstitial or replacement fibrosis in 55 patients (57%), and inflammatory cell infiltrates in 5 patients.

(Am J Cardiol 1987;60:1340–1355)

I diopathic dilated cardiomyopathy (IDC) is a well-recognized condition both clinically and morphologically. It is characterized by dilatation of both ventricular cavities and manifested clinically by chronic congestive heart failure (CHF), which usually becomes intractable and eventually fatal. Despite the relative frequency of this condition, few studies focusing on a large number of necropsy patients have been reported.

Herein, we describe certain clinical and morphologic features in 152 necropsy patients fulfilling a rigorous definition of IDC.

Patients Studied

Criteria for inclusion: All 152 patients were older than 15 years of age, all had dilated right and left ventricular cavities and all had hearts of increased weight (>350 g in women and >400 g in men). None had narrowing of any of the epicardial coronary arteries of >75% in cross-sectional area, none had a significant congenital cardiac anomaly, none had an anatomically abnormal cardiac valve (except for minimal focal thickening of the margins of the anterior mitral leaflet), none had a defect in the atrial or ventricular septum other than possibly a valvular competent patent foramen ovale, none had an infiltrative myocardial disease (such as amyloid, sarcoid, iron, calcium or glycogen), none had a systemic disease other than possibly adult-onset diabetes mellitus, none had a neurologic disease, none had extensive cystic or interstitial pulmonary parenchymal disease and none had a major grossly visible abnormality of the pericardium. During the last 3 months of life, the systemic arterial systolic pressure was <140 mm Hg and the systemic arterial diastolic pressure was <90 mm Hg. Additionally, none had clinical evidence in the past of hypertrophic cardiomyopathy and none had other family members who had hypertrophic cardiomyopathy. Patients with complete heart block from birth were excluded, and patients who had received a drug known to be capable of causing a dilated cardiomyopathy, such as doxorubicin, were excluded. Patients with a history of habitual alcoholism were included and considered to have idiopathic dilated cardiomyopathy.

From the Pathology Branch, National Heart, Lung, and Blood Institute, National Institutes of Health, Bethesda, Maryland. Manuscript received July 22, 1987, revised manuscript received and accepted August 18, 1987.

Address for reprints: William C. Roberts, MD, Building 10, Room 2N-258, National Institutes of Health, Bethesda, Maryland 20892.

Dr. Siegel's present address is Division of Cardiology, Department of Medicine, Cedars-Sinai Medical Center, Los Angeles, California.

Dr. McManus's present address is Cardiovascular Registry, Department of Pathology and Microbiology, University of Nebraska Medical Center, Omaha, Nebraska.

Selection of cases: All hearts and clinical and morphologic records of cases classified as IDC in the files of the Pathology Branch, National Heart, Lung, and Blood Institute, were reviewed. Of nearly 200 cases so classified, nearly 50 were eliminated from this study because they did not fulfill the aforementioned clinical and morphologic criteria. A total of 152 patients fulfilled the criteria and form the basis of this report. The clinical and necropsy records were reviewed in all 152 patients. Detailed data on the electrocardiograms recorded in the last 6 months of life were available in 101 of the 152 patients, and in 55 the electrocardiograms themselves were reexamined. All 152 hearts were examined initially by 1 of us (WCR) and most were examined later by RJS and BMM. All patients were studied at necropsy from 1959 through April 1981. The patients were studied clinically at 14 different hospitals, mainly those located in the Washington, DC, area, and the hearts were subsequently brought to one of us (WCR) for examination. In addition to the gross examination of each heart, at least 2 histologic sections of left ventricular wall extending from endocardium to epicardium and measuring ≥2 cm in circumferential length were examined in 96 of the 152 cases. A least 1 full-thickness histologic section of ventricular septum and right ventricular free wall also was examined in 80 and 88 of these 96 patients, respectively.

Statistics: Comparisons of all parametric data were made using the 2-tailed t test for independent samples when comparisons between 2 groups were made, and using a 1-way analysis of variance when comparisons among ≥3 groups were made. The level of significance was 0.05. Comparisons of nonparametric data were made using the chi-square method with a level of significance of 0.05. Correlations were tested using Spearman's rho and linear regression coefficients and calculated when deemed useful.

Clinical Findings

Age, race, sex and duration of congestive heart failure: The 152 patients ranged in age from 16 to 78

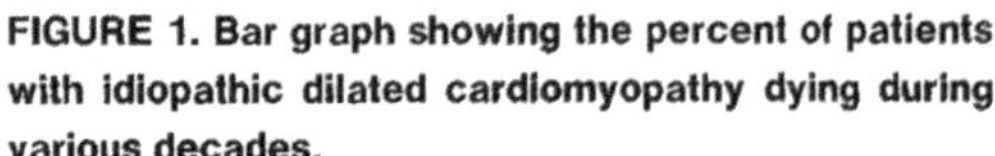

FIGURE 1. Bar graph showing the percent of patients with idiopathic dilated cardiomyopathy dying during various decades.

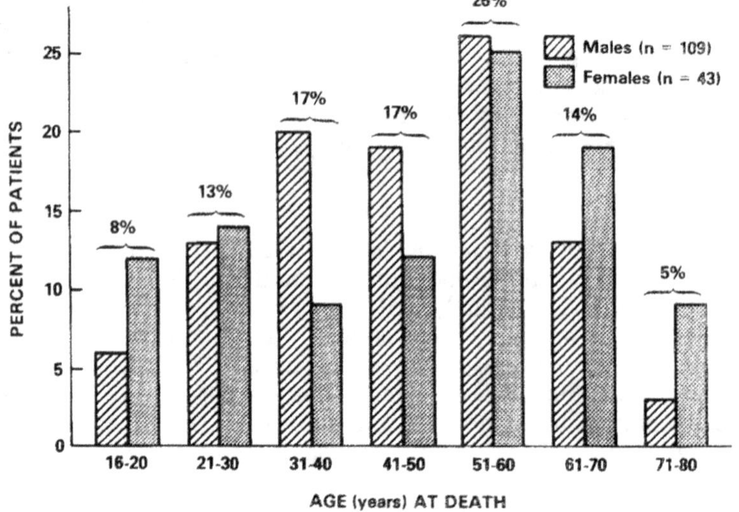

TABLE I   Certain Clinical and Necropsy Characteristics of 152 Patients with Idiopathic Dilated Cardiomyopathy and Comparisons Between 109 Men and 43 Women

	Total (n = 152)	Men (n = 109)	Women (n = 43)	p Value
Age (yr) (mean)	16–78 (45)	16–73 (45)	16–78 (49)	NS
Black:white	90:47 (1.9:1)	63:36 (1.8:1)	27:11 (2.5:1)	NS
Duration (mo) CHF	0–240 (54)	6–204 (43)	1–240 (69)	<0.05
Pulmonary edema	34/86 (40%)	21/61 (34%)	13/25 (52%)	NS
Angina pectoris	15/105 (14%)	11/75 (15%)	4/30 (13%)	NS
Nonanginal chest pain	40/114 (35%)	29/82 (35%)	11/32 (34%)	NS
"AMI" (history)	25/113 (22%)	17/80 (21%)	8/33 (24%)	NS
Alcoholism	49/136 (36%)	40/99 (40%)	9/37 (24%)	NS
Emboli				
Pulmonary, clinical	49/126 (39%)	31/89 (35%)	18/37 (49%)	NS
Pulmonary, necropsy	39/101 (39%)	29/72 (40%)	10/29 (34%)	NS
Systemic, clinical	24/122 (20%)	20/88 (23%)	4/34 (12%)	NS
Pulmonary, necropsy	23/90 (26%)	19/65 (29%)	4/25 (16%)	NS
Mode of death				
Chronic CHF	81/139 (58%)	55/98 (56%)	26/41 (63%)	NS
Sudden	38/139 (27%)	28/98 (29%)	10/41 (24%)	NS
Pulmonary embolus	12/139 (9%)	8/98 (8%)	4/41 (10%)	NS
Other	8/139 (6%)	7/98 (7%)	1/41 (2%)	NS
Heart weight (g)	400–940 (605)	400–940 (632)	360–860 (551)	<0.05
Intracavitary thrombi (T) only	42/148 (28%)	30/105 (29%)	12/43 (28%)	NS
Endocardial plaques (P) only	32/148 (22%)	22/105 (21%)	10/43 (23%)	NS
Both T and P	37/148 (25%)	28/105 (27%)	9/43 (21%)	NS
Transmural LV scars (gross)	9/148 (6%)	9/105 (9%)	5/43 (12%)	NS
LV replacement fibrosis (microscopic only)	71/96 (73%)	50/74 (68%)	21/22 (95%)	<0.05

AMI = acute myocardial infarction; CHF = chronic congestive heart failure; LV = left ventricular; NS = not significant (p >0.05); SD = sudden death.

years (mean 45) [Figure 1]. Of the 137 in whom race was known, 90 (66%) were black and 47 (34%) were white. Of the 152 patients, 109 (72%) were men and 43 (28%) were women. Comparison of various clinical and morphologic findings between the men and women is summarized in Table I. Of the 16 factors analyzed, 3 were significantly (p <0.05) different between the 2 groups. Compared with women, men had a shorter mean duration of chronic CHF (43 vs 69 months), a higher percentage of habitual alcoholism (40 vs 24%) and a higher mean heart weight (632 vs 551 g).

Relation to pregnancy: Of the 43 women, the relation of onset of symptoms of chronic CHF to pregnancy was known in 39. In 13 (33%) of them, symptoms of CHF appeared either during pregnancy (2 patients) or within 12 months after delivery (11 patients). In 7 of the latter 11 patients, the onset of symptoms of cardiac dysfunction was within 3 months of delivery. Comparison of findings in the 13 women with onset of CHF in the peripartum period to those in 26 women in whom the onset of CHF was known not to be related to pregnancy disclosed only 1 statistically significant factor (Table II): the mean age of the peripartum patients was younger (p <0.001) than that of the nonperipartum patients.

Habitual alcoholism: Information regarding habitual intake of alcohol was available in 128 of the 152 patients. At least 58 (45%) of the 128 patients were considered by their physicians to be "alcoholic." Comparison of 15 observations in the 58 known habitual alcoholics with those in the 70 nonalcoholic cases disclosed several factors to be significantly different (Table III). The male to female ratio among the alcoholics was 7.3:1 and in the nonalcoholics, 1.5:1 (p <0.05). The mean duration of symptoms of CHF was the same (50 months); the mean heart weight (631 vs 593 g) was significantly (p <0.05) greater in the alcoholics compared with the nonalcoholics, a reflection of the greater proportion of men in the alcoholic group.

Diabetes mellitus: Information regarding the presence or absence of diabetes mellitus was available in 110 of the 152 patients. Of that number, 8 patients (7%) (4 men, 4 women) had known diabetes mellitus beginning after age 35. Their ages at death ranged from 37 to 71 years (mean 55) and their ages at onset of diabetes from 36 to 64 years (mean 51). Two patients were treated with insulin and 4 with hypoglycemic agents; the type of diabetic treatment received in the other 2 patients is uncertain. Two of the 8 patients were habitual alcoholics. The duration of chronic CHF in the 8 patients ranged from 24 to 204 months (mean 105). At necropsy, 2 of the 8 patients had grossly visible left ventricular scars, and on histologic examination, none had abnormalities of the intramural coronary arteries.

Familial cardiomyopathy: At least 1 other family member had a similar fatal cardiac condition in 9 (6%) of the 152 patients. Of these 9 patients, at least 20 family members were affected by a similar cardiac condition, and all of the 20 affected relatives died before age 50 years, most before age 40 years. The 9 patients with familial dilated cardiomyopathy ranged in age from 17 to 58 years (mean 37); 7 were men and 2 were women. Only 2 were habitual alcoholics. The duration of the chronic CHF in 8 of the 9 patients ranged from 3 to 72 months (mean 46); the ninth patient had evidence of CHF for only 10 days. Six of the 9 patients died from chronic CHF and 3 died suddenly.

	Peripartum Onset (n = 13)	Nonperipartum Onset (n = 26)	p Value
Age (yr) (mean)	18–61 (32)	21–78 (57)	<0.001
Black:white	10:3	18:8	NS
Systemic hypertension	1 (8%)	8 (31%)	NS
Habitual alcoholism	2 (15%)	7 (27%)	NS
Duration CHF (mo) (mean)	2–264 (65)	1–240 (65)	NS
Embolic events	7 (54%)	18 (69%)	NS
Pulmonary	6 (46%)	13 (50%)	NS
Systemic	1 (8%)	5 (19%)	NS
Sudden death	3 (23%)	7 (26%)	NS
Heart weight (g) (mean)	370–770 (512)	360–810 (567)	NS
Transmural LV scars	1 (8%)	8 (31%)	NS
Intracardiac thrombi (only)	3 (23%)	8 (31%)	NS
Endocardial plaques (only)	3 (23%)	6 (22%)	NS
Both plaques and thrombi	2 (15%)	7 (27%)	NS
Either plaques or thrombi	8 (61%)	21 (81%)	NS

CHF = congestive heart failure; LV = left ventricular; NS = not significant.

TABLE III Clinical and Necropsy Characteristics of 58 Alcoholic and 70 Nonalcoholic Patients with Idiopathic Dilated Cardiomyopathy

	Alcoholic (n = 58)	Nonalcoholic (n = 70)	p Value
Age (yr) (mean)	21–78 (46)	16–75 (45)	NS
Male:female	51:7 (7.3:1)	42:28 (1.5:1)	<0.05
Black:white	37:14 (2.6:1)	34:29 (1.2:1)	NS
Duration (mo) CHF	0–144 (50)	1–168 (50)	NS
Pulmonary edema	9/33 (27%)	18/46 (39%)	<0.05
Angina pectoris	8/43 (19%)	7/59 (12%)	NS
"AMI" (history)	14/43 (32%)	8/61 (13%)	<0.05
Emboli			
Pulmonary, clinical	18/39 (46%)	24/59 (41%)	NS
Pulmonary, necropsy	16/36 (44%)	26/41 (63%)	<0.05
Systemic, clinical	12/41 (29%)	6/71 (8%)	<0.05
Systemic, necropsy	13/35 (37%)	8/38 (21%)	<0.05
Mode of death			
Chronic CHF	26/46 (57%)	39/67 (58%)	NS
Sudden death	14/46 (30%)	19/67 (28%)	NS
Pulmonary embolus	5/46 (11%)	5/67 (7%)	NS
Other	1/46 (2%)	4/67 (6%)	NS
Heart weight (g) (mean)	360–940 (631)	370–940 (593)	<0.05
Intracavitary thrombi (T) only	16/58 (28%)	18/70 (26%)	NS
Endocardial plaques (P) only	12/58 (21%)	14/70 (20%)	NS
Both T and P	16/58 (28%)	15/70 (21%)	NS
Transmural LV scars (gross)	8/58 (14%)	3/69 (4%)	NS
Replacement fibrosis (microscopic)	20/34 (59%)	19/31 (61%)	NS

AMI = acute myocardial function; CHF = congestive heart failure; LV = left ventricular; NS = not significant.

None of the 9 and none of the affected family members had evidence either clinically or morphologically of hypertrophic cardiomyopathy.

Congestive heart failure: Of the 152 patients, 148 (97%) had clinical evidence of chronic CHF; in 114 patients, it was the initial manifestation of their illness, and in most it became intractable and caused death. Good information on the interval from onset of chronic CHF to death was available in 120 of the 148 patients and it ranged from 1 to 264 months (mean 54) (Table I and Figure 2). From onset of CHF to death in these patients, 29 (24%) lived ≤12 months; 54 (45%), 13 to 60 months; 20 (17%) 61 to 120 months and 16 (14%), >120 months. These 120 patients were divided into 3 survival periods and 13 factors were compared (Table IV). Comparison of the 27 patients surviving >72 months after onset of chronic CHF to the 64 patients surviving ≤36 months disclosed a significantly (p <0.05) higher frequency in the longer survival group of older patients, of women, of habitual alcoholics, of patients with chest pain syndromes, diabetes mellitus and pulmonary emboli, of patients treated with warfarin and of patients with bigger hearts at necropsy.

Sudden death: Each of the 4 patients without clinical evidence of chronic CHF died suddenly and unexpectedly and sudden death in them was the initial manifestation of IDC. All 4 were men aged 23 to 43 years (mean 31) with hearts weighing 480 to 780 g

TABLE IV Duration of Survival in Idiopathic Dilated Cardiomyopathy: Clinical and Necropsy Findings

	Duration (mo) of Survival			
	≤36	>36–72	>72	p value
Number of patients	64 (53%)	29 (24%)	27 (23%)	—
Age (yr) (mean)	16–75 (40)	20–71 (49)	16–75 (51)	<0.05
Black:white	35/60(58%):25/60(42%)	16/27(59%):11/27(41%)	13/22(59%):9/22(41%)	NS
Male:female	49(77%):15(23%)	21(72%):8(28%)	13(48%):14(52%)	<0.05
Duration (mo) CHF (mean)	0–36 (15)	38–72 (58)	84–264 (131)	<0.05
Mode of death				
CHF	33 (52%)	17 (59%)	18 (67%)	<0.05
Sudden	12 (18%)	5 (17%)	3 (11%)	NS
Pulmonary emboli	6 (9%)	2 (7%)	4 (15%)	NS
Other	5 (7%)	4 (14%)	2 (7%)	NS
History				
Pulmonary edema	15 (21%)	9 (31%)	5 (36%)	<0.05
Angina pectoris	5 (7%)	4 (14%)	4 (20%)	<0.05
AMI	9 (14%)	5 (17%)	8 (33%)	<0.05
Hypertension	9 (14%)	2 (7%)	4 (17%)	NS
Diabetes mellitus	6 (8%)	3 (10%)	6 (26%)	<0.05
Emboli				
Pulmonary, clinical	21 (33%)	8 (28%)	13 (54%)	<0.05
Pulmonary, necropsy	23 (36%)	7 (24%)	9 (47%)	<0.05
Systemic, clinical	10 (16%)	6 (21%)	4 (17%)	NS
Systemic, necropsy	11 (17%)	4 (14%)	6 (32%)	NS
Warfarin therapy				
≥3 mo <12 mo	9 (14%)	5 (17%)	9 (33%)	<0.05
≥12 mo	3 (4%)	2 (7%)	6 (22%)	NS
Heart weight (g) (mean)	400–940 (586)	360–940 (615)	400–860 (625)	<0.05
LV scar				
Transmural	7 (11%)	3 (10%)	2 (7%)	NS
Subendocardial	9 (14%)	3 (10%)	5 (18%)	NS
Intracardiac				
Thrombi only	24 (36%)	7 (24%)	6 (22%)	NS
Plaques only	12 (18%)	3 (10%)	12 (44%)	<0.05
Both thrombi and plaques	14 (22%)	6 (21%)	7 (26%)	NS
Replacement fibrosis (microscopic)	7/25 (28%)	5/14 (36%)	3/18 (17%)	NS

Abbreviations as in Table III.

(mean 640). Three were habitual alcoholics. None had histories of systemic hypertension or evidence of diabetes mellitus. Thirty other patients died suddenly, but each of them previously had had CHF; of them, 19 had fatal cardiac arrest outside the hospital and the other 14 patients, while in the hospital.

Emboli: Information regarding the presence or absence of pulmonary or systemic emboli or both was available in 131 of the 152 patients, and of them 79 patients (60%) had either clinical or necropsy evidence or both of embolic events. Of the 79 patients, 40 (51%) had pulmonary emboli only, 13 (16%) had systemic emboli only and 26 (33%) had both. Thus, of the 79 patients, there were 66 (84%) with pulmonary emboli or infarcts and 39 (49%) with systemic emboli or infarcts. The manner in which the emboli were diagnosed, either clinically or morphologically or both, and their relation to intracardiac thrombi and to mural en-

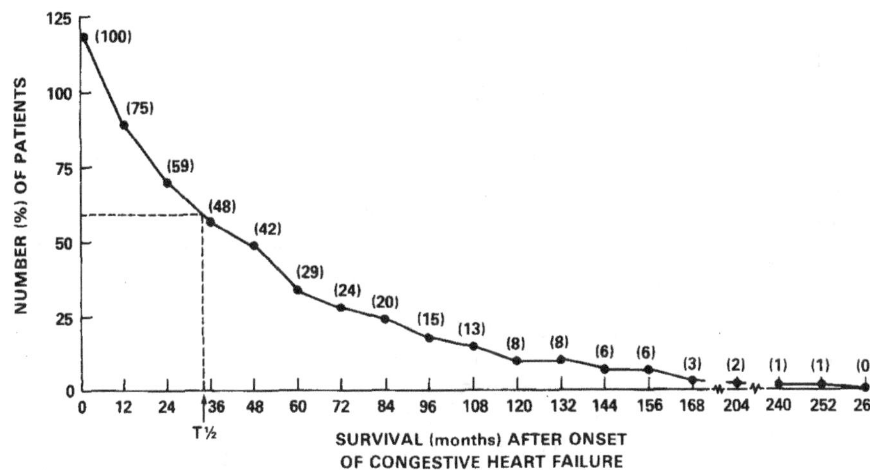

FIGURE 2. Cumulative survival of 118 patients with idiopathic dilated cardiomyopathy after onset of congestive heart failure. One-half of the patients were dead in <36 months ($T_{1/2}$).

TABLE V Frequency of Pulmonary and Systemic Emboli and Infarcts and Relation to Intracardiac Thrombi and Mural Endocardial Plaques in Idiopathic Dilated Cardiomyopathy

Present	Pt	Diagnosis			RV T Only	RV Plaques Only	Both	RAA T	RV or RAA T	Right-Sided T or Plaque	LV T Only	LV Plaques Only	Both	LAA T	LV or LAA T	Left-Sided T or Plaque	Either Right- or Left-Sided T or Plaque or Both	WS Rx
		Clinically Only	Necropsy Only	Both														
Pulmonary Emboli or Infarcts																		
+	66	19 (29%)	17 (20%)	30 (45%)	26 (39%)	8 (12%)	5 (8%)	20 (30%)	37 (56%)	45 (68%)	19 (29%)	11 (17%)	19 (29%)	10 (15%)	39 (59%)	50 (76%)	54 (82%)	12 (18%)
0	65	0	0	0	11 (17%)	4 (6%)	4 (6%)	15 (23%)	21 (32%)	26 (40%)	11 (17%)	14 (22%)	11 (17%)	11 (17%)	28 (43%)	45 (69%)	48 (74%)	11 (17%)
Systemic Emboli or Infarcts																		
+	39	15 (39%)	11 (28%)	13 (33%)	15 (22%)	7 (18%)	4 (10%)	13 (33%)	20 (51%)	29 (74%)	11 (28%)	8 (21%)	14 (36%)	6 (3%)	26 (66%)	34 (87%)	39 (100%)	10 (26%)
0	92	0	0	0	21 (23%)	5 (5%)	5 (5%)	20 (22%)	36 (39%)	40 (43%)	14 (15%)	22 (24%)	13 (14%)	13 (14%)	37 (40%)	59 (64%)	63 (68%)	13 (14%)
Total: Pulmonary or Systemic Emboli or Both																		
+	79	24 (30%)	20 (25%)	28* (35%)	29 (37%)	12 (15%)	6 (8%)	24 (30%)	41 (52%)	47 (59%)	33 (42%)	14 (18%)	28 (35%)	11 (14%)	64 (81%)	59 (75%)	67 (85%)	17 (22%)
0	52	0	0	0	8 (15%)	1 (27%)	3 (6%)	9 (17%)	15 (29%)	17 (33%)	9 (17%)	15 (29%)	8 (15%)	9 (17%)	20 (38%)	34 (65%)	36 (69%)	6 (12%)

* In an additional 2 patients with both pulmonary and systemic emboli, one was diagnosed clinically only and the other was diagnosed only at necropsy.

LAA = left atrial appendage; LV = left ventricular; RAA = right atrial appendage; RV = right ventricular; Rx = treatment; T = thrombus; WS = warfarin sodium.

docardial plaques (almost surely the result of organization of thrombi) are summarized in Table V. Comparison of the 66 patients with pulmonary emboli or infarcts to the 64 without disclosed a significantly higher frequency of right-sided intracardiac thrombi or endocardial plaques or both in the former (68 vs 40%, p <0.05). Comparison of the 39 patients with systemic emboli or infarcts to the 92 without also disclosed a significantly higher frequency of left-sided intracardiac thrombi or endocardial plaques or both in the former (87 vs 64%, p <0.05). Of the 79 patients with either pulmonary or systemic emboli or both, 67 (85%) had either right- or left-sided thrombi or mural endocardial plaques or both, whereas of the 52 without emboli, 36 (69%) had intracardiac thrombi or plaques (p <0.05). The numbers of patients treated with warfarin sodium were not large enough to make meaningful conclusions.

Electrocardiographic findings: Electrocardiographic observations during the last 6 months of life were available in 101 of the 152 patients and the findings are summarized in Table VI. Of the 101 patients, 25 had atrial fibrillation, and findings in them are summarized in Table VII and compared with observations in 25 age- and sex-matched patients with sinus rhythm: no significant differences were noted with regard to race, history of habitual alcoholism, duration of chronic CHF or mode of death. The patients with atrial fibrillation had a lower frequency of embolic events (64 vs 80%) and a lower frequency of intracardiac thrombi (13 vs 18 patients). The frequency of atrial thrombi among the 2 groups of patients was identical. P-wave abnormalities (in addition to their absence in 25% of the patients) were present in 49 of the 101 patients; left only in 35, right only in 6 and both in 8.

Either left ventricular (38 patients) or right (5 patients) ventricular hypertrophy or both (1 patient) were observed electrocardiographically in 44 patients. Complete bundle branch block occurred in 51 patients: left in 41, right in 6 and indeterminate intraventricular conduction delay in 4. Comparison of 32 patients with complete left bundle branch block to 33 with left ventricular hypertrophy and 15 with neither bundle branch block nor left ventricular hypertrophy disclosed that the patients with left bundle branch block had an older mean age (55 vs 45 years vs 42 years [p <0.05]), a longer mean duration of chronic CHF (83 vs 32 months vs 43 months [p <0.05]), larger mean heart weights (628 vs 605 vs 590 g [p <0.05]) and higher frequencies of grossly visible left ventricular scars (44 vs 21 vs 13% [p <0.05]). These observations are summarized in Table VIII and in Figure 3.

In 49 patients in whom electrocardiograms were recorded in the last year of life and available for reexamination, the QRS amplitude in all 12 leads was measured (Table IX, Figure 4). The total 12-lead QRS amplitude in the 35 men (mean age 46 years) ranged from 74 to 250 mm (10 mm = 1 mV) (mean 147) and in the 14 women (mean age 54 years), from 75 to 243 mm (mean 167). The heart weights in the 35 men ranged from 400 to 940 g (mean 620), and in the 14 women, from 400 to 860 g (mean 602). The maximal width of the QRS complex in the 35 men averaged 0.104 second and in 19 patients (54%) was ≥0.12 second; the width in the 14 women averaged 0.122 second and in 11 (79%) patients it was ≥0.12 second. The mean PR interval and QT interval were identical in both men and women (0.19 and 0.39 second, respectively).

The mean 12-lead QRS amplitude among 18 patients with complete left bundle branch block, in 22 patients with electrocardiographic evidence of left ventricular hypertrophy and in 10 patients with neither left bundle branch block nor electrocardiographic left ventricular hypertrophy did not correlate with heart weight (Figure 3). Comparison of total 12-lead QRS amplitude in all 12 leads to heart weight within each group, however, disclosed a striking positive correlation between total 12-lead QRS amplitude and heart weight in the group with complete left bundle

branch block (r = +0.81). Because the coefficient of determination was 0.66, approximately two-thirds of the total QRS amplitude in all 12 leads are presumed to be determined by heart weight in our patients with IDC and left bundle block branch. The correlation coefficients between total 12-lead QRS voltage and either voltage criteria of left ventricular hypertrophy or left bundle branch block or neither electrocardiographic criteria for left ventricular hypertrophy nor left bundle branch block were +0.09 and +0.15, re-

TABLE VI Electrocardiographic Findings in 101 Necropsy Patients with Idiopathic Dilated Cardiomyopathy*

	Number (= %)
Rhythm	
Sinus	76
Atrial fibrillation	25
QRS axis abnormality	50
Left (−30 to −90°)	43
Right (110 to 270°)	7
Atrial abnormality	49
Left[†]	35
Right[‡]	6
Both	8
Ventricular hypertrophy	44
Left[§] only	38
Without strain pattern	21
With[‖] strain pattern	17
Right[§] only	5
Both	1
Conduction abnormality[¶]	
Prolonged (>0.20 s) P-R interval	23
Second degree atrioventricular block	1
Complete atrioventricular block	1
Complete bundle branch block	51
Left	41
Right	6
Indeterminant intraventricular conduction delay	4
Arrhythmias, episodic	
Atrial premature complexes	12
Ventricular premature complexes	41
Supraventricular tachycardia	7
Ventricular tachycardia	5
Low voltage (sum QRS in I, II + III ≤ 15 mm)	22
Myocardial damage pattern	38
A. Poor R-wave progression precordial leads**	22
B. Q wave II, III, aVF	7
C. Q wave I, AVL, V_{4-6}	2
D. Combinations A. + B. =	5
B. + C. =	2
Nonspecific ST-T wave changes	12

* Based on analysis of electrocardiograms in 55 patients and detailed reports in 46 patients.

[†] P terminal force in V_1 is equal to or more negative than −0.04 mm-s.

[‡] P wave has height 2.5 mm in leads II, III or AVG.

[§] Criteria of Chou.

[‖] ST-segment depressed with upward convexity and final downward slope ends in an inverted T wave.

[¶] Eleven patients had neither complete bundle branch block nor left ventricular hypertrophy.

** R wave in lead V_3 ≤4 mm.

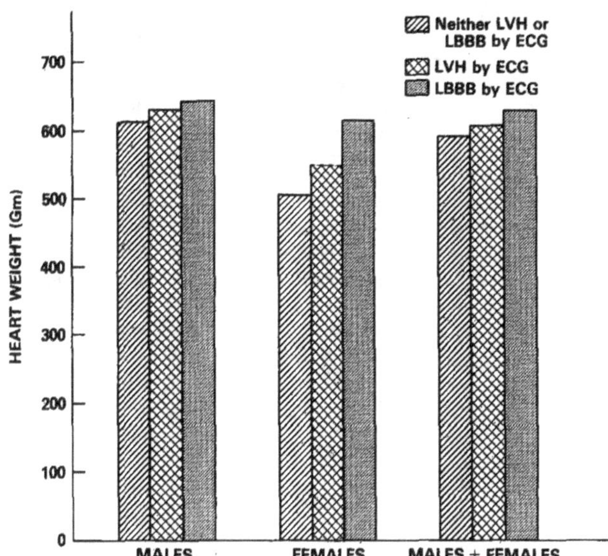

FIGURE 3. Bar graph showing relation of heart weight to electrocardiographic evidence of left ventricular hypertrophy (LVH) or left bundle branch block (LBBB) or neither in both sexes.

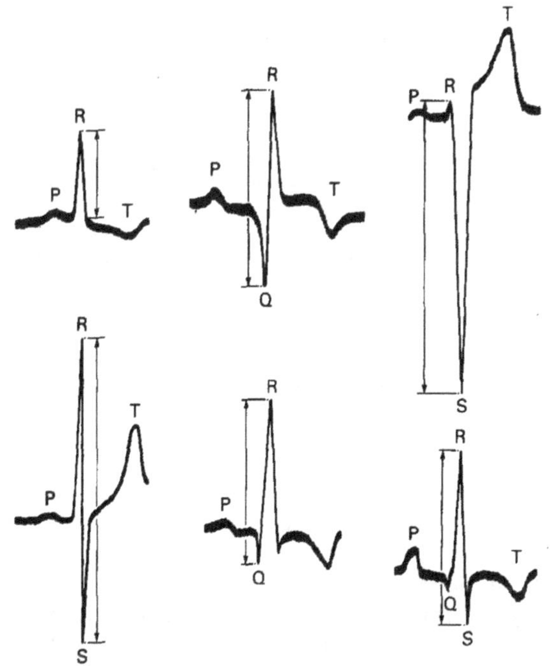

FIGURE 4. Various electrocardiographic QRS complexes showing how the voltage (in mm) was measured. Reproduced with permission from C.V. Mosby.[52]

TABLE VII Clinical and Necropsy Characteristics of 50 Patients with Idiopathic Dilated Cardiomyopathy: 25 with Atrial Fibrillation and 25 with Sinus Rhythm

	Sinus Rhythm (n = 25)	Atrial Fibrillation (n = 25)	p Value
Age (yr) (mean)	20–75 (49)	22–73 (53)	NS
Black:white	14:11 (56%:44%)	16:9 (64%:36%)	NS
Male:female	17:8 (68%:32%)	20:5 (80%:20%)	NS
Habitual alcoholism	12 (48%)	10 (40%)	NS
Duration (mo) CHF (mean)	8–168 (53)	1–264 (52)	NS
Mode of death			
CHF	17 (68%)	14 (60%)	NS
Emboli	3 (12%)	1 (4%)	NS
Sudden	4 (16%)	6 (26%)	NS
Other	1 (4%)	2 (8%)	NS
Emboli	20 (80%)	14 (64%)	NS
Pulmonary	15 (62%)	11 (44%)	NS
Systemic	10 (40%)	8 (32%)	NS
Electrocardiogram			
LV hypertrophy	3 (12%)	4 (16%)	NS
With strain	12 (48%)	2 (8%)	<0.01
Left BBB	9 (36%)	11 (44%)	NS
Right BBB	0	3 (12%)	NS
Heart weight (g)			
Total (mean)	400–940 (627)	370–770 (593)	NS
Male (mean)	440–940 (654)	390–760 (604)	NS
Female (mean)	400–860 (560)	370–770 (552)	NS
Cardiac thrombi			
RA-LA-RV-LV	10-6-12-15	10-6-6-7	<0.05
Thrombi only	7 (28%)	12 (48%)	NS
Mural plaque			
RA-LA-RV-LV	2-1-8-13	1-1-3-5	0.05
Plaque only	4 (16%)	4 (16%)	NS
Thrombi + plaque	11 (44%)	1 (4%)	0.001
Either:neither	22:3 (88%:12%)	17:8 (68%:32%)	NS
LV scars			
S:T	4:6	2:8	NS

BBB = bundle branch block; CHF = congestive heart failure; LA = left atrium; LV = left ventricular or left ventricle; NS = not significant; RA = right atrium; RV = right ventricle; S = subendocardial; T = transmural.

TABLE VIII Clinical and Necropsy Characteristics of Patients with Idiopathic Dilated Cardiomyopathy and Left Bundle Branch Block (BBB), Left Ventricular (LV) Hypertrophy or Neither by Electrocardiogram

	Left BBB (n = 32)	LV Hypertrophy (n = 33)	Neither (n = 15)
Ages (yr) (mean)	27–71 (55)	20–75 (45)	22–66 (42)
Male:female	21:11	27:6	8:7
Duration (mo) CHF (mean)	1–168 (83)	2–96 (32)	2–84 (43)
Heart weight (g) (mean)			
Male + female	400–860 (628)	400–870 (605)	370–940 (590)
Male only	400–860 (642)	400–870 (629)	410–940 (613)
Female only	460–800 (613)	440–650 (548)	370–680 (503)
Left ventricular scar			
Transmural (T):non-T	4:10 (12%:30%)	3:4 (9%:12%)	2:0 (13%:0)

spectively, indicating an insignificant relation between total 12-lead QRS amplitude and heart weight in these latter 2 groups.

Myocardial damage patterns unassociated with complete bundle branch block were observed by electrocardiogram in 38 (38%) of the 101 patients (Table VI). Thus, of the 50 patients without complete bundle branch block, 37 (76%) had myocardial damage patterns, including 22 with poor R-wave progression in the precordial leads, 7 with Q waves in leads II, III and aVF, 2 with Q waves in leads I, AVL and V_4 through V_6 and 7 with combinations of these 3. Comparison of the 38 patients to the 12 patients without a myocardial damage pattern on electrocardiogram (all 50 without complete bundle branch block) disclosed no significant differences in mean age, sex, mode of death, duration of CHF, frequency of chest pain syndromes, habitual alcoholism, diabetes mellitus, left ventricu-

TABLE IX   Electrocardiographic Measurements in 35 Necropsy Men and in 14 Necropsy Women with Idiopathic Dilated Cardiomyopathy

Pt	Age (yr) at ECG	Days ECG to Death	Heart Weight (g)	QRS Voltage (mm) Leads				QRS Width (s)	P-R Interval (s)	Q-T Interval (s)	QRS Axis (degrees)	Ventricular Rate (beats/min)
				All 12	I,II,III	A,L,F.	V_1–V_6					
							Men					
1	19	30	550	97	16	14	67	0.08	0.16	0.40	+120	80
2	20	3	610	250	35	29	186	0.08	0.16	0.40	+30	75
3	21	30	460	113	13	6	94	0.14	0.16	0.36	−45	110
4	22	9	700	109	13	12	84	0.08	0.22	0.36	+45	105
5	27	10	700	219	46	46	127	0.08	0.16	0.36	+30	115
6	28	240	540	197	24	20	153	0.08	0.16	0.36	−20	80
7	28	120	460	196	43	36	117	0.08	0.20	0.50	−15	65
8	32	990	—	133	15	16	102	0.08	0.19	0.40	−30	80
	35	5	940	114	10	9	95	0.06	0.20	0.48	−15	120
9	35	3	870	152	18	17	117	0.08	0.24	—	−20	105
10	36	60	750	135	10	8	107	0.08	0.18	0.32	+40	90
11	36	350	730	149	26	22	101	0.12	0.16	0.40	120	80
12	38	60	400	90	18	14	58	0.12	—	0.36	−30	80
13	41	426	—	145	16	13	116	0.10	0.23	0.40	0	76
	42	3	500	131	13	14	104	0.11	0.24	0.40	−90	90
14	42	9	630	103	13	12	78	0.12	0.14	0.44	—	90
15	42	117	550	188	21	19	148	0.08	0.22	0.36	−45	100
16	45	840	—	148	20	21	107	0.13	0.22	0.36	−90	120
	47	60	620	159	19	15	125	0.13	0.21	0.40	−90	105
17	46	60	500	144	22	17	105	0.08	0.24	0.40	−60	75
18	47	180	550	148	14	12	122	0.09	0.24	0.36	+30	90
19	47	30	760	281	28	19	234	0.08	0.22	0.40	−40	80
20	48	240	650	172	25	20	127	0.09	0.18	0.40	−15	75
21	50	15	650	112	12	11	89	0.08	0.20	0.36	−60	100
22	51	45	—	179	20	17	142	0.08	0.16	0.56	−20	50
	51	20	500	115	20	18	77	0.10	0.16	0.52	−40	45
23	51	71	650	74	9	10	55	0.09	0.22	0.40	−110	80
24	53	450	—	103	13	10	80	0.12	0.23	0.41	—	58
	54	3	—	106	14	14	78	0.13	0.10	0.32	—	110
25	54	1,500	—	164	24	19	121	0.09	0.16	0.40	+40	75
	58	6	610	107	12	13	82	0.14	0.24	0.40	−60	105
26	56	20	830	202	50	44	108	0.12	0.20	0.42	—	—
27	53	1,100	—	179	33	27	119	0.14	0.12	0.36	−80	75
	56	80	460	136	18	17	101	0.14	0.16	0.36	−75	110
28	58	90	440	114	15	11	88	0.08	0.16	0.36	−40	115
29	59	10	690	146	12	13	123	0.16	0.24	—	−60	95
30	62	450	—	178	22	16	140	0.12	0.16	0.40	−15	120
	63	37	700	185	19	15	151	0.16	0.18	0.38	−30	100
31	62	60	600	141	21	15	105	0.12	0.20	0.40	−40	100
32	63	9	500	123	27	28	68	0.12	0.21	0.40	−70	72
33	67	1	—	137	6	3	128	0.16	—	0.44	0	70
34	70	210	—	128	25	27	76	0.13	—	0.40	−40	77
35	73	4	725	182	31	26	125	0.08	—	0.40	−30	70
Mean	46	64*	620	147	21	18	109	0.104	0.192	0.39		90
							Women					
1	22	165	440	221	22	22	177	0.09	0.18	0.32	+60	90
2	32	12	650	195	18	17	160	0.08	0.16	0.36	+60	130
3	50	24	700	187	26	17	144	0.16	—	0.38	−45	75
4	51	270	570	75	16	13	46	0.06	—	0.36	−30	75
5	52	18	500	151	25	31	95	0.14	0.28	0.40	−80	110
6	53	20	400	155	18	17	120	0.08	0.18	0.42	0	70
7	54	900	—	154	15	13	126	0.13	0.20	0.36	+45	130
	57	9	550	108	12	8	88	0.14	0.22	0.40	+45	115
8	58	22	640	180	32	33	115	0.12	0.14	0.40	−40	110
9	58	180	—	196	55	54	87	0.18	0.22	0.40	−40	80
	58	30	860	241	48	48	145	0.20	0.24	0.44	−45	70
10	58	7	620	160	21	21	118	0.12	—	0.36	−70	120
11	59	15	750	243	25	18	200	0.14	0.20	0.42	−40	80
12	60	1	490	91	9	9	73	0.16	0.16	0.40	1	95
13	64	30	—	154	13	11	130	0.14	0.18	0.36	−60	90
14	75	7	650	182	28	26	128	0.08	0.21	0.40	−60	75
Mean	54	45*	602	167	22	21	124	0.122	0.195	0.39		93

* In the 9 patients with 2 ECGs analyzed, the mean utilizes the interval from the second ECG to death.

ECG = electrocardiogram. ,

| | | | Duration (mo) | | | Pressures (mm Hg) | | | | | | | | | | | | Thrombus | | |
| | | | | | | RA | | | RV | PA | PAW | | | LV | SA | | HW | | | |
Pt	Age (yr)	Sex	CHF	CHF → CC	CC → Death	a	v	m	(s/d)	(s/d)	a	v	m	(s/d)	(s/d)	CI	(g)	RV	LV	PE
1	17	M	36	9	27	9	8	5	26/10	26/14	20	22	16	100/14	100/60	4.1	585	0	+	0
2	18	F	5	2	3	—	—	—	—	36/22	—	—	—	80/25	80/40	—	—	0	0	+
3	20	M	46	4	2	10	8	5	26/7	26/12	10	12	9	102/13	115/60	3.0	610	0	0	+
4	22	M	12	1	11	—	—	—	—	—	—	—	—	100/26	100/50	—	600	+	+	+
5	26	M	16	4	12	9	4	2	17/13	17/10	8	12	5	110/10	110/75	1.4	700	0	+	0
6	26	M	4	1	3	—	—	—	—	27/14	—	—	14	100/12	100/60	1.4	460	0	0	0
7	26	M	5	4	1	—	—	13	—	45/20	—	—	32	—	—	1.5	—	0	+	—
8	29	F	108	103	5	—	—	—	90/-	90/-	—	—	32	90/25	90/60	—	460	0	+	+
9	30	M	5	3	2	18	17	13	70/22	70/26	26	22	18	150/28	140/70	1.5	410	0	0	+
10	32	M	96	84	12	2	3	2	26/2	24/17	—	—	22	120/27	120/70	—	550	+	+	+
11	37	F	23	22	5 days	16	18	17	51/23	51/37	—	—	28	—	—	—	—	0	0	+
12	37	M	36	22	14	AF	8	6	58/6	58/30	—	45	30	126/28	102/80	2.5	400	+	+	0
13	39	M	18	5	13	—	—	0	20/2	20/12	—	—	6	100/18	105/70	2.1	720	0	+	+
14	42	M	72	71	7 days	—	—	16	77/15	77/37	—	—	16	—	100/80	—	650	0	+*	+
15	42	M	30	25	5	30	27	23	40/20	43/32	—	—	35	—	100/60	1.6	550	+	+	0
16	42	M	24	11	13	—	—	7	55/10	55/30	—	—	35	95/35	95/60	1.6	510	0	0	+
17	47	M	12	6	6	9	6	5	45/7	45/20	26	38	25	85/25	85/60	1.5	550	0	+	+
18	48	M	60	48	12	—	—	—	45/8	45/30	—	—	30	85/30	85/55	—	—	0	+	0
19	49	M	48	41	7	AF	—	27	78/28	78/-	—	54	40	—	80/60	—	700	+	+	0
20	50	F	60	60	14 days	AF	30	25	74/24	70/40	—	45	36	100/30	110/75	1.1	700	+	+*	+
21	51	M	72	20	52	AF	10	9	50/9	52/24	—	—	15	120/20	120/75	1.85	570	0	0	0
22	55	M	60	59	1	AF	—	7	40/7	—	—	40	26	110/26	110/80	—	500	0	0	0
23	56	M	36	34	2	—	—	23	—	55/30	—	—	25	—	85/55	—	460	+	+	+
24	58	F	168	165	3	8	7	6	60/10	60/30	32	30	23	140/32	140/80	2.3	860	0	0	+
25	58	F	12	11	21 days	—	12	4	40/6	40/20	—	—	20	95/20	95/70	1.6	620	+	+*	+
26	62	F	62	24	1 day	—	—	4	55/24	55/35	—	—	25	108/23	110/90	2.4	760	0	0	+
27	63	M	—	—	5 days	AF	—	—	70/10	70/27	—	—	28	—	130/75	1.9	—	+	+	0
28	70	M	60	50	10	AF	—	4	60/10	60/20	—	9	7	150/8	150/60	—	580	+	+	+
Mean	41		44	33	8	12	12	11	51/12	50/25	20	30	28	108/23	106/67	2.0	587			

* Thrombus was not visualized on left ventricular angiogram performed 1 month or less before death.

a = a wave; AF = atrial fibrillation; CC = cardiac catheterization; CI = cardiac index (in liters/min/m^2); CHF ≈ congestive heart failure; HW = heart weight; LV = left ventricle; m = mean; PA = pulmonary artery; PE = pulmonary emboli (at necropsy); Pt = patient; RA = right atrium; RV = right ventricle; SA = systemic artery; s/d = peak systole/end diastole; V = V wave.

lar hypertrophy on electrocardiogram or intracardiac thrombi. The frequencies of atrial fibrillation and grossly visible left ventricular scars, however, were different. Of the 38 patients with myocardial damage patterns on electrocardiogram, 1.0 (26%) had atrial fibrillation and 10 (26%) had left ventricular scars; in contrast, all 12 patients without myocardial damage patterns were in sinus rhythm and none had left ventricular scars.

Hemodynamic data: Cardiac catheterization data were available in 28 of the 152 patients (Table X). The mean atrial or ventricular end-diastolic pressures or both were elevated in all 28 patients. The right ventricular end-diastolic pressure was >6 mm Hg in 18 (82%) of 22 patients, the left ventricular end-diastolic pressure was >12 mm Hg in 18 (86%) of 21 patients and the mean pulmonary arterial wedge pressure was >12 mm Hg in 22 (85%) of 26 patients. The pulmonary arterial systolic pressure was >30 mm Hg in 20 (77%) of 26 patients, including 8 in whom this pressure was ≥60 mm Hg. Of the 28 patients who had cardiac catheterization, 17 had necropsy evidence of pulmonary emboli or infarcts, and 12 (71%) had pulmonary arterial systolic pressures >30 mm Hg, including 10 (59%) in whom this pressure was >50 mm Hg. A left ventricular to aortic peak systolic pressure gradient of 23 mm Hg was observed in 1 patient, and this patient at necropsy had a thrombus in the left ventricular outflow tract. The cardiac indexes were <2.5 liters/min/m^2 in 14 (82%) of 17 patients. Left ventricular angiograms in 18 patients disclosed global hypokinesia in all 18 and mitral regurgitation in 6 of 13 in whom it was mentioned. No significant correlation was observed between total duration of chronic CHF or duration of CHF from the time of catheterization to death and the pulmonary arterial systolic pressure (r = +0.39 and r = −0.20), but a significant correlation was observed between the total duration of CHF and the mean pulmonary arterial wedge pressure (r = +0.65) (p <0.002). The left ventricular end-diastolic pressure did not correlate with heart weight (r = −0.08), total duration of CHF (r = −0.14) or duration of CHF from catheterization to death (r = −0.17).

Necropsy Findings

Heart weights and chamber sizes: The hearts at necropsy ranged in weight from 360 to 940 g (mean 615): in the women the range was from 360 to 860 g (mean 551) and in the men, from 400 to 940 g (mean 632) (p <0.05). By definition, both right and left ventricular cavities were dilated in all patients (Figures 5 through 7). So were both atria. The frequency of intracavity thrombi and mural endocardial plaques have been described previously.

Ventricular scars: Grossly visible left ventricular or right ventricular scars or both (excluding isolated papillary muscle scars) were found in 22 (14%) patients: 21 scars involved, at some point, greater than the inner one-half of the myocardial wall, that is, transmural, and 1 was limited to the inner one-half, that is, subendocardial. The scars were small in 14 patients, moderate in 4 and large in 4. The scars involved left ventricular free wall in all 22 patients, the ventricular septum also in 20 and the right ventricular free wall in 5. The frequency of intraventricular thrombi and endocardial plaques was similar in the patients with and without grossly visible ventricular wall scars. The 22 patients with ventricular scars ranged in age from 17 to 67 years (mean 56), which is an average of 13 years older than the mean (43 years) of the 130 patients without grossly visible left ventricular scars (p <0.05). Of these 22 patients, 21 had chronic CHF an average of 44 months, which is significantly (p <0.05) less than the mean duration (65 months) of chronic CHF in the 99 patients in whom no grossly visible ventricular scars were present and information on the duration of chronic CHF was available. Of the 22 patients, 4 had clinical events during life considered to be compatible with "acute myocardial infarction." None, of course, had significantly (>75% in cross-sectional area) narrowed coronary arteries at necropsy. Of the 22 patients, 11 had histories of habitual alcoholism and 2 had adult-onset diabetes mellitus. Electrocardiograms, available in 21 of the 22 patients, disclosed voltage criteria for left ventricular hypertrophy in 6 (29%), complete bundle branch block in 9 (43%) and myocardial infarct or damage patterns in 6 (29%). The mean heart weight (available in 19 patients) in the patients

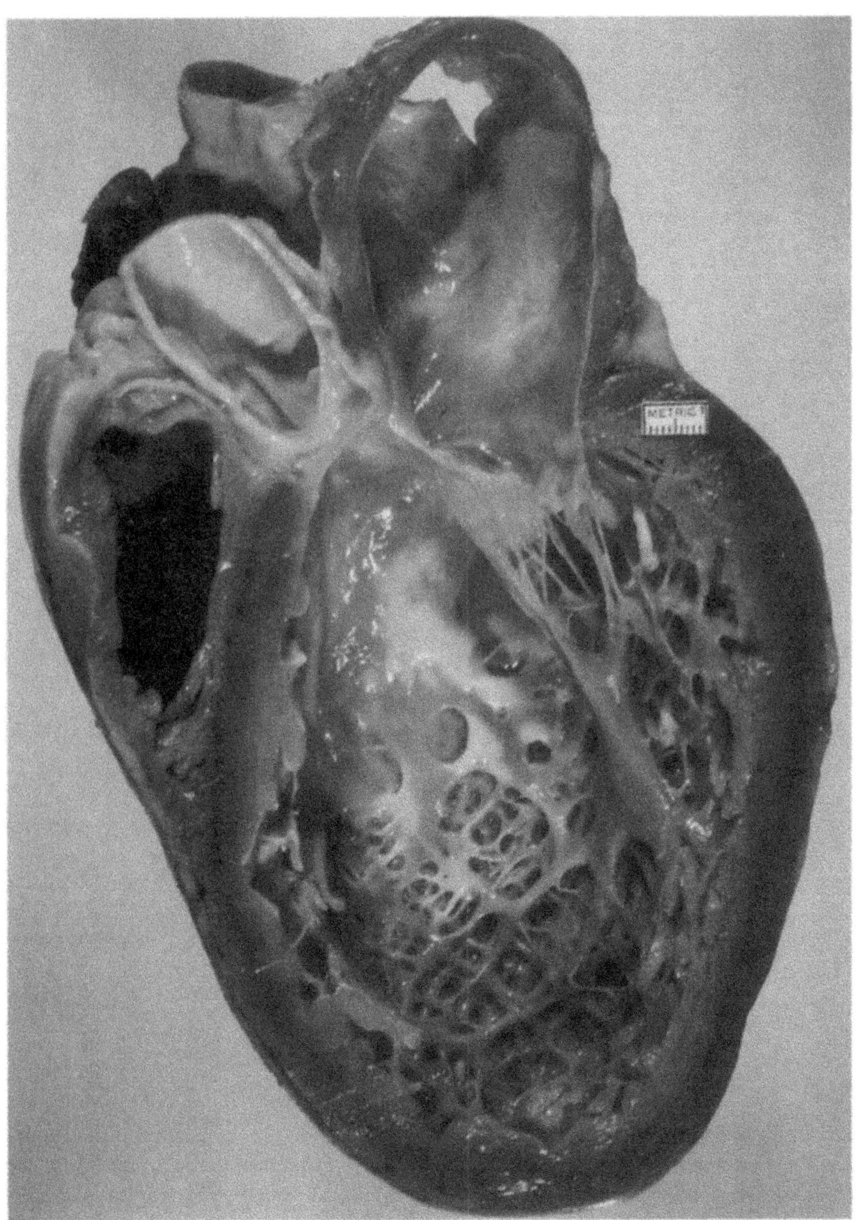

FIGURE 5. Longitudinal view of left side of the heart from a 54-year-old man (SH A81-57) with idiopathic dilated cardiomyopathy. Shown is the outflow portion of right ventricle and much of the left ventricle. The white plaques on the left ventricular aspect of the ventricular septum probably are residua of organization of thrombi. The mitral valve occupies a small portion of the very dilated left ventricular cavity. The heart weighed 920 g. Congestive heart failure had been present for 3.5 years.

with grossly visible scars was similar to that in the patients without (607 vs 615 g).

Histology of ventricular myocardium: A total of 1,422 histologic sections of myocardial wall from 96 patients were examined: 508 sections of left ventricle, 215 of ventricular septum, 355 of right ventricle and 344 of atrium. Additionally, 967 sections of cross-sections of major (right, left main, left anterior descending and left circumflex) epicardial coronary arteries were examined. The ventricular myocardium contained multiple patchy areas of replacement fibrosis in 29 (35%) of 83 sections of right ventricle and in 55 (57%) of 96 sections of left ventricle from the 96 patients. The replacement fibrosis often was accompanied by in-

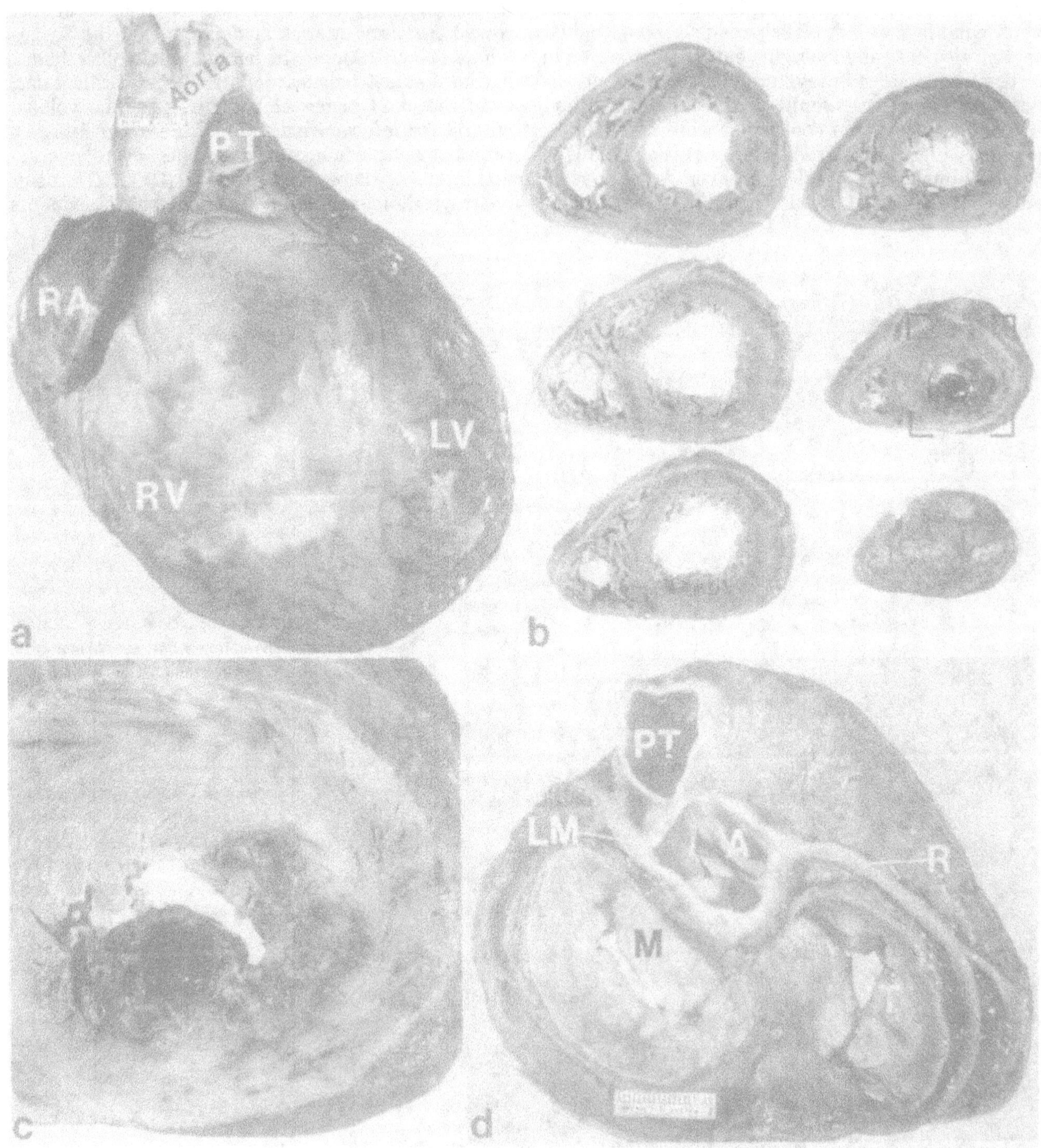

FIGURE 6. Heart from a 58-year-old woman (SH A78-7) with congestive heart failure for 10 years due to idiopathic dilated cardiomyopathy. *A*, exterior view of the heart. LV = left ventricle; PT = pulmonary trunk; RA = right atrium; RV = right ventricle. *B*, sections of the dilated cardiac ventricles after transverse sectioning. *C*, close-up view of the section shown in brackets in *B*. A thrombus is present. *D*, view of the mitral (M), tricuspid (T) and aortic (A) valves and of pulmonary trunk after removal of the atrial walls. R = right; LM = left main coronary arteries.

creased perivascular fibrous tissue and perimyocytic fibrosis in the left ventricle: it was present in 22 (23%) of 96 and 27 (28%) of 96 patients, respectively (Figure 8). In addition, in 13 (16%) of 83 sections of right ventricle and in 32 (33%) of 96 sections of left ventricle extensive subendocardial scarring was present. Interstitial inflammatory cell infiltrates were present in ventricular myocardium in 5 patients: 4 had prominent mononuclear infiltrates without associated myocardial necrosis and 1 had multiple small foci of necrotizing inflammation. One patient with lymphoid infiltrates and patchy replacement fibrosis had a progressive 5-week course of CHF with positive serology for Coxsackie B_3 virus. Tiny collections of perivascular "sentinal" mononuclear cells were seen in many patients. Seven (8%) of 83 patients had small foci of coagulation necrosis in the right ventricle and 11 (11%) of 96 in the left ventricle.

Myocytes had variable degrees of hypertrophy and atrophy. Two patients had small foci of myofiber disorganization in ventricular septum or left ventricular free wall or both. Another 2 patients had occasional calcified myocytes in ventricular myocardium and another 2 had subendocardial left ventricular foci of colliquative myocytolysis. Platelet aggregate was present in an intramural coronary artery in 1 patient. No infectious organisms were identified in any section.

Discussion

Josserand and Gallavardin[1] in 1901 apparently were the first to describe a patient with what appears to have been IDC, although they used the term "idiopathic hypertrophy of the heart." Another 24 years elapsed before another case of what appears to have been IDC was described by Laubry and Walser.[2] Whit-

tle[3] in 1929 added another case. By 1944, Levy and Von Glahn[4] reported 10 necropsy cases of "cardiac hypertrophy of unknown cause" and they described the usual clinical features: "marked cardiac hypertrophy; occurrence of various types of arrhythmia; frequent emboli to the pulmonary and systemic circulations; rapidly progressive course after the onset of symptoms; and death from gradual cardiac failure or in sudden fashion." In 1955 Serbin and Chojnacki[5] reported 3 more cases of "idiopathic cardiac hypertrophy" and collected 46 previously published cases. Spodick and Littman[6] in 1958 described 8 necropsy cases of "idiopathic myocardial hypertrophy" and summarized findings in 72 previously published necropsy cases of "unexplained large hearts." Of the previously reported cases, 42% survived <12 months and 65% for <24 months. The heart weight in all but 1 patient was ≥400 g. Of the 72 cases, 62 (86%) were younger than 50 years at death.

Since 1958, numerous publications[7-47] have described various clinical features in patients with IDC, but none have focused on findings at necropsy. Massumi et al[11] in 1965 described clinical features of 50 cases of "primary myocardial disease" seen in a 41-month period; 13 died and necropsies were performed in 10. Goodwin[13] in 1970 studied 70 patients with IDC; 41 (55%) had died and the average duration from onset of symptoms to death was 3.5 years; necropsies were performed in 26 patients and all had heart weights ≥400 g. Hamby[14] in 1970 described clinical features in 100 cases; 44 died in a 5-year period, and necropsies were performed in 23. Shugoll et al[17] followed 50 patients for 3 to 72 months (mean 30); 10 died and necropsies were performed in 5. Hatle et al[22] followed up 106 patients for 2 to 12 years; 50 died and necropsies were

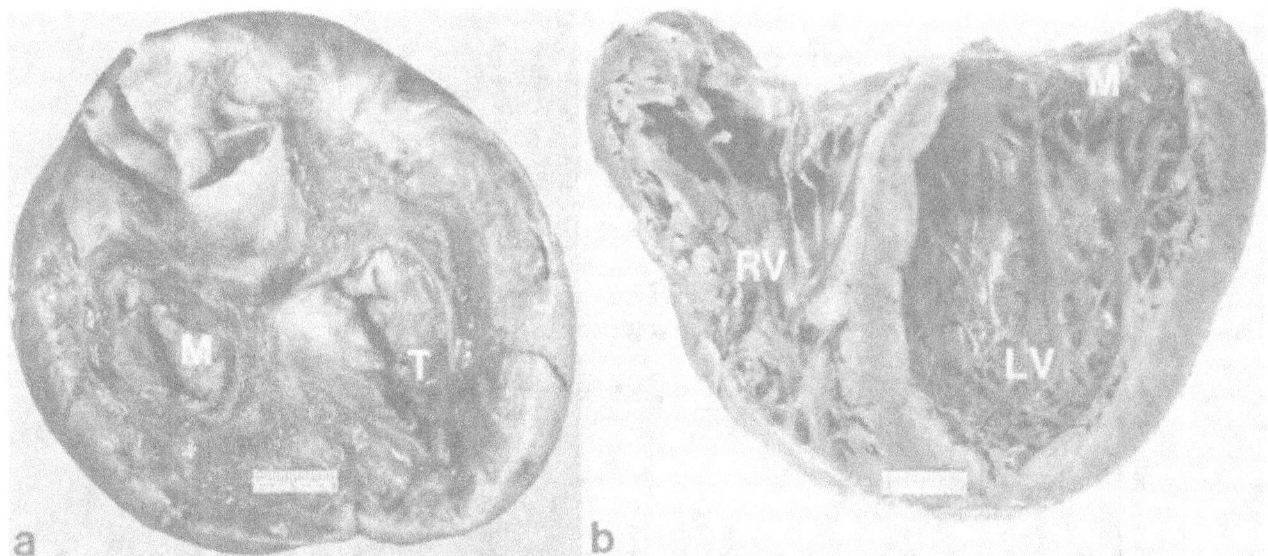

FIGURE 7. Heart (*A* and *B*) from a 34-year-old woman (DCGH 74A-65) with congestive heart failure for 5 years from idiopathic dilated cardiomyopathy. The mitral (M) anulus is only mildly dilated, whereas the tricuspid (T) valve anulus is considerably dilated, as are both ventricular cavities. The usual mechanism of tricuspid regurgitation in patients with idiopathic dilated cardiomyopathy is dilatation of the tricuspid valve anulus. In contrast, the usual mechanism of mitral regurgitation in idiopathic dilated cardiomyopathy is altered papillary muscle anchoring due to dilatation of the left ventricular cavity, mainly in its more central portion. The heart in this patient weighed 870 g.

TABLE XI Certain Reported Studies Since 1960 in Idiopathic Dilated Cardiomyopathy

	First Author	Year	No. Cases (males)	Period Patients Seen	Age Range (yr) (mean) When First Seen or When Studied	Age (yr) at Death (mean)	Race B	Race W	Range of Follow-up (mo) (mean)	Duration (mo) S → Death (mean)	History of Alcoholism	Peri-partum (no. women)	Familial	Diabetes Mellitus	No. Having Coronary Angiography	No. Died in Follow-Up	No. Having Necropsy
1	Fowler et al[7,8]	1962	29 (25)	—1964	8–62 (36)	18–68 (45)	10	19	1–312 (—)	6–312 (120)	8/23	1 (4)	1	0	0	26	26
2	Dye et al[9,10]	1963	32 (32)	—	20–68 (43)	—	14	18	—48 (—)	—(44)	21	0 (0)	—	—	0	12	9
3	Massumi et al[11]	1965	50 (40)	1960–1963	20–79 (—)	28–79 (54)	45	5	—41 (—)	—(10)	30	—(10)	0	—	0	13	10
4	Alexander[12]	1966	83 (83)	1949–1960	19–67 (44)	——(47)	—	—	—	—(2)	24	0 (0)	—	—	0	27	—
5	Goodwin[13]	1970	70 (—)	—	—	—	—	—	—	—(42)	16	7 (—)	—	—	9	41	26
6	Hamby[14]	1970	100 (71)	1954–1968	20–61 (45)	—(45)	71	29	2–60 (15)	—(55)	40	—(29)	—	3	24	35	23
7	McDonald and Rahimtoola[15]	1971	48 (47)	1959–1969	21–57 (38)	—	42	6	0.2–108 (52)	—(45)	48	0 (1)	—	—	0	19	14
8	Demakis[16]	1971	27 (0)	—	—	—	—	—	12–252 (97)	—	0	27 (27)	0	—	0	13	—
9	Shugoll et al[17]	1972	50 (50)	—1961	22–50 (—)	—	46	4	3–72 (30)	12–108 (38)	31	0 (0)	0	—	23	10	5
10	Kreulen et al[18]	1973	33 (24)	—	20–69 (43)	—	—	—	—	—	7	—(9)	—	—	33	9	—
11	Feild et al[19]	1973	36 (23)	—	18–66 (46)	—	—	—	—56 (—)	3–144 (38)	5	—(13)	0	5	15	19	5
12	Damakis et al[20]	1974	57 (49)	1962–1970	23–50 (41)	—	47	10	4–96 (41)	—(36)	57	0 (8)	—	—	4	24	7
13	Bashour et al[21]	1975	65 (56)	1969–1974	21–66 (42)	—	—	—	—(21)	—	65	—(9)	—	—	—	—	—
14	Hatle et al[22,23]	1976	91 (—)	1962–1972	<10–>60 (—)	—	—	—	2–12 (—)	—	2	—(—)	5	0	81	50	36
15	Hess et al[24]	1976	30 (24)	—	—(43)	—	—	—	10–34 (24)	—	—	—(6)	—	—	30	8	—
16	Segal et al[25]	1978	115 (71)	1961–1976	1–65 (—)	1–65 (46)	37	78	60–192 (96)	—(74)	0	0 (44)	0	0	—	77	48
17	Shirey et al[26]	1980	113 (—)	—	—	—	—	—	—96 (60)	0.5–90 (25)	8	—(—)	—	12	113	44	—
18	Koide et al[27]	1980	36 (29)	1965–1978	(44 ± 13)	—(53)	—	—	1–216 (—)	—(53)	10	3 (7)	3	—	—	17	11
19	Convert et al[28]	1980	132 (110)	1969–1977	15–71 (46)	—	—	—	(40 ± 24)	<6–>36 (—)	77	—(22)	—	—	79	48	—
20	Fuster et al[29]	1981	104 (64)	1960–1973	—(49)	—	—	—	72–240 (132)	—	22	3 (40)	—	0	46	80	39
21	Lengyel and Kokeny[30]	1981	98 (88)	1973–1979	17–66 (41)	17–66 (40)	—	—	6–70 (18)	6–60 (13)	34	2 (10)	5	—	15	39	15
22	Engler et al[31]	1982	18 (—)	—	32–71 (54)	—	—	—	6–49 (25)	—	—	—(—)	—	—	18	—	—
23	Kuhn et al[32]	1982	258 (187)	1971–1980	8–68 (44)	(44 ± 10)	—	—	(36 ± 24)	(60 ± 36)	40	—(71)	—	—	258	69	18
24	Franciosa et al[33]	1983	87 (—)	1974–1981	—	—	—	—	1–41 (12)	(45 ± 43)	—	—(—)	—	—	22	30	—
25	Huang et al[34]	1983	35 (24)	1976–1980	22–72 (51)	—	—	—	4–74 (34)	—	—	—(11)	—	—	35	4	—
26	von Olshausen et al[35]	1984	60 (54)	1981–1982	18–60 (45)	—	—	—	1–18 (12)	—	—	—(6)	—	—	60	7	—
27	Meinertz et al[36,37]	1984	74 (—)	—	—	—(50)	—	—	2–21 (11)	(60 ± 37)	0	—(—)	—	—	74	19	—
28	Poll et al[38]	1984	11 (6)	1975–1983	27–74 (49)	—	—	—	—(21)—	—	—	—(5)	—	—	—	4	—
29	Unverferth et al[39,40]	1984	69 (49)	1979–1982	19–79 (45)	19–79 (45)			—12 (—)	(31 ± 46)	15	2 (20)	4	5	69	24	—
30	Wallis et al[41]	1984	50 (32)	1981–1983	11–68 (47)	—	—	—	1–26 (11)	—	—	—(18)	—	—	47	10	—
31	Holmes et al[42]	1985	15 (12)	1981–1983	34–66 (50)	—	—	—	6–21 (11)	—	3	1 (3)	0	0	5	5	5
32	Anderson et al[43,44]	1985	50 (33)	1981–1984	25–75 (50)	—	—	—	1–38 (19)	—	0	—	—	—	All > 30	11	—
33	Sanderson et al[45]	1985	20 (9)	—	—(34)	—	—	—	—	—	—	—	—	—	<9	—	—
34	Michels et al[46]	1985	169 (119)	1976–1982	<50	—	—	—	—	—	—	—	11	—	~80	—	—
35	O'Connell et al[47]	1986	69 (—)	—	—(44)	—	—	—	—	—	—	14 (—)	—	—	—	—	—

B = black; M = men; S = symptoms of cardiac dysfunction; W = white; — = no information available.

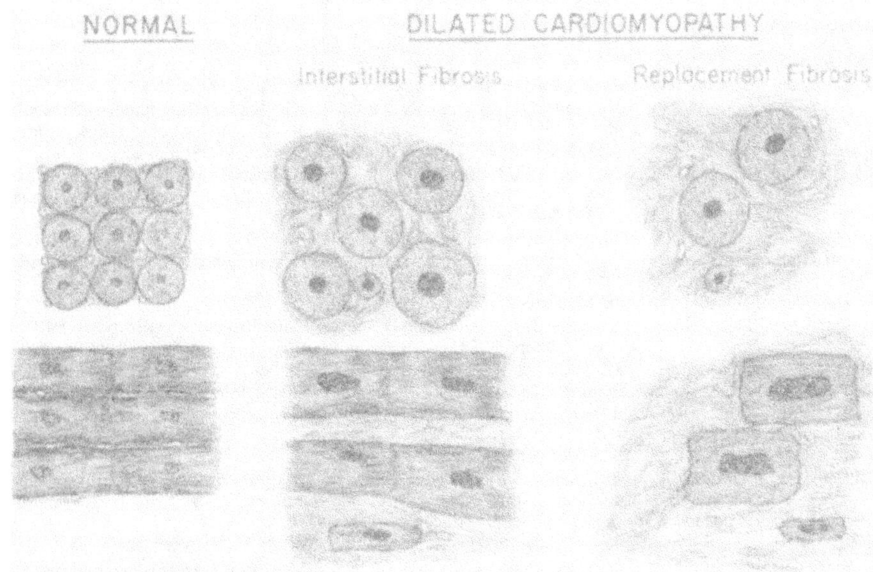

FIGURE 8. Diagram showing the various findings commonly observed in sections of left ventricular wall in the patients with idiopathic dilated cardiomyopathy. Some myocardial cells are larger than normal, others are smaller than normal and others have been replaced by fibrous tissue, which also is increased in the interstitum between the myocardial cells.

performed in 36. Segal et al[25] followed 115 patients with presumed IDC for a minimum of 5 years (median 8); 77 died and necropsies were performed in 48. Only 35 of the 48 had cardiomegaly at necropsy, an observation suggesting that some of the cases may not have been IDC. Shirey et al[26] studied 113 patients with IDC (only 48 of whom had CHF), following them up to 8 years (mean 5); 44 died but the number who had necropsy is unclear. Fuster et al[29] followed 104 patients from 6 to 20 years (median 11); 80 died and necropsy was performed in 39. Franciosa et al[33] followed 87 patients from 1 to 41 months (mean 12); 30 died but the number who had necropsy is unclear. These studies and many others are summarized in Table XI.

In contrast to the studies just mentioned, the starting point in the present study was the finding at necropsy of cardiac abnormalities fulfilling a rigorous definition of IDC. All 152 patients had hearts that were enlarged (>350 g in women and >400 g in men), all had dilated cardiac ventricular cavities, all had anatomically normal cardiac valves and pericardia, all had insignificant narrowing of the epicardial coronary arteries and none had an abnormality of a noncardiac body organ sufficient to cause the cardiac abnormalities. None during life had a systemic arterial indirect pressure >140/90 mm Hg during their last 3 months of life. Of the 148 patients with chronic CHF, the diagnosis of IDC was either made or suspected clinically. In the 4 patients whose initial manifestation of IDC was sudden death, diagnosis of IDC, of course, was not made until necropsy.

The findings in the present study are shown in detail in Tables I through X. This study provides the most extensive data for the natural history of IDC thus far presented. Clues to the cause of the IDC were not provided by this morphologically based study. Despite current interest in myocardial biopsy for identification of inflammatory myocardial injury in patients with IDC, this technique if applied shortly before death in the 152 patients included in this study probably would not have produced a diagnosis of "myocarditis" in a single patient. Our findings are in keeping with other observations regarding the infrequency of significant inflammatory cells in ventricular myocardium in patients with IDC.[48,49]

Although numerous reports have described electrocardiographic changes in patients with IDC (see references compiled by Perloff[50]), the present study is the first to describe total 12-lead QRS voltage in patients with IDC. A recent study by Odom et al[51] provided total 12-lead QRS voltage in a group of necropsy patients with no evidence of cardiac or pulmonary dysfunction or myocardial ischemia during life and all had normal-sized hearts at necropsy. Only 1 of the 30 subjects with normal-sized hearts had total 12-lead QRS voltage >175 mm (10 mm = 1 mV). The total 12-lead QRS voltage in 49 patients with IDC included in this study ranged from 75 to 250 mm (mean 153), a mean number within normal limits despite a mean heart weight for the group of >550 g. For comparison, Siegel and Roberts[52] determined total 12-lead QRS voltage in 50 patients aged 16 to 65 years with severe and fatal isolated aortic valve stenosis. The total 12-lead QRS voltage in these 50 patients ranged from 144 to 417 mm (mean 260), and the heart weights were similar to those in the present study of patients with IDC. In a study of total 12-lead QRS voltage in 30 patients with severe and fatal cardiac amyloidosis, Roberts and Waller[53] found total 12-lead QRS voltage to range from 60 to 199 mm (mean 104) despite a mean heart weight of the 30 patients of 532 g. Thus, by total 12-lead QRS voltage criteria, few IDC patients in the present study or patients with severe cardiac amyloidosis have "left ventricular hypertrophy" despite the occurrence of considerable cardiomegaly at necropsy.

References

1. Josserand E, Gallavardin L. De l' a systolie progressive des jeunes sujets par myocardite subaigue primitive. Arch Gen Med 1901;6:513–548.
2. Laubry C, Walser J. Sur un cas d'insuffisance cardiaque primitive. Les

myocardies. *Bull Mem Soc Med Hop Paris* 1925;49:409-418.

3. Whittle CH. "Idiopathic" hypertrophy of heart in young man. *Lancet* 1929;1:1354-1355.

4. Levy RL, Von Glahn WC. *Cardiac hypertrophy of unknown cause. A study of the clinical and pathologic features in ten adults. Am Heart J 1944;28:714-741.*

5. Serbin RA, Chojnacki B. *Idiopathic cardiac hypertrophy. Report of 3 cases. N Engl J Med 1955;252:10-13.*

6. Spodick DH, Littman D. *Idiopathic myocardial hypertrophy. Am J Cardiol 1958;1:610-623.*

7. Fowler NO, Gueron M, Rowlands DT Jr. *Primary myocardial disease. Dis Chest 1962;41:593-602.*

8. Fowler NO, Gueron M. *Primary myocardial disease. Circulation 1965;32:830-836.*

9. Dye CL, Rosenbaum D, Lowe JC, Behnke RH, Genovese PD. *Primary myocardial disease: part I. Clinical features. Ann Intern Med 1963;58:426-441.*

10. Dye CL, Genovese PD, Daly WJ, Behnke RH. *Primary myocardial disease. Part II. Hemodynamic alterations. Ann Intern Med 1963;58:442-453.*

11. Massumi RA, Rios JC, Gooch AS, Nutter D, De Vita VT, Datlow DW. *Primary myocardial disease. Report of fifty cases and review of the subject. Circulation 1965;31:19-41.*

12. Alexander CS. *Idiopathic heart disease: I. Analysis of 100 cases, with special reference to chronic alcoholism. Am J Med 1966;41:213-228.*

13. Goodwin JF. *Congestive and hypertrophic cardiomyopathies. A decade of study. Lancet 1970;1:732-739.*

14. Hamby RI. *Primary myocardial disease. A prospective clinical and hemodynamic evaluation in 100 patients. Medicine 1970;49:55-78.*

15. McDonald CD, Burch GE, Walsh JJ. *Alcoholic cardiomyopathy managed with prolonged bed rest. Ann Intern Med 1971;74:681-691.*

16. Demakis JG, Rahimtoola SH. *Peripartum cardiomyopathy. Circulation 1971;44:964-968.*

17. Shugoll GI, Bowen PJ, Moore JP, Lenkin ML. *Follow-up observations and prognosis in primary myocardial disease. Arch Intern Med 1972;129:67-72.*

18. Kreulen TH, Gorlin R, Herman MV. *Ventriculographic patterns and hemodynamics in primary myocardial disease. Circulation 1973;47:299-308.*

19. Feild BJ, Baxley WA, Russell RO Jr, Hood WP Jr, Holt JH, Dowling JT, Rackley CE. *Left ventricular function and hypertrophy in cardiomyopathy with depressed ejection fraction. Circulation 47:1022-1031.*

20. Demakis JG, Proskey A, Rahimtoola SH, Jamil M, Sutton GC, Rosen KM, Gunnar RM, Tobin JR Jr. *The natural course of alcoholic cardiomyopathy. Ann Intern Med 1974;80:293-297.*

21. Bashour TT, Fahdul H, Cheng TO. *Electrocardiographic abnormalities in alcoholic cardiomyopathy. A study of 65 patients. Chest 1975;68:24-27.*

22. Hatle L, Orjavik O, Storstein O. *Chronic myocardial disease. I. Clinical picture related to long-term prognosis. Acta Med Scand 1976;199:399-405.*

23. Hatle L, Stahe G, Storstein O. *Chronic myocardial disease. II. Hemodynamic findings related to long-term prognosis. Acta Med Scand 1976;199:407-411.*

24. Hess OM, Turina J, Goebel NH, Krayenbuhl HP. *Clinical course of congestive cardiomyopathy. Schweiz Med Wochenschr 1976;106:1577-1579.*

25. Segal JP, Stapleton JF, McClellan JR, Waller BF, Harvey WP. *Idiopathic cardiomyopathy: clinical features, prognosis and therapy. Curr Probl Cardiol 1978;3:1-49.*

26. Shirey EK, Proudfit WL, Hawk WA. *Primary myocardial disease. Correlation with clinical findings, angiographic and biopsy diagnosis. Follow-up of 139 patients. Am Heart J 1980;99:198-207.*

27. Koide T, Kato A, Takabatake Y, Iizuka M, Uchida Y, Ozeki K, Morooka S, Kakihana M, Serizawa T, Tanaka S, Ohya T, Momomura S, Murao S. *Variable prognosis in congestive cardiomyopathy. Role of left ventricular function, alcoholism, and pulmonary thrombosis. Jpn Heart J 1980;21:451-463.*

28. Convert G, Delaye J, Beaune J, Biron A, Gonin A. *Prognosis of primary nonobstructive cardiomyopathies. Arch Mal Coeur 1980;73:227-237.*

29. Fuster V, Gersh BJ, Giuliani ER, Tajik AJ, Brandenburg RO, Frye RL. *The natural history of idiopathic dilated cardiomyopathy. Am J Cardiol 1981; 47:525-531.*

30. Lengyel M, Kokeny M. *Follow-up study in congestive (dilated) cardiomyopathy. Acta Cardiol 1981;36:35-48.*

31. Engler R, Ray R, Higgins CB, McNally C, Buxton WH, Bhargava V, Shabetai R. *Clinical assessment and follow-up of functional capacity in patients with chronic congestive cardiomyopathy. Am J Cardiol 1982;49:1832-1837.*

32. Kuhn H, Becker R, Fischer J, Curtius JM, Losse B, Hort W, Loogen F. *Studies on the etiology, the clinical course and the prognosis of patients with dilated cardiomyopathy (DCM). Z Kardiol 1982;71:497-508.*

33. Franciosa JA, Wilen M, Ziesche S, Cohn JN. *Survival in men with severe chronic left ventricular failure due to either coronary heart disease or idiopathic dilated cardiomyopathy. Am J Cardiol 1983;51:831-836.*

34. Huang SK, Messer JV, Denes P. *Significance of ventricular tachycardia in idiopathic dilated cardiomyopathy: observations in 35 patients. Am J Cardiol 1983;51:507-518.*

35. Von Olshausen K, Schäfer A, Mehmel HC, Schwarz F, Senges J, Kübler W. *Ventricular arrhythmias in idiopathic dilated cardiomyopathy. Br Heart J 1984;51:195-201.*

36. Meinertz T, Hofmann T, Kasper W, Treese N, Bechtold H, Stienen U, Pop T, Leitner E-RV, Andresen D, Meyer J. *Significance of ventricular arrhythmias in idiopathic dilated cardiomyopathy. Am J Cardiol 1984;53:902-907.*

37. Meinertz T, Treese N, Kasper W, Geibel A, Hofmann T, Zehender M, Bohn D, Pop T, Just H. *Determinants of prognosis in idiopathic dilated cardiomyopathy as determined by programmed electrical stimulation. Am J Cardiol 1985;56:337-341.*

38. Poll DS, Marchlinski FE, Buxton AE, Doherty JU, Waxman HL, Josephson ME. *Sustained ventricular tachycardia in patients with idiopathic dilated cardiomyopathy; electrophysiologic testing and lack of response to antiarrhythmic drug therapy. Circulation 1984;70:451-456.*

39. Unverferth DV, Mehegan JP, Magorien RD, Unverferth BJ, Leier CV. *Regression of myocardial cellular hypertrophy with vasodilator therapy in chronic congestive heart failure associated with idiopathic dilated cardiomyopathy. Am J Cardiol 1983;51:1392-1398.*

40. Unverferth DV, Magorien RD, Moeschberg ML, Baker PB, Fetters JK, Leier CV. *Factors influencing the one-year mortality of dilated cardiomyopathy. Am J Cardiol 1984;54:147-152.*

41. Wallis DE, O'Connell JB, Henkin RE, Costanzo-Nordin MR, Scanlon PJ. *Segmental wall motion abnormalities in dilated cardiomyopathy: a common finding and good prognostic sign. JACC 1984;4:674-679.*

42. Holmes J, Kubo SH, Cody RJ, Kligfield P. *Arrhythmias in ischemic and nonischemic dilated cardiomyopathy: prediction of mortality by ambulatory electrocardiography. Am J Cardiol 1985;55:146-151.*

43. Anderson JL, Lutz JR, Gilbert EM, Sorensen SG, Yanowitz FG, Menlove RL, Bartholomew M. *A randomized trial of low-dose beta-blockade therapy for idiopathic dilated cardiomyopathy. Am J Cardiol 1985;55:471-475.*

44. Anderson JL, Carlquist JF, Lutz JR, DeWitt CW, Hammond EH. *HLA A, B and DR typing in idiopathic dilated cardiomyopathy: a search for immune response factors. Am J Cardiol 1984;53:1326-1330.*

45. Sanderson JE, Koech D, David I, Ojiambo HP. *T-lymphocyte subsets in idiopathic dilated cardiomyopathy. Am J Cardiol 1985;55:755-758.*

46. Michels VV, Driscoll DJ, Miller FA Jr. *Familial aggregation of idiopathic dilated cardiomyopathy. Am J Cardiol 1985;55:1232-1233.*

47. O'Connell JB, Costanzo-Nordin MR, Subramanian R, Robinson JA, Wallis DE, Scanlon PJ, Gunnar RM. *Peripartum cardiomyopathy: clinical, hemodynamic, histologic and prognostic characteristics. JACC 1986;8:52-56.*

48. Cassling RS, Linder J, Sears TD, Waller BF, Rogler WC, Wilson JE, Kugler JD, Kay HD, Dillon JC, Slack JD, McManus BM. *Quantitative evaluation of inflammation in biopsy specimens from idiopathically failing or irritable hearts: experience in 80 pediatric and adult patients. Am Heart J 1985; 110:713-720.*

49. Tazelaar HD, Billingham ME. *Leukocytic infiltrates in idiopathic dilated cardiomyopathy. Am J Surg Pathol 1986;10:405-412.*

50. Perloff JK. *The cardiomyopathies: dilated and restrictive. Circulation 1981;63:1189-1198.*

51. Odom H II, Davis JL, Dinh H, Baker BJ, Roberts WC, Murphy ML. *QRS voltage measurements in autopsied men free of cardiopulmonary disease: a basis for evaluating total QRS voltage as an index of left ventricular hypertrophy. Am J Cardiol 1986;58:801-804.*

52. Siegel RJ, Roberts WC. *Electrocardiographic observations in severe aortic valve stenosis: correlative necropsy study to clinical, hemodynamic, and ECG variables demonstrating relation of 12-lead QRS amplitude to peak systolic transaortic pressure gradient. Am Heart J 1982;103:298-301.*

53. Roberts WC, Waller BF. *Cardiac amyloidosis causing cardiac dysfunction: analysis of 54 necropsy patients. Am J Cardiol 1983;52:137-146.*

Usefulness of Total 12-Lead QRS Voltage Compared with Other Criteria for Determining Left Ventricular Hypertrophy in Hypertrophic Cardiomyopathy: Analysis of 57 Patients Studied at Necropsy

ALLEN L. DOLLAR, M.D., WILLIAM C. ROBERTS, M.D. *Bethesda, Maryland*

PURPOSE: The sensitivity of electrocardiographic indicators of left ventricular (LV) hypertrophy is known to be rather poor. To date, no study has undertaken a comparison of the various electrocardiographic criteria for LV hypertrophy among patients with hypertrophic cardiomyopathy (HC). In this study, we compared the sensitivity of the total 12-lead QRS amplitude with the sensitivity of certain standard electrocardiographic criteria for LV hypertrophy in necropsy patients with HC.

MATERIALS AND METHODS: A total of 57 hearts were studied. The last technically satisfactory electrocardiogram available from each necropsy patient was used. Electrocardiographic criteria employed to diagnose LV hypertrophy included the Sokolow and Lyon index, the Romhilt-Estes voltage criteria, the Romhilt-Estes point score, the ratio of RV6:RV5 greater than 1 proposed by Holt and Spodick, and a method utilizing the sum of the amplitudes of the QRS complexes of all 12 leads.

RESULTS: The total 12-lead QRS amplitude ranged from 66 to 339 mm (mean: 197 mm) (10 mm = 1 mV). Using 175 mm as the upper limit of normal, this technique yielded a sensitivity of 53%, which was the highest sensitivity of any criteria tested. The Sokolow-Lyon index had a sensitivity of 39%; the Romhilt-Estes voltage criteria, 37%; the Romhilt-Estes point score system, 49%; and the criterion of RV6 more than RV5, 39%. No correlation was found between total 12-lead QRS voltage and heart weight, LV free wall thickness, LV peak systolic and end-diastolic pressures, or LV outflow tract peak systolic pressure gradient. The 10 patients (18%) with transmural LV scars had significantly lower total 12-lead QRS voltage than did the 48 patients (78%) without such scars (155 mm versus 205 mm, p = 0.02).

CONCLUSION: Total 12-lead QRS amplitude more than 175 mm is a useful indicator of LV hypertrophy and, among patients with HC, it is more sensitive than other more commonly employed criteria.

From the Pathology Branch, National Heart, Lung, and Blood Institute, National Institutes of Health, Bethesda, Maryland. Requests for reprints should be addressed to Pathology Branch, Building 10, Room 2N258, National Institutes of Health, Bethesda, Maryland 20892. Manuscript submitted March 9, 1989, and accepted in revised form July 10, 1989.

Electrocardiographic indicators of left ventricular (LV) hypertrophy are known to be relatively nonspecific and insensitive. The sensitivity of these criteria also varies with the various etiologies of LV hypertrophy [1]. Although many studies have described electrocardiographic abnormalities in hypertrophic cardiomyopathy (HC) [2–12], none have compared the various electrocardiographic criteria for LV hypertrophy among patients with HC. In this investigation, we describe electrocardiographic findings in 57 patients with HC studied both clinically and at necropsy and determine which electrocardiographic criteria are most sensitive for LV hypertrophy in these patients.

MATERIALS AND METHODS

From July 1959 to July 1988, the hearts of 210 patients with HC were studied in the Pathology Branch, National Heart, Lung, and Blood Institutes (NHLBI), Bethesda, Maryland. Of this number, 179 were 12 years of age or older and, of these, electrocardiograms obtained during the last year of life were available in 57. Most of the other 122 patients had not been seen at the National Institutes of Health (NIH) during their last year of life or they had never been studied at NIH and only their hearts had been submitted to the Pathology Branch (NHLBI). Various clinical, electrocardiographic, and morphologic observations in these 57 patients are summarized in **Table I**. Of the 57 patients, 31 died shortly after a cardiac operation, and the other 26 never had a cardiac operation. Of these 26, 13 died suddenly outside the hospital, six of progressive congestive heart failure, two of consequences of strokes, and five of noncardiac causes. The last technically satisfactory electrocardiogram available from each patient was analyzed. The interval from the studied electrocardiogram until death ranged from 0 to 327 days (average, 37 days). In the 31 patients who died perioperatively, the immediate preoperative 12-lead electrocardiogram was analyzed.

The amplitudes of the QRS complexes were measured from the peak of the R wave to the nadir of either the Q wave or the S wave, whichever was deeper, according to the method of Siegel and Roberts [13] **(Figure 1)**. The electrocardiographic criteria used to diagnose LV hypertrophy included the Sokolow and Lyon index [14] (sum of SV1 plus the larger of RV5 or RV6 greater than 35 mm), the Romhilt-Estes voltage criteria [15] (either tallest limb-lead R or deepest limb-lead S greater than 20 mm or tallest RV4-6 or deepest SV1-3 greater than 25 mm), the Romhilt-Estes point score [15] (a system utilizing ST-T segment changes, QRS axis, left atrial abnormality, QRS duration, and duration of the intrinsicoid deflection in addition to electrocardiographic voltage criteria), the ra-

TABLE I

Clinical, Electrocardiographic, and Morphologic Observations in 57 Patients with HC

Patient	Age (years)	Interval ECG-Death (days)	HR (beats/minute)	Rhythm	QRS Axis (o)	PR	Interval(s) QRS (BBB)	QTc	P Wave Abnormality	Romhilt-Estes Score	Sokolow-Lyon Index	Total QRS Voltage (mm)	HW (g)	Thickness (mm) VS	Thickness (mm) LV	Transmural LV Scar	Interval CC-Death (days)	RV (s/d)	LV (s/d)	SA (s/d)	LV-SA psg (rest)	LV-SA psg (p)	CI
Women																							
1	36	1	80	S	−90	0.20	0.12 (R)	0.34	1	6	3	68	500	22	15	+	—	—	—	—	—	—	—
2	65	0	80	AF	−45	—	0.16 (L)	0.42	—	4	13	87	475	19	24	—	210	75/20	190/8	195/90	0	100	1.4
3	30	9	125	S	−60	0.24	0.14 (R)	0.46	1	6	3	111	510	15	18	+	—	—	—	—	—	—	—
4	45	7	50	S	70	0.16	0.08	0.40	1	3	24	131	290	15	15	—	26	20/4	110/12	105/60	5	115	2.9
5	46	10	100	S	−60	0.22	0.12 (L)	0.46	1	3	23	134	460	18	17	+	—	—	—	—	—	—	—
6	61	2	60	S	−30	0.20	0.12 (L)	0.46	—	3	32	136	580	28	17	—	192	30/6	110/30	100/70	10	125	2.4
7	21	120	78	S	90	0.20	0.12	0.55	1	4	7	144	390	27	18	—	270	30/6	170/18	90/—	80	105	—
8	54	10	72	S	−45	0.22	0.10	0.48	1	6	26	150	455	20	20	—	30	55/5	230/18	120/65	120	—	3.4
9	65	21	100	S	30	0.12	0.06	0.39	1	1	27	151	430	19	15	—	6	65/12	260/45	110/65	150	—	2
10	62	48	72	S	30	0.20	0.10	0.44	—	2	23	153	450	19	15	—	60	40/4	225/14	135/90	90	150	2.8
11	52	19	55	S	−30	0.20	0.12	0.48	1	6	27	158	470	22	20	—	21	65/8	140/28	120/70	20	80	—
12	19	5	85	S	−20	0.16	0.08	0.45	b	1	40	160	360	25	20	—	30	50/12	210/28	130/80	80	110	—
13	65	1	54	S	60	0.20	0.10	0.42	—	2	26	166	615	25	20	—	5	85/24	240/25	120/80	140	—	1.5
14	25	33	90	S	0	0.22	0.10	0.44	1	4	23	171	720	38	25	—	—	—	—	—	—	—	—
15	20	68	52	S	−90	0.16	0.12	0.48	—	4	14	173	1230	45	32	+	—	—	—	—	—	—	—
16	59	3	67	S	−30	0.20	0.16 (L)	0.55	1	6	31	182	610	23	23	+	6	98/10	275/30	100/60	160	—	1.5
17	87	8	85	S	−30	0.16	0.10	0.38	—	4	32	190	460	26	20	—	—	—	—	140/50	—	—	—
18	19	12	80	S	0	0.20	0.12	0.44	1	4	34	195	730	—	—	—	120	28/8	260/14	98/75	162	—	3.1
19	25	265	67	S	0	0.20	0.16 (R)	0.49	1	4	26	198	650	18	15	+	—	—	—	—	—	—	—
20	70	15	120	AF	0	—	0.08	0.40	—	4	51	205	450	31	29	—	2	—	160/20	95/70	65	—	1.9
21	56	2	65	S	45	0.18	0.10	0.42	—	8	37	206	310	18	19	—	7	—	165/14	115/70	40	90	—
22	61	1	65	S	0	0.20	0.08	0.46	1	3	39	207	500	19	16	—	90	26/11	188/10	108/80	80	115	2.5
23	58	327	82	S	0	0.22	0.12	0.47	1	7	31	214	900	—	—	—	—	—	—	—	—	—	—
24	65	18	70	S	20	0.18	0.10	0.43	1	8	45	219	410	26	22	—	5	32/—	210/20	110/60	100	140	—
25	35	41	78	S	60	0.16	0.08	0.43	—	1	42	232	600	35	20	—	—	—	—	—	—	—	—
26	40	2	82	S	45	0.20	0.10	0.51	1	7	48	240	475	18	18	—	5	24/9	208/12	104/—	104	115	—
27	70	5	70	S	120	0.20	0.12	0.48	—	4	25	263	664	29	24	—	4	115/20	245/20	120/65	125	—	1.2
28	58	23	90	S	90	0.18	0.12	0.39	1	8	44	265	490	22	15	—	300	—	205/5	108/53	100	—	2.5
29	64	2	130	S	45	0.12	0.08	0.41	—	4	44	266	355	30	25	—	1	42/6	230/12	160/70	60	—	—
30	81	1	60	S	0	0.12	0.20 (L)	0.44	1	7	55	272	550	25	13	—	—	—	—	—	—	—	—
31	59	115	95	S	30	0.20	0.12	0.45	1	8	58	277	460	20	15	—	450	—/14	135/19	75/58	60	84	1.8
32	62	3	68	S	−45	0.14	0.12	0.47	1	9	38	281	730	30	25	—	90	22/2	160/10	140/70	20	68	2.3
33	25	1	73	S	−30	0.20	0.12	0.42	1	3	38	286	400	22	22	—	270	—	130/38	130/80	0	0	—
34	64	4	70	S	−25	0.20	0.12 (L)	0.45	1	7	44	290	670	22	21	—	5	36/18	180/22	145/50	35	84	2
35	56	18	42	S	15	0.16	0.12	0.42	1	8	64	314	680	33	25	—	180	50/3	230/25	105/60	130	—	3
36	61	10	60	S	15	0.19	0.08	0.44	—	4	60	327	665	25	18	—	8	80/10	200/26	110/60	90	—	1.7
Mean	51	34	77		4	0.19	0.11	0.43		5	33	201	547	25	20	—	92	51/10	195/20	118/68	78	99	2.2

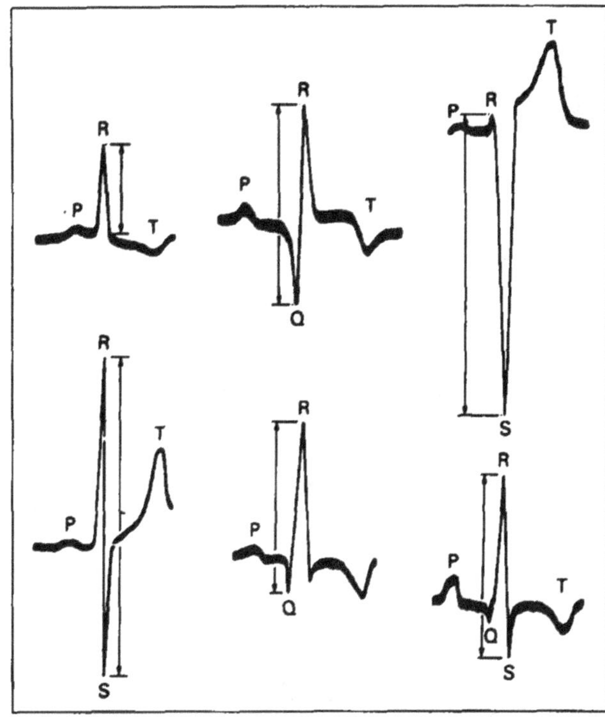

Figure 1. Various electrocardiographic QRS complexes showing how the voltage (in mm) was measured. Reproduced with permission from [13].

tio of RV6:RV5 greater than 1 as proposed by Holt and Spodick [16], and a method utilizing the sum of the amplitudes of the QRS complexes of all 12 leads. Patients with bundle branch block were included in all analyses. Amplitudes were standardized to 10 mm equaling 1 mV.

At necropsy, the heart weight used was that of the formalin-fixed heart. The fixation period before the heart was weighed varied from about two to 20 days, a period during which heart weight of the fresh specimen is the same as the fixed specimen.

Statistical methods included linear regression analysis, unpaired two-tailed Student's t-test, and chi-square analysis applied where appropriate. Significance was determined if the p value was <0.05.

RESULTS

The 57 patients ranged in age from 14 to 87 years (mean: 49 years). Of these, 21 (37%) were men and 36 (63%) were women; 53 (93%) were white and four (7%) were black. Heart weights ranged from 290 to 1,230 g (mean: 593 g). The LV free wall thicknesses ranged from 1.2 to 3.2 cm (mean: 2.0 cm), and the ventricular septa, from 1.5 to 4.5 cm (mean: 2.4 cm). Cardiac catheterization data within two years of death were available in 42 patients. Left ventricular to aortic (or another systemic artery) peak systolic pressure gradients greater than 10 mm Hg were present at rest in 32 (77%) patients and with provocation in 35 patients (85%). The resting peak systolic gradients ranged from 12 to 162 mm Hg (mean: 79 mm Hg), and the provoked gradients, from 40 to 190 mm Hg (mean: 104 mm Hg). There were no differences between patients with and without LV-to-systemic arterial peak systolic gradients at rest with regards to heart weight, ventricular

Men																							
1	59	1	57	J	130	—	0.18 (L)	0.47	—	1	13	107	670	20	16	—	720	55/—	—	—	0	0	—
2	33	13	74	S	−60	0.18	0.10	0.44	l	7	11	110	450	27	13	—	14	—	—	—	0	0	2
3	60	54	87	S	−90	0.18	0.16 (R)	0.46	l	6	12	112	475	16	12	+	—	—	—	100/65	—	—	—
4	45	122	87	AF	−60	—	0.20	0.55	—	3	21	120	760	20	15	+	515	—	120/25	120/75	0	0	—
5	56	99	150	S	−30	0.14	0.12 (L)	0.44	l	4	23	134	680	25	18	—	630	44/8	220/12	130/80	90	190	2
6	55	27	60	S	30	0.16	0.10	0.44	l	5	25	151	790	22	20	—	—	31/10	200/35	145/85	50	75	—
7	54	96	150	S	0	0.16	0.06	0.44	l	1	27	161	515	20	25	—	671	40/—	—	—	80	—	—
8	41	2	75	AF	30	—	0.10	0.45	—	2	25	162	700	25	21	—	4	—	—	—	—	—	—
9	57	219	90	AF	−30	—	0.12	0.44	—	4	21	163	580	20	18	—	—	—	—	—	—	—	—
10	50	2	95	S	20	0.22	0.12	0.38	l	5	43	168	655	25	16	—	—	—	150/15	136/85	40	100	—
11	51	18	110	S	30	0.12	0.16 (L)	0.49	—	5	32	170	890	20	20	—	90	41/8	115/12	115/60	0	120	2.2
12	68	2	85	S	−30	0.16	0.08	0.45	l	5	28	170	540	21	24	—	14	32/9	189/4	163/69	26	100	—
13	58	66	55	S	−45	0.22	0.16	0.46	l	10	12	183	585	20	15	+	—	49/9	180/40	110/80	70	110	2.6
14	63	15	85	S	0	0.24	0.12	0.48	—	2	36	207	735	25	20	—	180	52/13	—/24	120/80	50	80	—
15	29	2	70	S	0	0.22	0.10	0.43	l	8	46	228	995	21	21	—	30	—	160/13	125/65	30	130	—
16	24	4	56	S	−90	0.24	0.16 (R)	0.46	l	9	30	232	750	33	24	—	30	28/7	188/8	110/60	76	110	1.9
17	55	45	60	S	−45	0.20	0.16 (L)	0.50	l	10	56	237	735	30	25	—	90	40/5	110/12	110/65	0	0	2.8
18	41	6	50	S	20	0.18	0.10	0.38	l	5	38	266	750	28	19	+	396	22/5	140/24	128/70	12	55	—
19	29	17	72	S	−60	0.28	0.12	0.42	—	3	28	279	450	28	20	—	150	100/15	118/24	118/70	0	40	4.1
20	21	38	60	S	−45	0.28	0.12 (R)	0.44	l	10	30	281	1070	33	24	—	30	40/9	—	—	—	—	3
21	14	18	55	S	60	0.12	0.08	0.38	l	7	48	339	325	17	12	—	30	44/9	—	—	—	—	—
Mean	46	41	80		−13	0.19	0.12	0.45		5	29	190	671	33	19		225	44/9	158/19	124/72	33	79	2.6

+ = present; AF = atrial fibrillation; b = biatrial enlargement; BBB = bundle branch block; bpm = beats per minute; CC = cardiac catheterization; CI = cardiac index in $L/minute/m^2$; HR = heart rate; HW = heart weight; I = intraventricular conduction delay; J = junctional; L = left; l = left atrial abnormality; p = peak; psg = peak systolic gradient; QTc = QT interval corrected for heart rate; R = right; S = sinus; s/d = peak systole/end diastole; SA = systemic artery; VS = ventricular septum.

The cardiac rhythm was sinus in 51 patients (89%), atrial fibrillation in five (9%), and junctional in one (2%). A history of atrial fibrillation was present in 17 (30%) patients. Left atrial abnormality was present in 37 (73%) of the 51 patients in sinus rhythm and biatrial abnormality in one (2%). The QRS complex width was 0.12 seconds or greater in 33 patients (58%), with a left bundle branch block pattern in 10 (18%), a right bundle branch block pattern in six (11%), and a nonspecific conduction delay in 17 (30%).

The total 12-lead QRS amplitude in the 57 patients ranged from 66 to 339 mm (mean: 197 mm). (The upper limit of normal for total QRS amplitude of 175 mm was first suggested by Roberts and Day [17] and validated by Odom *et al* [18] who found that this upper limit yielded a specificity of 93% in a group of normal hearts.) Of the criteria examined, the total 12-lead QRS amplitude had the highest sensitivity (53%) (**Table II**). Although the total 12-lead QRS amplitude was the most sensitive criterion tested, there was no correlation of heart weight with the total 12-lead QRS amplitude (**Figure 2**). This observation was demonstrated both by linear regression analysis and by comparison of the mean heart weights for those patients with total 12-lead QRS amplitudes greater than 175 mm to those with amplitudes equal to or less than 175 mm, and there was no difference in mean heart weights (605 and 579 g, respectively, p = 0.6). Total QRS amplitude also was compared to ventricular wall thicknesses, LV peak systolic and end-diastolic pressures at rest, and provoked LV outflow tract gradients using linear regression analysis. No comparison was significant.

Transmural (involving all the inner one half and a portion of the outer one half of the LV free wall or ventricular septum) scars were present in 10 of the 57 patients (six women, four men). The mean heart weight of the group with transmural LV or septal scars was not significantly different from that of the group without scars. There was, however, a significantly lower total 12-lead QRS amplitude in the group with transmural scars (155 mm versus 205 mm, p = 0.02) and a lower mean Sokolow-Lyon index (11.6 versus 13.2, p = <0.001). The mean Romhilt-Estes score was not statistically different in the two groups.

COMMENTS

This study examined total 12-lead QRS voltage and other more standard electrocardiographic criteria for diagnosing LV hypertrophy in patients with HC studied at necropsy (Table II). The highest sensitivity among the criteria for LV hypertrophy in patients with HC was achieved by the total 12-lead QRS voltage (53%). In the patients with HC, the voltage criteria of Romhilt and Estes and the Sokolow-Lyon index were relatively insensitive (37% and 39%, respectively). The criterion of RV6 greater than RV5 proposed by Holt and Spodick [16] was 39% sensitive. Koito and Spodick [19] reported an overall 52% sensitivity of the criterion of RV6 greater than RV5 in a group of patients with LV hypertrophy of various etiologies but noted that there was a trend toward less sensitivity of this criterion in patients with HC. Several previous studies have evaluated the sensitivity of these criteria in patients with HC [4–6,9–11], and they are summarized in **Table III**.

Our study is the first to examine total 12-lead QRS

TABLE II

Sensitivity of Electrocardiographic Criteria for Diagnosing LV Hypertrophy in 57 Necropsy Patients with HC

Electrocardiographic Criteria	Number (%) of Patients Above Normal Limit
Total 12-lead QRS amplitude >175 mm	30 (53)
Romhilt-Estes Point Score ≥5	28 (49)
Sokolow-Lyon Index (SV1 + RV5 or RV6 [larger] > 35 mm)	22 (39)
RV6:RV5 > 1	22 (39)
Romhilt-Estes Voltage Criteria (either tallest limb-lead R or deepest limb-lead S > 20 mm or tallest RV1-3 or deepest SV1-3 > 25 mm)	21 (37)

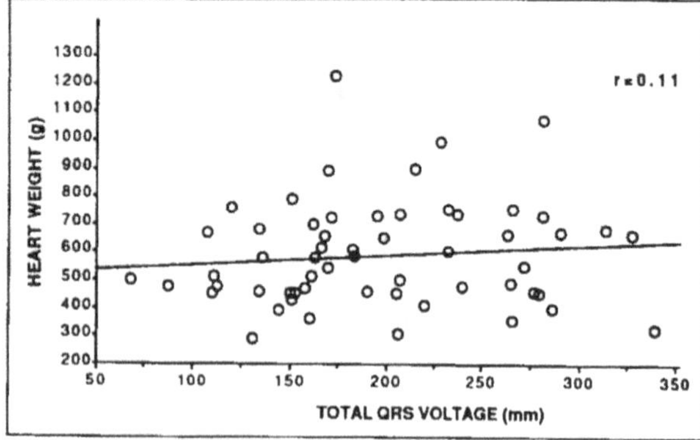

Figure 2. Relation between total QRS amplitude and heart weight at necropsy in 57 patients with HC who had an electrocardiogram recorded within one year of death.

TABLE III

Comparison of Previous Studies Determining the Sensitivity of Various Criteria for LV Hypertrophy in HC

References	Number of Patients Meeting Criteria for LV Hypertrophy/Number of Patients Studied (Sensitivity)
Sokolow-Lyon Index	
Braunwald *et al* [4]	47/64 (73%)
Harmjanz *et al* [5]	9/25 (36%)
McKenna *et al* [9]	45/100 (45%)
Dollar and Roberts (present study)	22/57 (39%)
Romhilt-Estes Point Score (≥5 points)	
Walston *et al* [6]	22/33 (67%)
Maron *et al* [10]	72/153 (47%)
Alcini *et al* [11]	8/20 (40%)
Dollar and Roberts (present study)	28/57 (49%)

septal thickness, total QRS amplitude, and Romhilt-Estes scores. The Sokolow-Lyon index was significantly different in the patients with and without obstruction: the mean index was 37 in the obstructive group and 28 in the non-obstructive group (p <0.02). Mean values for age, heart rate, axis, electrocardiographic intervals, total 12-lead QRS amplitude, ventricular wall thickness, LV outflow tract gradient, and heart weight were compared between men and women. Only mean heart weight was significantly different between the two groups: mean heart rate of men equal to 671 g and that of women equal to 547 g (p <0.02).

TABLE IV

Comparison of the Sensitivity of Total QRS Voltage in Identifying LV Hypertrophy of Various Etiologies

	Valvular Aortic Stenosis (n = 30)	Aortic Regurgitation (n = 12)	HC (n = 57)	Idiopathic Dilated Cardiomyopathy (n = 49)	Amyloid (n = 30)	Normal (n = 30)
Age (years)	52 ± 5	52 ± 6	49 ± 17	48 ± 15	58 ± 17	56 ± 10
Heart weight (g)	630 ± 14	745 ± 132	593 ± 189	614 ± 126	532 ± 139	393 ± 57
Total QRS voltage (mm)	245 ± 56	274 ± 87	197 ± 67	153 ± 48	104 ± 36	127 ± 29
Number > 175 mm (%)	43 (93)	27 (90)	30 (53)	16 (33)	2 (7)	2 (7)

voltage in patients with HC. Several studies, however, have evaluated the relation between the total 12-lead QRS voltage and heart weight at necropsy in other cardiac diseases (**Table IV**) [13,17,18,20,21]. Measurement of the total 12-lead QRS voltage provides a sensitive marker for LV hypertrophy among patients with aortic stenosis and aortic regurgitation (93% and 90%, respectively). Among patients with HC, this criterion is moderately sensitive (53%), albeit the most sensitive of the criteria examined. Total QRS amplitude in patients with idiopathic dilated cardiomyopathy identified 33% as having LV hypertrophy. As expected, a low total amplitude was observed in patients with cardiac amyloidosis severe enough to cause cardiac dysfunction.

REFERENCES

1. Murphy ML, Thenabadu PN, de Soyza N, Meade J, Doherty JE, Baker BJ: Sensitivity of electrocardiographic criteria for left ventricular hypertrophy according to type of cardiac disease. Am J Cardiol 1985; 55: 545–549.

2. Braunwald E, Morrow AG, Cornell WP, Aygen MM, Hilbish TF: Idiopathic hypertrophic subaortic stenosis. Clinical, hemodynamic and angiographic manifestations. Am J Med 1960; 29: 924–945.

3. Estes EH Jr, Whalen RE, Roberts SR Jr, McIntosh HD: The electrocardiographic and vectorcardiographic findings in idiopathic hypertrophic subaortic stenosis. Am Heart J 1963; 65: 155–161.

4. Braunwald E, Lambrew CT, Rockoff SD, Ross J Jr, Morrow AC: Idiopathic hypertrophic subaortic stenosis. I. A description of the disease based upon an analysis of 64 patients. Circulation 1964; 30 (suppl IV): IV-3–IV-119.

5. Harmjanz D, Bottcher D, Schertlein G: Correlations of electrocardiographic pattern, shape of ventricular septum and isovolumetric relaxation time in irregular hypertrophic cardiomyopathy (obstructive cardiomyopathy). Br Heart J 1971; 33: 928–937.

6. Walston A II, Behar VS, Wagner GS, Greenfield JC Jr: Electrocardiographic and hemodynamic correlations in patients with idiopathic hypertrophic subaortic stenosis. Am Heart J 1976; 91: 11–17.

7. Savage DD, Seides SF, Clark CE, et al: Electrocardiographic findings in patients with obstructive and nonobstructive hypertrophic cardiomyopathy. Circulation 1978; 58: 402–408.

8. McKenna W, Deanfield J, Faruqui A, England D, Oakley C, Goodwin J: Prognosis in hypertrophic cardiomyopathy: role of age and clinical, electrocardiographic and hemodynamic features. Am J Cardiol 1981; 47: 532–538.

9. McKenna WJ, Borggrefe M, England D, Deanfield J, Oakley CM, Goodwin JF: The natural history of left ventricular hypertrophy in hypertrophic cardiomyopathy: an electrocardiographic study. Circulation 1982; 66: 1233–1240.

10. Maron BJ, Wolfson JK, Ciro E, Spirito P: Relation of electrocardiographic abnormalities and patterns of left ventricular hypertrophy identified by 2-dimensional echocardiography in patients with hypertrophic cardiomyopathy. Am J Cardiol 1983; 51: 189–194.

11. Alcini E, Mottironi P, Martinelli MM, Ale E, Aratari D: Hypertrophic cardiomyopathy: electrocardiographic and 2-dimensional echocardiographic correlations. Panminerva Med 1984; 27: 165–173.

12. Nair CK, Kudesia V, Hansen D, et al: Echocardiographic and electrocardiographic characteristics of patients with hypertrophic cardiomyopathy with and without mitral annular calcium. Am J Cardiol 1987; 59: 1428–1430.

13. Siegel RJ, Roberts WC: Electrocardiographic observations in severe aortic valve stenosis: correlative necropsy study to clinical, hemodynamic, and ECG variables demonstrating relation of 12-lead QRS amplitude to peak systolic transaortic pressure gradient. Am Heart J 1982; 103: 210–221.

14. Sokolow M, Lyon TP: The ventricular complex in left ventricular hypertrophy as obtained by unipolar precordial and limb leads. Am Heart J 1949; 37: 161–186.

15. Romhilt DW, Estes EH Jr: A point-score system for the ECG diagnosis of left ventricular hypertrophy. Am Heart J 1968; 75: 752–758.

16. Holt DH, Spodick DH: The RV6:RV5 voltage ratio in left ventricular hypertrophy. Am Heart J 1962; 63: 65–66.

17. Roberts WC, Day PJ: Electrocardiographic observations in clinically isolated, pure, chronic, severe aortic regurgitation: analysis of 30 necropsy patients aged 19 to 65 years. Am J Cardiol 1985; 55: 432–438.

18. Odom H II, Davis JL, Dinh H, Baker BJ, Roberts WC, Murphy ML: QRS voltage measurements in autopsied men free of cardiopulmonary disease: a basis for evaluating total QRS voltage as an index of left ventricular hypertrophy. Am J Cardiol 1986; 58: 801–804.

19. Koito H, Spodick DH: Accuracy of the RV6:RV5 voltage ratio for increased left ventricular mass. Am J Cardiol 1988; 62: 985–987.

20. Roberts WC, Waller BF: Cardiac amyloidosis causing cardiac dysfunction: analysis of 54 necropsy patients. Am J Cardiol 1983; 52: 137–146.

21. Roberts WC, Siegel RJ, McManus BM: Idiopathic dilated cardiomyopathy: analysis of 152 necropsy patients. Am J Cardiol 1987; 60: 1340–1355.

Usefulness of Total 12-Lead QRS Voltage in Diagnosing Left Ventricular Hypertrophy in Clinically Isolated, Pure, Chronic, Severe Mitral Regurgitation

Brian N. Glick, MD,* and William C. Roberts, MD

Electrocardiographic criteria for diagnosing left ventricular (LV) hypertrophy are known to be relatively nonspecific and insensitive. Several studies from this laboratory[1–7] and elsewhere[8–10] have described total 12-lead QRS voltage in various cardiac diseases, and most have found this criterion to be more sensitive than previously described criteria. We examined total 12-lead QRS voltage in 24 necropsied patients with chronic, pure, isolated mitral regurgitation, and compared its sensitivity to the Sokolow-Lyon and Romhilt-Estes criteria for diagnosis of LV hypertrophy.

From the Pathology Branch, National Heart, Lung, and Blood Institute, National Institutes of Health, Bethesda, Maryland 20892. Manuscript received April 24, 1992; revised manuscript received and accepted May 28, 1992.

*Cardiology Fellow, Georgetown University Medical Center, Washington, D.C.

The 24 patients ranged in age from 21 to 84 years (mean 42); 13 (54%) were women and 11 (46%) were men (Table I). All 24 patients had clinical evidence of mitral regurgitation for >5 months. None had clinical or hemodynamic evidence of associated mitral stenosis, and none had evidence of aortic valve dysfunction. Additionally, all 24 patients had New York Heart Association functional class III or IV congestive heart failure, and 9 (38%) had mitral valve replacement or repair from 1 to 120 days (mean 25) before death. Cardiac catheterization was performed in 19 (79%) of the 24 patients and the recorded pressures are listed in Table I. To be included in this study, 1 or more 12-lead electrocardiograms recorded within 400 days of death (always before a mitral valve operation) had to be available for examination. The amplitude of the QRS was measured from the peak of the R wave to the nadir of either the Q wave or

TABLE I Clinical and Hemodynamic Data in the 24 Patients with Clinically Isolated, Pure, Chronic Mitral Regurgitation

| | | | | | | | | Pressures (mm Hg) | | | | |
| | | | | | | | | LA | | | | |
Case No.	Necropsy No.	Age (yr)	Gender	Valvular Etiology	Duration of Cardiac Symptoms (yrs)	MVR	Interval MVR to Death (days)	m	v	LV (s/d)	SA (s/d)	RV (s/d)
1	A63–234	21	F	Rheumatic	11	+	2	15	30*	—	120/70	40/3
2	A56–200	23	F	Rheumatic	12	0	—	31	55*	—	125/75	60/7
3	A60–208	23	F	Rheumatic	8	0	—	30	45*	—	125/75	48/12
4	A70–221	24	M	Rheumatic	5	+	17	16	28*	90/8	100/60	30/6
5	A69–240	30	F	Rheumatic	6	+	2	30	65*	102/14	110/78	58/12
6	A60–131	30	M	Rheumatic	5	+	1	30	48	115/20	135/80	—
7	A57–150	31	F	Rheumatic	7	0	—	23	44*	—	118/74	—
8	A58–213	33	F	Rheumatic	3/4	0	—	—	—	—	115/80	—
9	A60–270	38	F	Rheumatic	9	0	—	32	60	115/15	120/70	—
10	A62–232	38	M	Rheumatic	2	+	7	20	39	108/16	120/84	48/8
11	A59–39	39	F	Rheumatic	6	0	—	30	55	125/20	150/65	35/4
12	A64–98	41	F	Rheumatic	6	+	1	—	—	106/15	106/60	34/10
13	A67–178	43	M	Rheumatic	3	0	—	16	28	148/13	150/84	43/4
14	A54–21	49	M	Rheumatic	3	0	—	26	60*	—	170/100	64/0
15	A63–24	28	M	MVP-RCT	1	0	—	—	—	—	130/80	23/5
16	312579	60	F	MVP-RCT	6	0	—	—	—	—	120/70	—
17	A69–62	65	M	MVP-RCT	3/4	+	120	—	—	—	—	—
18	226434	84	M	MVP-RCT	20	0	—	—	—	—	135/80	—
19	A56–59	41	M	MVP+RCT	2	0	—	32	39*	—	150/70	110/21
20	A70–244	56	M	MVP+RCT	7	+	28	25	40	100/12	110/65	42/6
21	A70–280	60	M	MVP+RCT	4	+	50	17	20*	118/17	120/80	110/21
22	A62–19	24	F	IE+RCT	3/4	0	—	27	66	108/11	108/85	—
23	A75–63	54	F	IE+RCT	2	0	—	—	—	110/15	120/70	50/10
24	A72–8	64	F	IE+RCT	12	0	—	38	50*	120/20	120/70	85/18
	Mean	42	—	—	6	—	25	23	43	113/14	125/75	55/9

*Pulmonary arterial wedge rather than left atrial pressures.
ECG = electrocardiogram; IE = infective endocarditis; LA = left atrium; LV = left ventricle; m = mean; MVP = mitral valve prolapse; MVR = mitral valve replacement; RCT = ruptured chordae tendineae; RV = right ventricle; SA = systemic artery; s/d = peak systole/end-diastole; v = v wave.

the S wave, whichever was deeper, according to the method of Siegel and Roberts[1] (Figure 1). The electrocardiographic criteria used to diagnose LV hypertrophy included the Sokolow and Lyon Index[11] (sum of SV_1 plus the larger of RV_5 or RV_6 >35), the Romhilt-Estes point score[12] (a system using ST-T-segment changes, QRS axis, left atrial abnormality, QRS duration and duration of the intrinsicoid deflection in addition to electrographic voltage criteria), and a method using a sum of the amplitudes of the QRS complexes of all 12 leads. Amplitudes were standardized to 10 mm equaling 1 mV.

The hearts at necropsy were examined by WCR and the etiologic classification was made by him.[13] In no patient was the mitral regurgitation the result of myocardial ischemia. Although 3 patients (nos. 13, 17 and 21, Table I) had narrowing (in each case by atherosclerotic plaque) of a single (left anterior descending in each) major epicardial coronary artery, none had LV fibrosis or necrosis as a result. Only 1 (no. 20) of the 24 patients at necropsy had a grossly visible myocardial lesion, namely necrosis; the lesion was secondary to a coronary embolus in the early postmitral valve replacement period, and the electrocardiogram analyzed was that recorded just before the mitral valve operation. Therefore, none of the 24 patients had grossly visible LV lesions when the electrocardiograms used in this study

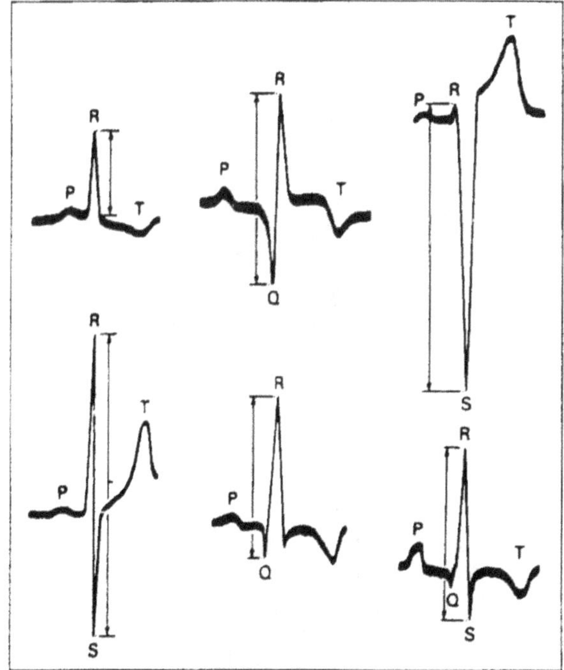

FIGURE 1. Various electrocardiographic QRS complexes showing how the voltage (in mm) was measured. (Reproduced with permission from Am Heart J.[1])

TABLE II Electrocardiographic Findings in the 24 Patients with Clinically Isolated, Pure, Chronic Mitral Regurgitation

Case No.	Days ECG Recorded Before Death	Chronic AF	VR (beats/min)	QRS Axis	Leads												Total QRS	R-E Score	S-L Index	S Wave V_1	R Wave V_5 or V_6	HW (g)
					I	II	III	AVR	AVL	AVF	V_1	V_2	V_3	V_4	V_5	V_6						
1	5	+	85	30	10	12	16	6	15	13	8	27	28	24	37	23	219	4	38	8	30	400
2	14	+	85	120	14	16	10	16	11	13	13	40	42	40	38	37	290	4	30	4	26	600
3	15	+	60	60	5	17	18	8	7	17	7	15	33	32	33	36	228	4	39	6	33	400
4	68	+	75	75	5	25	27	15	13	26	12	38	39	30	44	42	316	4	44	10	34	520
5	3	+	140	45	7	9	10	7	8	10	10	15	26	25	23	13	163	1	33	10	23	480
6	13	+	70	30	5	15	11	8	4	11	20	40	50	18	54	58	294	5	78	20	58	600
7	50	+	85	90	4	10	9	5	6	10	8	14	33	34	35	19	187	4	33	7	26	675
8	9	0	90	60	7	18	13	14	8	18	30	40	30	26	36	30	270	5	55	22	33	490
9	213	+	80	60	5	12	17	5	7	15	9	15	32	18	38	32	205	4	44	6	38	450
10	43	+	80	30	5	17	15	10	5	15	24	50	62	40	80	41	364	5	87	7	80	675
11	39	+	60	90	4	15	15	7	7	16	15	30	24	20	30	18	201	4	40	14	26	450
12	2	+	70	60	4	14	17	6	7	15	8	23	31	33	25	13	196	1	25	3	22	470
13	154	+	65	80	2	5	7	5	4	6	5	21	40	22	18	14	149	1	25	7	18	550
14	16	+	65	0	5	15	10	8	5	12	10	17	38	35	45	30	230	4	48	10	38	700
15	11	0	120	120	10	17	26	4	17	21	5	26	43	52	44	24	289	4	15	5	10	600
16	330	+	70	60	4	8	6	5	4	7	5	12	15	35	28	25	154	4	36	6	25	440
17	400	0	110	−45	10	8	8	7	8	9	28	38	26	23	46	48	259	9	70	22	48	640
18	50	+	75	60	5	13	8	8	4	9	12	9	11	18	18	17	111	1	29	12	17	400
19	5	+	140	110	14	25	18	16	12	20	22	20	40	50	40	33	310	3	26	4	22	775
20	30	+	90	−45	6	6	8	4	7	8	14	19	19	10	14	14	129	4	28	14	14	750
21	57	0	65	120	10	10	12	6	9	10	8	44	40	34	36	21	240	4	25	5	20	710
22	9	0	120	90	3	7	8	5	7	8	6	17	23	10	9	11	114	1	14	4	10	350
23	260	+	70	45	6	8	5	7	5	7	9	10	22	27	28	15	149	1	29	9	20	500
24	8	+	100	120	4	12	14	6	7	11	10	26	44	40	24	10	208	4	18	10	8	430
Mean	75		86		6.4	13.1	12.8	7.8	7.8	12.8	12.4	25.3	33.0	29.0	34.3	26.0	220	3.5	38	9	28	544

AF = atrial fibrillation; ECG = electrocardiogram; HW = heart weight; R–E = Romhilt-Estes; S-L = Sokolow-Lyon; VR = ventricular rate.

were recorded. The hearts of the 11 men ranged in weight from 400 to 750 g (mean 629) (normal ≤400), and those of the 13 women, 350 to 675 g (mean 472) (normal ≤350).

The electrocardiographic findings are summarized in Table II. Nineteen patients (79%) had chronic atrial fibrillation. Left atrial abnormality was present in 1 of the 5 patients in sinus rhythm. The QRS complex width was ≥0.12 second in 1 patient (no. 19, Table II), and he had a right bundle branch pattern. All 24 patients were being treated with digoxin at the time of the study electrocardiogram. The total 12-lead QRS amplitude in the 24 patients ranged from 111 to 364 mm (mean 220). (The upper limit of normal for total QRS amplitude of 175 mm was first suggested by Roberts and Day[3] and validated by Odom et al[5] who found that the upper limit yielded a specificity of 100% in subjects whose hearts weighed <400 g.) Of the criteria examined, the total 12-lead QRS amplitude had the highest sensitivity (71%) (Table III). Although the 12-lead QRS amplitude was more sensitive than the other 2 criteria examined, heart weight did not correlate with the total 12-lead QRS amplitude (Figure 2).

TABLE III Sensitivity of Electrocardiographic Criteria for Diagnosing Left Ventricular Hypertrophy in 24 Necropsy Patients with Clinically Isolated, Pure, Chronic, Severe, Mitral Regurgitation

Electrocardiographic Criteria	No. (%) of Patients Above Normal Limit
Total 12-lead QRS amplitude <175 mm	17 (71%)
Sokolow-Lyon index (SV$_1$ + RV$_5$ or RV$_6$ (larger) >35mm)	11 (46%)
Romhilt-Estes point score ≥ 5	4 (17%)

This study examined total 12-lead QRS voltage and other more standard electrocardiographic criteria for diagnosing LV hypertrophy in patients with clinically isolated, pure, chronic, severe mitral regurgitation. The highest sensitivity among the criteria for LV hypertrophy in our study group was the total 12-lead QRS voltage (71%). In these patients, the criteria of Romhilt and Estes and Sokolow-Lyon index were relatively insensitive (17 and 46%, respectively).

This study is the first to examine total 12-lead QRS voltage in patients with mitral regurgitation. Several

TABLE IV Comparison of the Sensitivity of Total QRS Voltage in Identifying Left Ventricular Hypertrophy of Various Etiologies

	Normal (n = 17)*	Aortic Stenosis (n = 50)	Aortic Regurgitation (n = 30)	Hypertrophic Cardiomyopathy (n = 57)	Idiopathic Dilated Cardiomyopathy (n = 49)	Amyloid (n = 30)	Mitral Regurgitation (n = 24)
Age (years) (mean)	41–74 (54)	16–65 (48)	19–65 (45)	14–87 (49)	19–75 (48)	21–93 (58)	21–84 (42)
Heart weight (g) (range)	288–392	380–880	375–1110	290–1230	400–940	370–900	350–900
Mean	351	606	696	593	614	532	550
Total QRS voltage (mm) (range)	84–159	144–417	109–428	66–339	74–281	58–199	111–364
Mean	124	257	270	197	153	104	220
Patients with 12-lead QRS voltage >175 mm	0 (0%)	47 (94%)	27 (90%)	30 (53%)	20 (41%)	2 (7%)	17 (71%)

*Patients with heart weights <400 g.

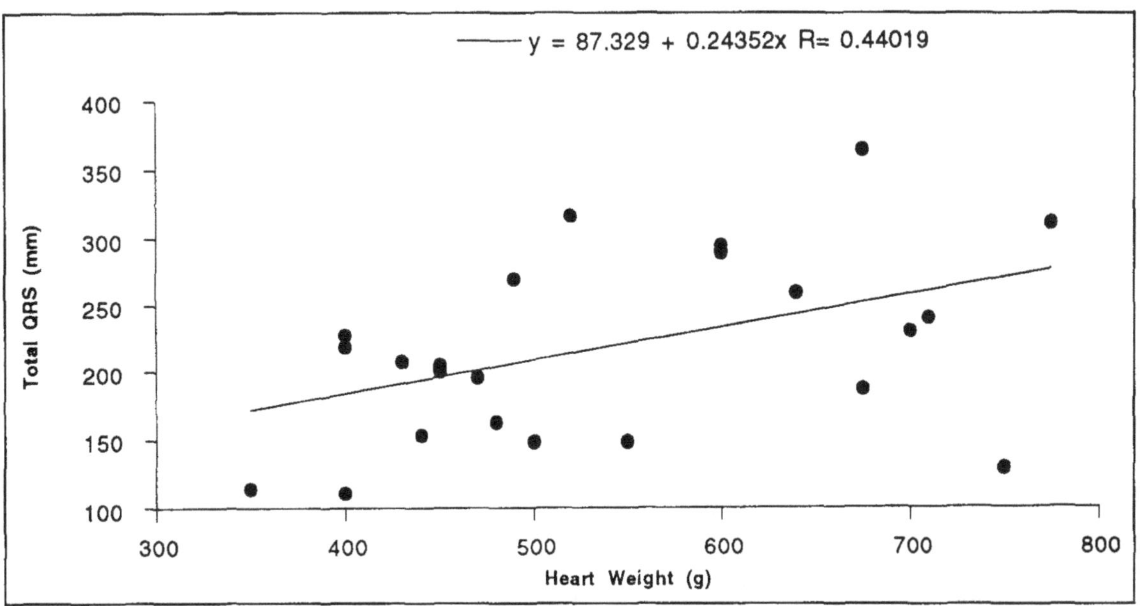

FIGURE 2. Relation between total QRS amplitude and heart weight at necropsy in 24 patients with isolated pure, chronic, severe mitral regurgitation.

studies, however, have evaluated the relation between the total 12-lead QRS voltage and heart weight at necropsy in other cardiac diseases (Table IV).[1-3,5-7]

1. Siegel RJ, Roberts WC. Electrocardiographic observations in severe aortic valve stenosis: correlative necropsy study to clinical, hemodynamic, and ECG variables demonstrating relation of 12-lead QRS amplitude to peak transaortic pressure gradient. *Am Heart J* 1982;103:210–221.

2. Roberts WC, Waller BF. Cardiac amyloidosis causing cardiac dysfunction: analysis of 54 necropsy patients. *Am J Cardiol* 1983;52:137–146.

3. Roberts WC, Day PJ. Electrocardiographic observations in clinically isolated, pure, chronic, severe aortic regurgitation: analysis of 30 necropsy patients aged 19 to 65 years. *Am J Cardiol* 1985;55:432–438.

4. Ross E, Roberts WC. The carcinoid syndrome: comparison of 21 necropsy subjects with carcinoid heart disease to 15 necropsy subjects without carcinoid heart disease. *Am J Med* 1985;79:339–354.

5. Odom H II, Davis JL, Dinh H, Baker BJ, Roberts WC, Murphy ML. QRS voltage measurements in autopsied men free of cardiopulmonary disease: a basis for evaluating total QRS voltage as an index of left ventricular hypertrophy. *Am J Cardiol* 1986;58:801–804.

6. Roberts WC, Siegel RJ, McManus BM. Idiopathic dilated cardiomyopathy: Analysis of 152 necropsy patients. *Am J Cardiol* 1987;60:1340–1355.

7. Dollar A, Roberts WC. Usefulness of total 12-lead QRS voltage compared with other criteria for determining left ventricular hypertrophy in hypertrophic cardiomyopathy: analysis of 57 patients studied at necropsy. *Am J Med* 1989;87:377–381.

8. Lanti M, Puddu PE, Menotti A. Voltage criteria of left ventricular hypertrophy in sudden and nonsudden coronary artery disease mortality: the Italian section of the Seven Countries Study. *Am J Cardiol* 1990;66:1181–1185.

9. Pelliccia F, Critelli G, Cianfrocca C, Nigri A, Reale A. Electrocardiographic correlates with left ventricular morphology in idiopathic dilated cardiomyopathy. *Am J Cardiol* 1991;68:642–647.

10. Rodriguez P. Usefulness of total 12-lead QRS voltage for determining the presence of left ventricular hypertrophy in systemic hypertension. *Am J Cardiol* 1991;68:261–262.

11. Romhilt DW, Estes EH Jr. A point score system for the ECG diagnosis of left ventricular hypertrophy. *Am Heart J* 1968;75:1752–1758.

12. Sokolow M, Lyon TP. The ventricular complex in left ventricular hypertrophy as obtained by unipolar precordial and limb leads. *Am Heart J* 1949;37:161–186.

13. Roberts WC. Morphologic aspects of cardiac valve dysfunction. *Am Heart J* 1992;123:1610–1632.

Clinical, Electrocardiographic and Morphologic Features of Massive Fatty Deposits ("Lipomatous Hypertrophy") in the Atrial Septum

JAMSHID SHIRANI, MD, WILLIAM C. ROBERTS, MD, FACC*

Bethesda, Maryland

Objectives. This study examined the morphologic features and the clinical significance of massive fatty deposits in the atrial septum of the heart.

Background. Large deposits of adipose tissue in the atrial septum were first described in 1964 and have been referred to as "lipomatous hypertrophy" of the atrial septum. A relation between these fatty deposits and atrial arrhythmias has been suggested.

Methods. The thickness of the atrial septum cephalad to the fossa ovalis ranged from 1.5 to 6 cm in 91 patients and was ≥2 cm in 80 patients. This report focuses primarily on the latter 80 patients.

Results. The thickness of the atrial septum in the 80 patients correlated with body weight and the thickness of the adipose tissue in the atrioventricular groove and that covering the right ventricle. In 53 patients (67%), one or more of the four major epicardial coronary arteries were narrowed >75% in cross-sectional area by atherosclerotic plaque. Atrial arrhythmias were present in 31 patients (40%). Patients with larger deposits of fat (atrial septal thickness ≥3 cm) had a higher frequency of atrial arrhythmias (60% vs. 34%, p < 0.01). The atrial septum was significantly thicker in patients with atrial arrhythmia compared with those without atrial arrhythmias (2.9 vs. 2.3 cm, p < 0.01). Of the 28 patients with available electrocardiograms, 20 (71%) showed atrial arrhythmias (nine atrial premature complexes, seven atrial fibrillation, three atrial tachycardia, one ectopic atrial rhythm and one junctional rhythm).

Conclusions. Massive fatty deposits in the atrial septum are associated with large deposits of fat elsewhere in the body and other parts of the heart. They are frequently associated with atrial arrhythmias and atherosclerotic coronary artery disease.

(J Am Coll Cardiol 1993;22:226–38)

In the western world there is an expectation among many that people gain weight with age. The increase in weight is primarily due to the deposition of fat in various locations in the body. The heart is not spared from the fatty deposits. Most often the fat in the heart is in the subepicardial adipose tissue, particularly in the areas where the epicardial coronary arteries are located. Another location for fatty deposits in the heart is the atrial septum. When the fatty deposits in the atrial septum are large, such deposits have been called "lipomatous hypertrophy of the atrial septum." Since the initial description of this entity in 1964 (1), several reports (2–20) describing relatively few cases have appeared. Some reports (2–4) have suggested that some cardiac arrhythmias, particularly those of atrial origin, may be a consequence of this fatty deposition in the atrial septum. This report analyzes a large group of patients with massive infiltration of the atrial septum by fat to discern if there were specific clinical or electrocardiographic features that could be attributed to these fatty infiltrates.

From the Pathology Branch, National Heart, Lung, and Blood Institute, National Institutes of Health, Bethesda, Maryland.

Manuscript received September 3, 1992; revised manuscript received November 20, 1992, accepted December 1, 1992.

*Present address: Baylor Cardiovascular Institute, Baylor University Medical Center, 3500 Gaston Avenue, Dallas, Texas 75246.

Address for correspondence: Jamshid Shirani, MD, Department of Medicine, Division of Cardiology, Medical College of Virginia, MCV Station, Box 123, Richmond, Virginia 23298.

Methods

Sources of patients. The files of the Pathology Branch, which include essentially only cases with cardiovascular disease, were searched for cases coded as "lipomatous hypertrophy of the atrial septum" or "atrial septal lipoma." Although the files include cases entered as early as 1953, the first case of lipomatous hypertrophy of the atrial septum was not coded until 1975. Since that time, 91 cases have been so coded and approximately 7,000 cases >15 years of age were accessioned in the Pathology Branch from 1975 to July 1992.

The hearts from all 91 patients were originally examined and coded by one of the authors (W.C.R.) and subsequently 74 of the 91 hearts were examined by the other author (J.S.). The hearts in the 91 cases were submitted by 19 different medical centers, including 26 from Suburban Hospital (Bethesda, Maryland), 14 from the District of Columbia Veterans Affairs Hospital, 11 from the National Naval Medical Center, 9 from Georgetown University Medical Center, 9 from the District of Columbia Medical Examiners' Office, 5 from the Washington Hospital Center, 3 from Franklin Square Hospital (Baltimore, Maryland), 2 from the Clinical Center of the National Institutes of Health, 2 from Sibley Hospital (Washington, D.C.) and 1 each from each of 10 other medical centers. The medical records from each of the 91 cases were reviewed and the actual electrocardiograms were obtained in 29 cases.

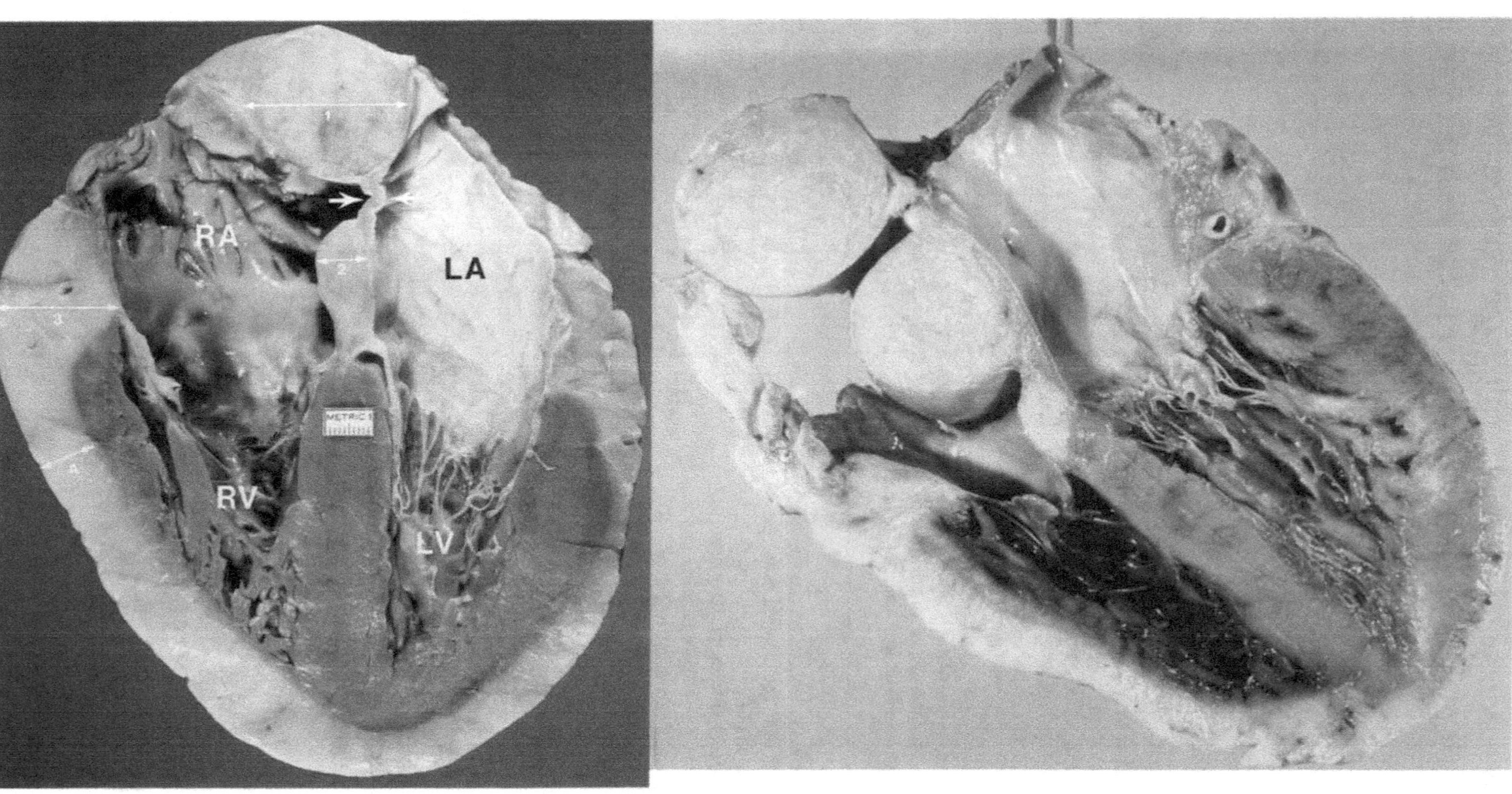

Figure 1 (left). Four-chamber view of the heart of a 70-year old man (NNMC# A86-42), showing the method used to measure the thickness of the cephalad portion of the atrial septum [1], the caudal portion of the atrial septum [2], the fat in the right atrioventricular groove [3] and the fat overlying the right ventricular wall [4]. LA = left atrium; LV = left ventricle; RA = right atrium; RV = right ventricle. The **double arrowheads** point to the fossa ovalis.

Figure 2 (right). Four-chamber view of the heart of a 74-year old woman (GT# 774-42). The caudal portion of the atrial septum is thicker than that in any of the other 90 cases.

Table 1. Clinical and Morphologic Findings in 11 Patients With Fatty Deposits in the Atrial Septum and an Atrial Septal Thickness <2 cm

Pt No.	Age (yr)/ Gender	HD in Life	AP	AMI	AA*	Htn	DM	Fatal CAD	HW (g)	Heart Floats	Thickness of Atrial Septum (cm)	≥1 CA With >75% ↓ in CSA by Plaque	LV Fibrosis	LV Necrosis
1	49/M	+	0	0	0	+	0	0†	580'	0	1.6	0	0	0
2	53/F	0	0	0	0	0	0	0	300‡	+	1.7	0	0	0
3	57/M	0	0	0	0	+	0	+	355	+	1.8	+	0	0
4	67/M	+	+	+	+	+	0	+	530	+	1.8	+	0	+
5	71/M	0	0	0	0	0	0	0	465	+	1.8	+	0	0
6	72/M	+	+	+	+	0	+	+	555	0	1.7	+	+	0
7	76/F	+	0	+	+	0	0	+	610	+	1.8	+	0	+
8	79/M	+	+	+	+	0	0	+	410	+	1.5	+	0	+
9	79/F	0	0	0	0	+	0	0	420	+	1.5	+	0	0
10	80/F	0	0	0	0	+	0	0	425	+	1.5	0	0	0
11	89/F	+	+	+	+	0	+	+	520	+	1.8	+	+	0
Total or mean value	70	6	4	5	5	5	2	6	470	9	1.7	8	2	3

*None had ventricular arrhythmias. †Died of aortic valve infective endocarditis. ‡Patient had cachexia and died of metastatic breast cancer. AA = atrial arrhythmia; AMI = acute myocardial infarction; AP = angina pectoris; CA = coronary artery; CAD = atherosclerotic coronary artery disease; CSA = cross-sectional area; DM = diabetes mellitus; F = female; HD = heart disease; Htn = systemic hypertension; HW = heart weight; LV = left ventricular; M = male; Pt = patient; 0 = absent; + = present; ↓ = decrease.

Methods of examining the hearts. Each heart was weighed on very accurate scales after fixation in formalin from 3 to 14 days and after carefully removing all portions of parietal pericardium and after removing the pulmonary trunk and ascending aorta by transverse incisions approximately 2-cm cephalad to the sinotubular junctions. Hearts received completely intact were placed in a large container of water to see whether or not they floated. (A floating heart is indicative of a very fatty heart [21].)

Each of the four major coronary arteries (right, left main, left anterior descending, left circumflex) was examined by transverse incisions, each about 5 mm apart, and the maximal degrees of cross-sectional area narrowing of each was recorded (0% to 25%, 26% to 50%, 51% to 75%, 76% to 100%). The cardiac ventricles were not opened in an entirely uniform fashion; they were opened by coronal, sagittal or transverse incisions, or a combination of these incisions. The maximal thickness of the fat in the right atrioventricular (AV) groove and that covering the right ventricular myocardium was measured as illustrated in Figure 1.

The atria were opened by a coronal incision, such that the midportion of the fossa ovalis of the atrial septum was incised. Measurements of the maximal thicknesses of the atrial septum both cephalad and caudal to the fossa ovalis were made after the incision through the midportion of the fossa ovalis (Fig. 1).

Statistical analysis. For each variable, the mean value and standard deviation was determined. Correlations were calculated between the thickness of the atrial septum and body weight, 12-lead QRS voltage and thickness of adipose tissue inferior to fossa ovalis, in the AV groove and overlying the right ventricular wall. Statistical analysis of the noncontinuous variables was done by the chi-square method. Continuous data were analyzed by the Student *t* test. A probability < 0.05 was considered significant.

Results

Atrial septal thickness cephalad versus caudal to the fossa ovalis. In all 91 patients, the thickness of the atrial septum cephalad to the fossa ovalis was always greater than that of the atrial septum caudal to the fossa ovalis. Either none or only minimal amounts of adipose tissue were present in the fossa ovalis. The maximal thickness of the cephalad portion of atrial septum ranged from 1.5 to 6 cm (mean 2.4) and that of the caudal portion of septum from 0.3 to 2.4 cm (mean 0.9). The 91 cases were divided into two groups on the basis of the maximal thickness of the cephalad portion of the atrial septum. One group consisted of 11 patients in whom the maximal atrial septal thickness ranged from 1.5 to 1.8 cm, and pertinent clinical and morphologic findings in these patients are detailed in Table 1.

The other group consisted of 80 patients in whom the maximal right to left thickness of the cephalad portion of atrial septum ranged from 2 to 6 cm (mean 2.5). The remainder of this report focuses on these 80 patients. Of the 80 patients, 69 (86%) had an atrial septum with a maximal thickness of 2 to 3 cm and 11 patients (14%) had an atrial septum with a maximal thickness >3 cm. Certain clinicopathologic findings in the patients with an atrial septum ≥2 cm are summarized in Table 2 and illustrated in Figures 1 to 11. The 80 patients (52 men, 28 women) ranged in age from 48 to 91 years (mean 69). Only 1 patient was <50 years of age and only 1 was >90 years of age; 12 patients were aged 51 to 60 years, 5 patients 81 to 90 years and 61 patients (76%) 61 to 80 years of age.

Table 2. Clinical and Morphologic Findings in 80 Patients With Massive Fatty Deposits in the Atrial Septum

	All Patients (n = 80)	Men (n = 52)	Women (n = 28)
Age (yr), range (mean)	48–91 (69 ± 9)	48–91 (68 ± 9)	53–86 (71 ± 9)
White/black	72/3	47/5	25/3
Heart disease in life	47/77 (61%)	30/49 (61%)	17 (61%)
Angina pectoris	19/77 (25%)	16/49 (33%)	3 (11%)
Myocardial infarction	20/77 (26%)	14/49 (29%)	6 (32%)
Congestive heart failure	21/77 (27%)	11/49 (22%)*	10 (36%)*
Sudden death	26/79 (33%)	21/51 (41%)*	5 (18%)*
Arrhythmias			
Supraventricular	31/77 (40%)	18/49 (37%)	13/28 (48%)
Ventricular	6/78 (8%)	6/50 (12%)	0 (0%)
Systemic hypertension	46/77 (60%)	31/49 (63%)	15 (54%)
Habitual alcoholism	10/76 (13%)	9/48 (19%)	1 (4%)
Diabetes mellitus	19/77 (25%)	15/49 (31%)	4 (14%)
Corticosteroid therapy	10/76 (13%)	6/48 (13%)	4 (14%)
Cancer			
All	28/78 (36%)	17/50 (34%)	11 (39%)
Fatal	22/28 (79%)	15/17 (88%)	7/11 (64%)
Body weight (kg), range (mean)†	55–125 (79 ± 14)	57–118 (82 ± 13)	55–125 (75 ± 16)
Height (cm), range (mean)†	145–193 (168 ± 12)	150–193 (173 ± 10)*	145–193 (162 ± 12)*
Cause of death			
Cardiac	37 (46%)	27 (52%)	10 (36%)
Vascular	10 (13%)	6 (11%)	4 (14%)
Noncardiovascular	33 (41%)	19 (37%)	14 (50%)
Death outside hospital	13/75 (17%)	10/47 (21%)	3 (9%)
Heart weight (g), range (mean)	300–915 (545 ± 125)	345–915 (566 ± 118)	300–880 (505 ± 134)
Heart floats in water	52/69 (75%)	35/48 (73%)	17/21 (81%)
No. of coronary arteries with >75% ↓ in CSA by plaque			
4	3 (4%)	2 (4%)	1 (4%)
3	13 (16%)	9 (18%)	4 (14%)
2	18 (23%) } 53 (67%)	16 (31%) } 41 (80%)*	2 (7%) } 12 (43%)*
1	19 (24%)	14 (27%)	5 (18%)
0	27 (33%)	10 (20%)	16 (57%)
Coronary arteries with >75% ↓ in CSA by plaque			
Left main	4 (5%)	2 (4%)	2 (7%)
Left anterior descending	47 (59%)	38 (73%)*	9 (32%)*
Left circumflex	21 (26%)	14 (27%)	7 (25%)
Right	34 (43%)	27 (52%)*	7 (25%)*
Left ventricular fibrosis	22 (28%)	18 (35%)*	4 (14%)*
Left ventricular necrosis	15 (19%)	10 (19%)	5 (18%)
Mitral annular calcium	21 (26%)	14 (27%)	7 (25%)
Thickness of atrial septum (cm), range (mean)			
Cephalad portion	2–6 (2.5 ± 0.7)	2–5 (2.4 ± 0.5)*	2–6 (2.8 ± 0.9)*
Caudal portion	0.3–2.4 (1.0 ± 0.3)	0.4–1.5 (0.9 ± 0.2)	0.3–2.4 (1.0 ± 0.5)
Thickness of fat in atrioventricular groove, range (mean) (cm)	0.7–2.6 (1.7 ± 0.5)	0.7–2.6 (1.6 ± 0.5)	0.7–2.5 (1.8 ± 0.6)
Thickness of fat over the right ventricle, range (mean) (cm)	0.2–1.5 (0.7 ± 0.2)	0.3–1.5 (0.7 ± 0.2)	0.2–1.3 (0.7 ± 0.3)

*p ≤ 0.05. †Data available in 40 patients. Abbreviations as in Table 1.

Small versus large septum. Comparison of the 59 patients with a smaller septum (2 to 2.9 cm) with the 21 patients with a larger septum (≥3 cm) disclosed significant differences in the frequency of male gender (73% vs. 43%), atrial arrhythmias (34% vs. 60%), systemic hypertension (71% vs. 55%), mean heart weight (520 vs. 565 g) (despite the smaller percent of men in the group with a larger heart) and a smaller quantity of cardiac fat overall as evidenced by the percent of hearts that floated in water (70% vs. 94%) (Table 3). Neither diabetes mellitus nor corticosteroid therapy had an effect on the thickness of the atrial septum. The average thickness of the septum in the 19 patients with diabetes mellitus was 2.4 cm and that in the 58 patients without diabetes was 2.6 cm. The mean thickness of the septum was 2.8 cm in the 10 patients on corticosteroid therapy and 2.5 cm in those not receiving corticosteroid therapy.

Coronary artery disease. Comparison of the 53 patients with significant coronary artery disease (one or more major epicardial coronary arteries narrowed >75% in cross-sectional area by atherosclerotic plaque at necropsy) with

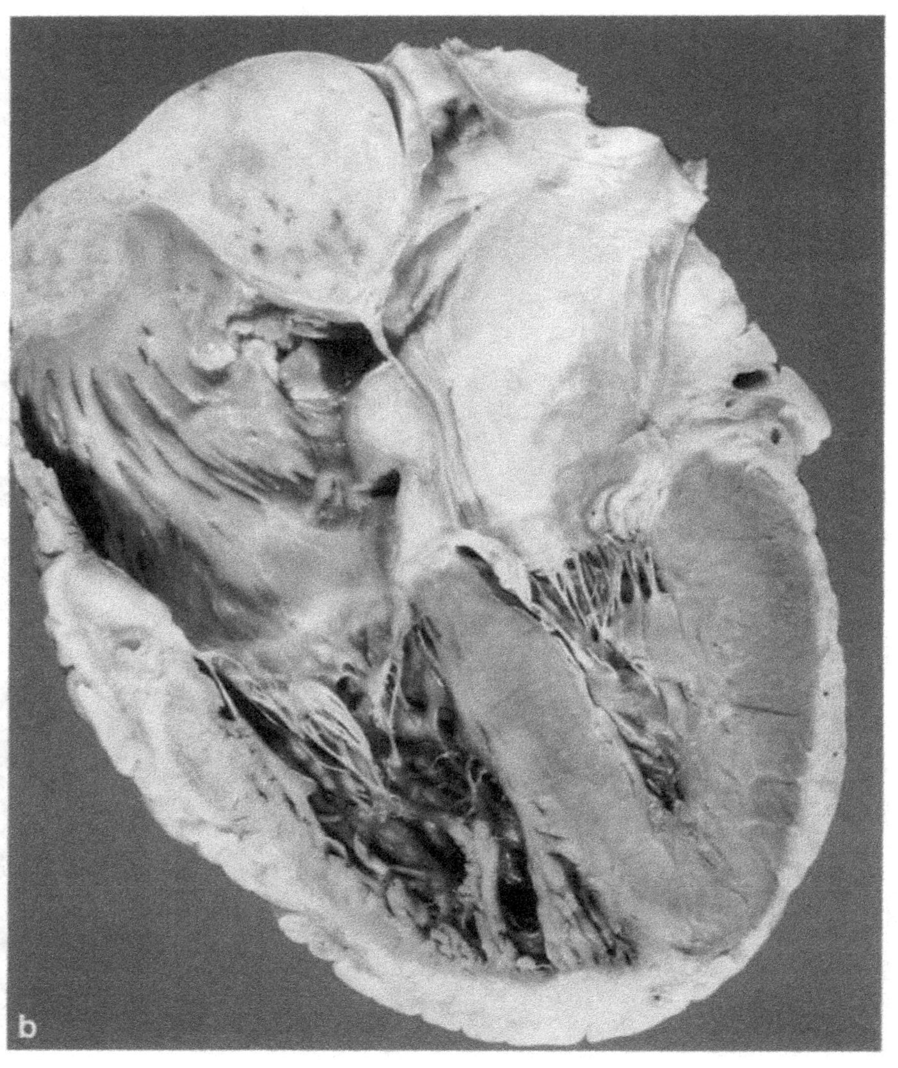

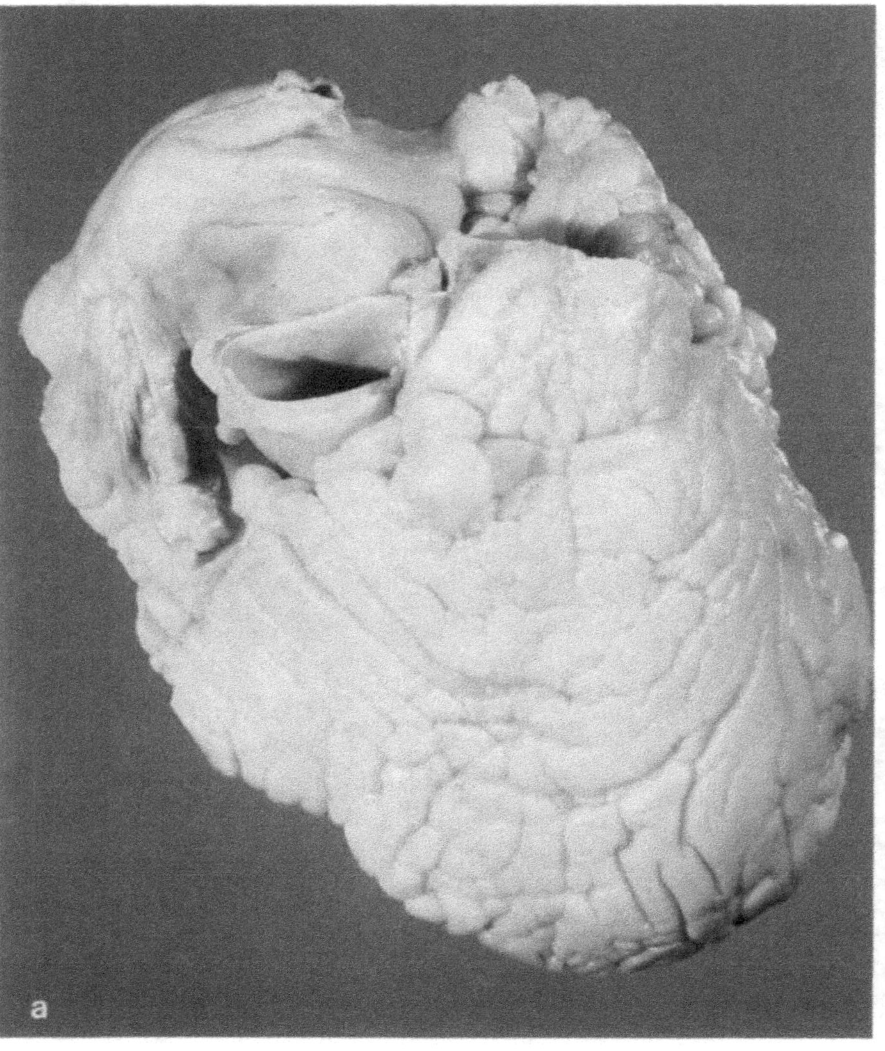

Figure 3. Exterior (a) and four-chamber (b) view of the heart of an 83-year old woman (NNMC# A88-43), showing massive amounts of epicardial adipose tissue covering the entire surface of both ventricles.

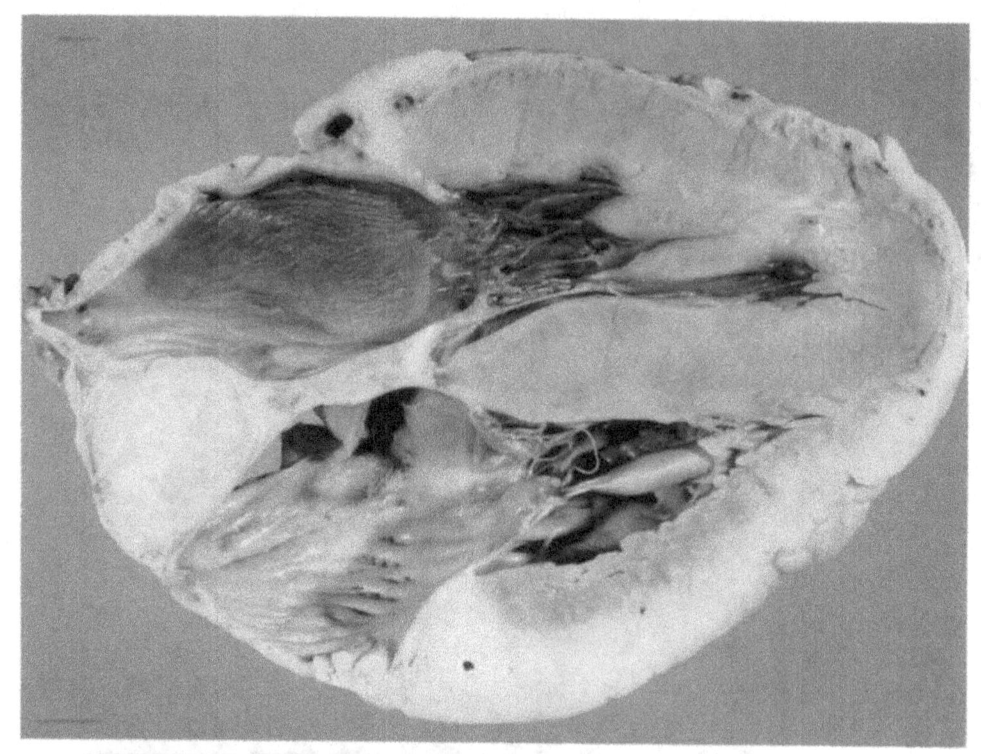

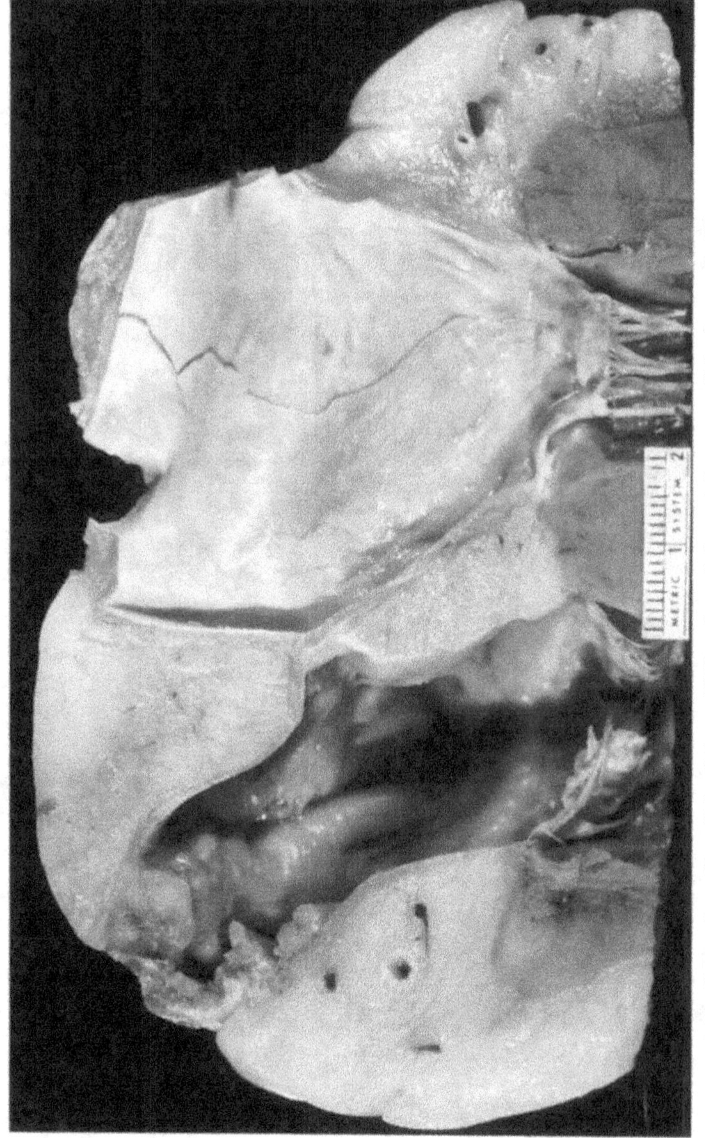

Figure 4 (left). Coronal section of the right and left atria and the atrial septum of the heart of a 71-year old woman (SV# 7/78).

Figure 5 (right). Four-chamber view of the heart of a 77-year old woman (NNMC# A89-33). The coronal section through the atrial septum is made slightly anterior to the fossa ovalis.

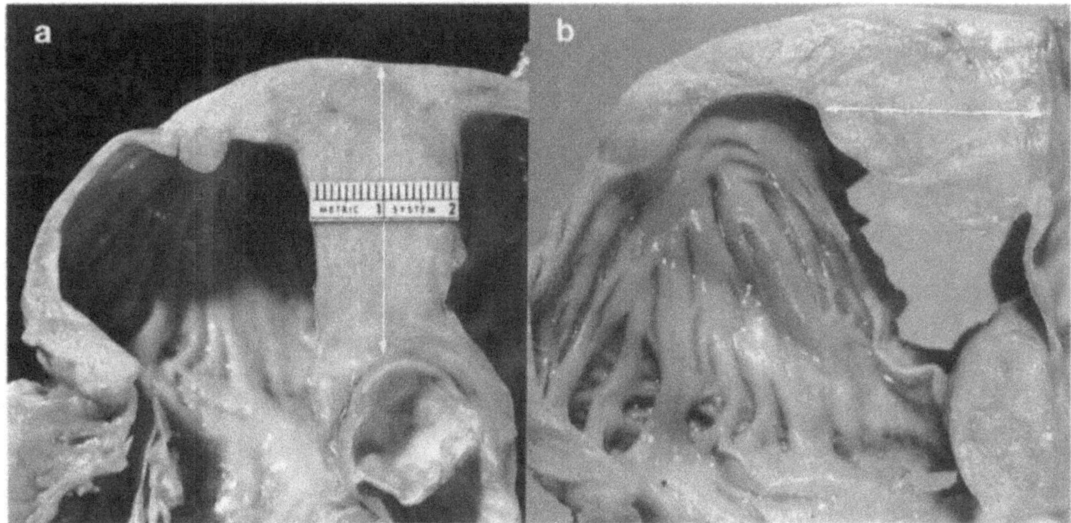

Figure 6. Close-up of the right atrium and atrial septum in a four-chamber view of the heart of a 76-year old woman (NNMC# A75-32). The coronal section is anterior to the fossa ovalis in a and at the level of the fossa ovalis in b. If the atrial septum is measured from its cephalad to its caudal extension as shown in a (between the arrows), the thickness of the septum would be nearly twice that of the cephalad portion at the level of the fossa ovalis as shown in b. Measurements in the present study were all done as shown in b.

the 27 patients with insignificant coronary narrowing disclosed a significantly higher proportion of men (77% vs. 41%), a lesser frequency of fatal cancer (21% vs. 42%) and a smaller mean thickness of the atrial septum (2.4 vs. 2.9 cm). No significant difference in the frequency of atrial arrhythmias between the two groups was observed (41% vs. 38%).

Fatal cancer. Comparison of the 22 patients with fatal cancer with the 56 patients without cancer disclosed a significantly lower frequency of coronary artery disease in the cancer group (50% vs. 73%) and a smaller mean heart weight among the women (405 vs. 545 g). The mean thickness of the atrial septum was similar between these two groups (2.5 vs. 2.6 cm).

Atrial arrhythmias and conduction disturbances. Comparison of the 31 patients with atrial arrhythmias with the 46 patients without such arrhythmias disclosed a thicker atrial

Figure 7. Postmortem radiograph (a) and four-chamber view (b) of the heart of a 73-year old man (SH# A92-12). The needle (enclosed by perpendicular lines) in the atrial septum (arrows) measures 2.8 cm in length.

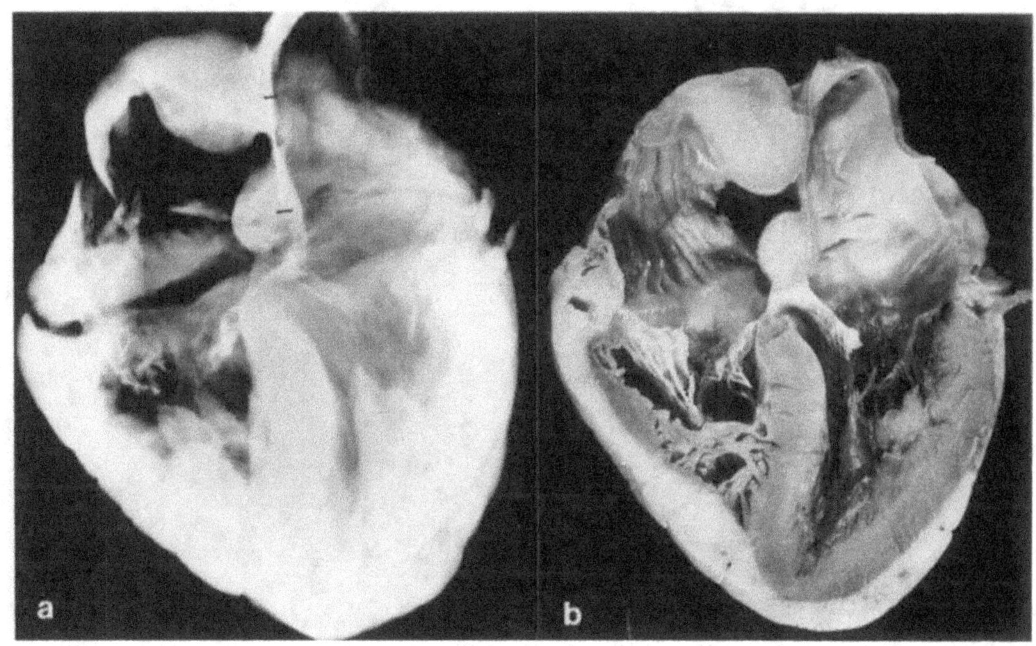

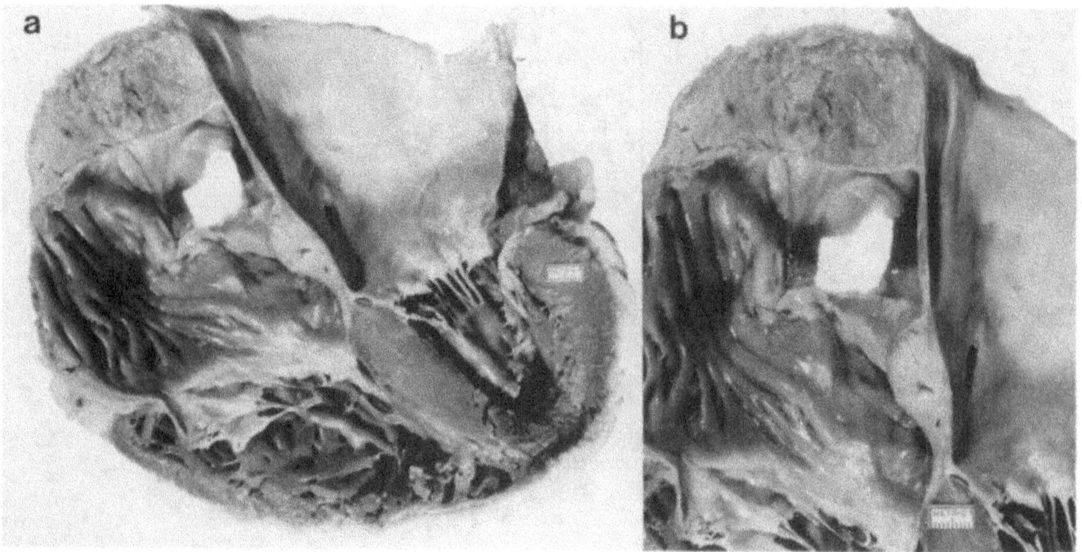

Figure 8. Four-chamber view of the heart of a 71-year old woman (a) and close-up of the right and left atria and atrial septum (b) (FSH# A-4088). Both atria are very dilated. The portion of the atrial septum cephalad to the fossa ovalis is 6 cm thick.

septum in the patients with arrhythmia (2.9 vs. 2.3 cm), a heavier heart in the women (545 vs. 470 g) and a higher frequency of signs and symptoms of congestive heart failure (42% vs. 17%) (Table 4). No significant differences occurred in the frequency of significant coronary artery disease (68% vs. 67%) or of myocardial infarction (45% vs. 37%) (Table 4).

Various electrocardiographic measurements were performed in 28 of the 80 patients with an atrial septum ≥ 2 cm in thickness (Table 5). Twelve (43%) of the 28 patients with an electrocardiogram had chronic atrial arrhythmias (atrial fibrillation in 8). Of the 18 patients with sinus, junctional or ectopic atrial rhythm, 9 (50%) had atrial premature complexes. Six patients (21%) had major conduction disturbances, but four of them had myocardial infarction. Total

Figure 9. Four-chamber view of the heart of a 78-year old man (a) and close-up of the right atrium and atrial septum (b).

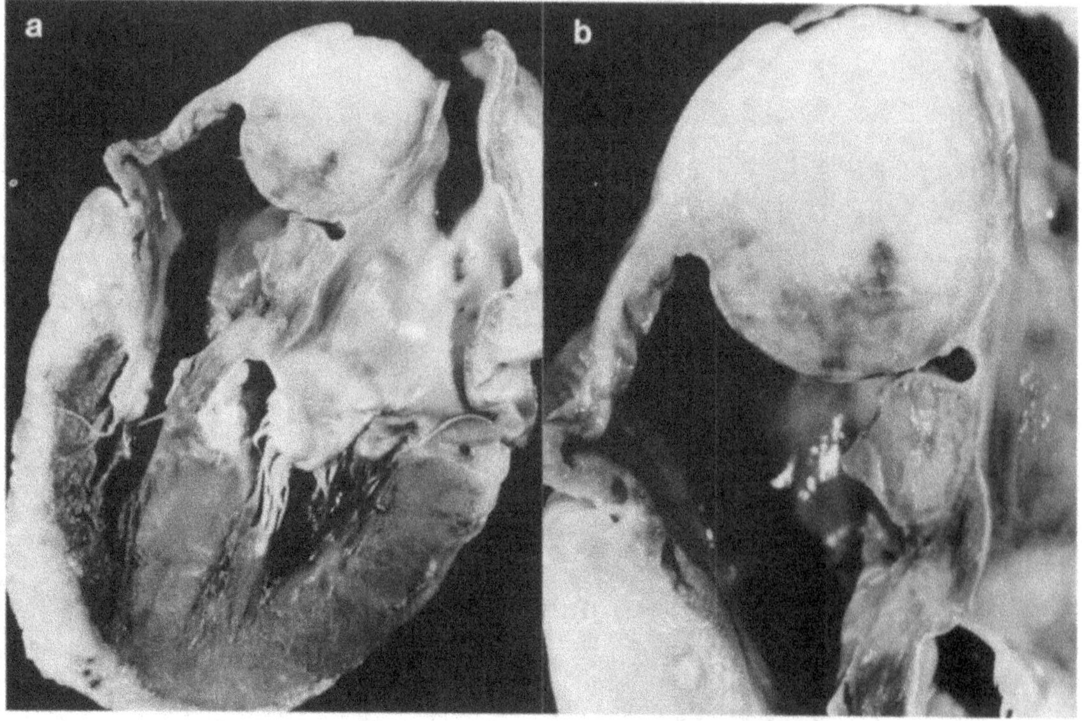

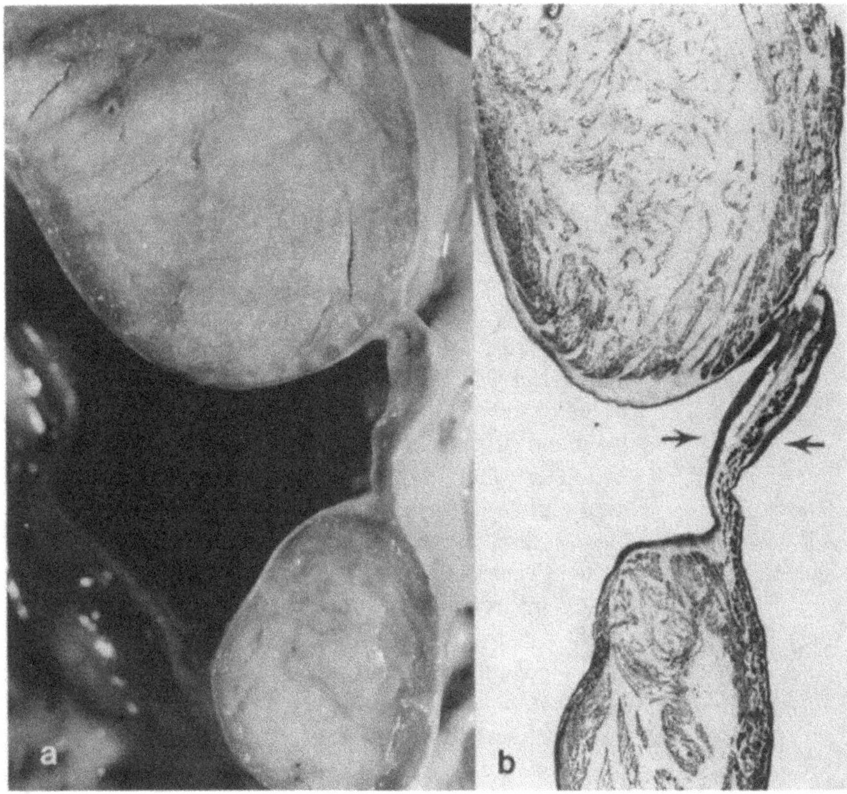

Figure 10. Gross (a) and histologic (b) section of the atrial septum of the heart of a 60-year old woman. Only minimal amounts of adipose tissue are present in the fossa ovalis (**arrows**). Movat stain ×25 (b).

12-lead QRS voltage measured by the method of Siegel and Roberts (22) ranged from 59 to 266 mm (mean 131 ± 51). Patients with an atrial septum ≥3 cm had a significantly higher frequency of atrial arrhythmias (75% vs. 18%) and larger total 12-lead QRS voltages (150 vs. 115 mm) than those of patients with an atrial septum <3 cm (Table 6).

Discussion

Measurement of atrial septal thickness. One difference in our study from those published previously on this subject is

Figure 11. Normal atrial septum (DCMEO 78-04-284) with a maximal thickness of 6 mm in its cephalad portion and no fatty deposit. The fossa ovalis membrane (**arrows**) measures <1 mm in thickness. LA = left atrium; RA = right atrium.

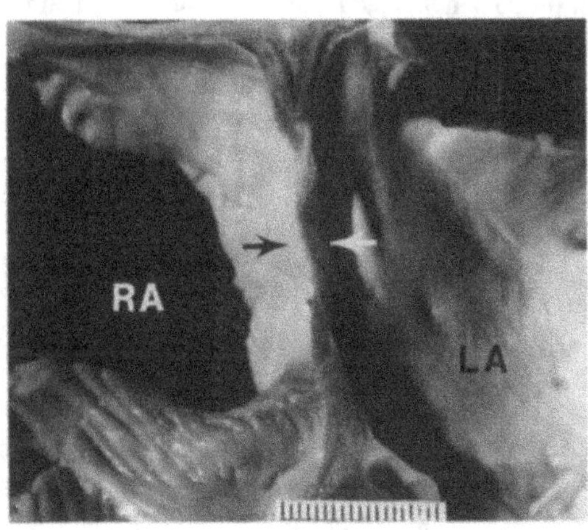

Table 3. Comparison of the Clinical and Morphologic Findings in Patients With Small (septal thickness <3 cm) and Large (septal thickness ≥3 cm) Fatty Deposits in the Atrial Septum

	Atrial Septal Thickness <3 cm (n = 59)	Atrial Septal Thickness ≥3 cm (n = 21)
Age (yr), range (mean)	48–91 (68)	51–85 (71)
Men	43 (73%)*	9 (43%)*
Atrial arrhythmias	19/56 (34%)*	12/20 (60%)*
Systemic hypertension	31/56 (55%)*	15/21 (71%)*
Body weight (kg), range (mean)	55–95 (78)	55–125 (84)
Heart weight (g), range (mean)	300–915 (520)*	335–880 (565)*
Heart floats in water	37/53 (70%)*	15/16 (94%)*
No. of coronary arteries with >75% ↓ in CSA by plaque		
4	2 (4%) ⎤	1 (5%) ⎤
3	10 (17%) ⎟ 42 (71%)	3 (14%) ⎟ 11 (52%)
2	15 (25%) ⎟	3 (14%) ⎟
1	15 (25%) ⎦	4 (19%) ⎦
0	17 (29%)	10 (48%)
LV fibrosis	17 (29%)	5 (24%)
LV necrosis	12 (20%)	3 (14%)
Thickness of atrial septum (cm) range (mean)		
Cephalad portion	2.0–2.9 (2.1)*	3.0–6.0 (3.6)*
Caudal portion	0.3–1.3 (1.0)	0.6–2.4 (1.2)
Thickness of fat in atrioventricular groove (cm), range (mean)	0.7–2.6 (1.7)	0.9–2.5 (1.9)
Thickness of fat over the right ventricle (cm), range (mean)	0.2–1.3 (0.7)	0.4–1.5 (0.8)

*p < 0.05. Abbreviations as in Table 1.

Table 4. Comparison of Patients With Massive Fatty Deposits in the Atrial Septum With and Without Atrial Arrhythmias

	Atrial Arrhythmia	
	Present (n = 31)	Absent (n = 46)
Age (yr), range (mean)	52–84 (72)	48–91 (67)
Male/female	18 (58)/13 (42%)	31 (67)/15 (33%)
Systemic hypertension	18 (58%)	28 (61%)
Angina pectoris	9 (29%)	10 (22%)
Congestive heart failure	13 (42%)*	8 (17%)*
Diabetes mellitus	9 (29%)	10 (22%)
Corticosteroid therapy	5 (16%)	5/44 (11%)
Cancer	14 (45%)	14 (30%)
≥1 CA with >75% ↓ in CSA by plaque	21 (68%)	31 (67%)
Heart weight (g), range (mean)		
Men	410–915 (605)	345–800 (585)
Women	315–880 (545)*	300–680 (470)*
Heart floats	17/25 (68%)	34/42 (81%)
Maximal thickness of the atrial septum (cm)	2.0–5.5 (2.9)*	2.0–6.0 (2.3)*
Mitral annular calcium	8 (26%)	12 (26%)
Myocardial infarction		
Healed	8 (26%)	9 (20%)
Acute	4 (13%) } 14 (45%)	6 (13%) } 18 (40%)
Both healed and acute	2 (6%)	3 (7%)

*$p < 0.05$. Abbreviations as in Table 1.

the method chosen to measure the thicknesses of the atrial septum. In the present study, the atrial septum was incised in a coronal fashion, with the incision extending through the midportion of the fossa ovalis, which contains minimal amounts, if any, of fat and therefore is only ≈1 cm thick. By incising the atrial septum using the fossa ovalis as the landmark, the thickness of the cephalad portion was always greater than the thickness of the caudal portion of the septum. With this method of measuring the thickness of the atrial septum, 6 cm was the thickest and 1.5 cm was the thinnest atrial septum. Previous publications (5) have described larger atrial septa, but the method of measurement was never described precisely. If we had determined the thickness of the atrial septum by measuring, for example, the longitudinal thickness either anterior or posterior to the fossa ovalis, measurements two or more times as large as our maximal measurements would have resulted. The use of the fossa ovalis as the landmark for measuring atrial septal thickness also allows comparison of the necropsy measurements with those recorded by echocardiography-computed tomography and nuclear magnetic resonance (NMR) imaging.

Normally the atrial septum both cephalad and caudal to the fossa ovalis is <1 cm thick. In the present study, we focused primarily on patients with a maximal atrial septal thickness ≥2 cm. Because previous reports have included cases with <2 cm atrial septal thickness, we also included cases with maximal septal thickness ranging from 1.5 to 1.9 cm, so that these cases could be compared with others previously reported (Table 1).

Adipose tissue in other portions of the heart. When the atrial septum is massively infiltrated by fatty deposits, the amount of adipose tissue is always increased in other portions of the heart, mainly the subepicardial adipose tissue, particularly over the right ventricular wall and in the AV sulci. The fatty deposits may be so extensive that every square centimeter of ventricular myocardium is covered by adipose tissue. The huge deposits of fat in all portions of the heart made the heart in many of our patients lighter than water, such that 75% (52 of 69) of the hearts floated in water. The actual weight of the fat, measured in five of our patients, constituted 32% to 52% (mean 41%) of the total weight of the heart. The maximal thickness of the atrial septum in our patients with septa ≥2 cm correlated with the thickness of the subepicardial adipose tissue over the right ventricular myocardial wall ($r = 0.61$) and that in the AV sulcus ($r = 0.79$). Among our 80 patients, the body weight was available in 40 and the maximal thickness of atrial septum in these patients correlated with body weight ($r = 0.84$).

The adipose tissue in the heart may be the last site to disappear with weight loss. Support for this view is gained by the presence of huge quantities of cardiac fat in the 22 patients with fatal cancer, a number of whom were cachectic at necropsy. The maximal thickness of the atrial septum in the 22 patients with cancer was similar to that in the 56 patients without known cancer (2.5 vs. 2.6 cm).

In addition to the constant association of the massive atrial septal fatty deposits with massive deposits of fat in other portions of the heart and usually in other portions of the body, there also was near universal increase in heart weight: 77 (96%) of the 80 patients had an increased heart weight (>350 g in women, >400 g in men). Systemic hypertension, as might be expected because of the high prevalence of obesity, was present in 46 (60%) of 77 patients (Table 2). Significant atherosclerotic coronary artery disease was also common. Of the 80 patients, 53 (66%) had >75% narrowing in cross-sectional area of one or more major epicardial coronary arteries by atherosclerotic plaque and 33 (62%) of the 53 patients died from consequences of coronary artery disease.

Presence of atrial arrhythmias. Whether the frequency of atrial arrhythmias is greater in patients with massive atrial septal fatty deposits than in patients of similar age and gender without these deposits has been controversial. Among 122 cases of atrial septal fatty deposits reported by others (1–20), atrial arrhythmias of some type, including atrial premature complexes, were present in 56 (45%). Among our 80 patients with septa ≥2 cm thick, 31 (40%) had supraventricular arrhythmias. (This number and percent excludes atrial premature complexes.) In our patients, the frequency of atrial arrhythmias increased with increasing thickness of the atrial septa, such that 60% of the patients with an atrial septum ≥3 cm had atrial arrhythmias com-

Table 5. Electrocardiographic Findings in 28 Men and Women With Lipomatous Hypertrophy of the Atrial Septum

| Pt No. | Age at Death (yr)/Gender | Interval From ECG to Death (days) | Heart Rate (beats/min) | Heart Rhythm | Interval (ms) | | | Conduction Abnormality | QRS Voltage (mm) | | | APC | LAA | HW (g) | LV Fibrosis | LV Necrosis | Thickness of Atrial Septum (cm) | ≥1 CA >75% ↓ in CSA by Plaque | Cause of Death |
					PR	QRS	QTc		12-Lead	I,II, III,R, L,F	V_1–V_6								
								Men											
1	48/M	94	56	S	14	8	42	0	97	34	63	0	0	490	0	0	2.5	+	CAD
2	51/M	7	85	S	18	8	36	0	170	59	111	0	+	630	0	+	2.0	+	CAD
3	57/M	57	110	S	16	8	37	0	155	54	101	+	0	685	0	0	3.0	0	Cancer
4	64/M	23	82	S	15	9	28	0	139	59	80	+	+	470	0	0	2.5	0	Suicide
5	65/M	10	80	AF	—	12	—	Left BBB	241	95	146	–	–	450	+	+	3.0	+	CAD
6	68/M	1	56	S	18	10	44	0	93	34	59	+	+	490	0	0	2.0	+	CAD
7	70/M	3	72	J	17	14	44	Right BBB	118	53	65	0	+	520	0	+	2.5	+	CAD
8	70/M	1	124	AF	—	10	30	0	147	60	87	–	–	795	0	0	5.0	0	Infection
9	72/M	11	170	AT	—	11	26	IVCD	134	49	85	–	–	710	+	0	2.0	+	CAD
10	73/M	41	95	S	18	15	37	Right BBB,LPFB	94	49	45	+	+	690	+	0	2.9	+	Cancer
11	73/M	89	84	EA	22	13	41	Left BBB	112	50	62	+	–	550	0	0	3.4	+	AAA
12	84/M	5	120	AT	—	8	—	0	157	43	114	–	–	410	0	0	3.5	+	Cancer
Subtotal	67 ± 10/12M	29 ± 9	95 ± 30	6S	18 ± 2	10 ± 2	37 ± 6	5	140 ± 43	54 ± 17	87 ± 29	5 (63%)	6/7	576 ± 129	3	3	2.9 ± 0.9	9 (75%)	
								Women											
13	59/F	6	136	S	16	8	36	0	90	49	41	+	+	410	+	0	2.0	+	Cancer
14	60/F	1	125	S	16	9	36	0	91	20	71	0	0	680	+	+	3.0	+	CAD
15	70/F	43	82	S	17	10	44	0	127	60	67	+	+	550	0	+	2.0	+	CAD
16	71/F	9	89	S	18	9	38	0	125	52	67	0	+	630	0	+	2.2	+	CAD
17	72/F	15	85	S	20	10	40	0	93	23	70	0	+	330	0	0	2.0	0	Cancer
18	73/F	3	80	AF	—	9	40	0	158	52	106	–	–	680	0	0	2.7	+	CAD*
19	74/F	130	78	AF	—	9	—	0	133	51	82	–	–	540	0	0	3.5	0	Cancer
20	76/F	11	120	AT	—	8	—	0	266	80	186	–	–	450	0	0	3.0	0	—
21	77/F	6	146	AF	—	8	27	0	75	20	55	–	–	530	+	0	3.0	+	Infection
22	77/F	16	105	S	19	8	28	0	138	40	98	+	+	440	0	0	2.0	0	Leukemia
23	78/F	13	117	S	20	7	—	0	121	41	80	0	+	410	0	0	2.5	0	COPD
24	78/F	2	155	AF	—	10	—	0	110	34	76	–	–	540	0	0	3.3	0	Cancer
25	79/F	11	92	S	21	9	42	LAFB	88	50	38	0	+	420	0	0	2.0	+	COPD
26	79/F	455	100	S	20	8	38	0	217	71	146	0	+	500	0	0	3.5	0	Stroke
27	80/F	3	120	S	20	7	32	0	59	27	32	+	0	350	0	0	2.0	+	Cancer
28	83/F	39	132	AF	—	7	27	0	89	26	63	–	–	575	0	0	4.0	+	COPD
Subtotal	74 ± 7/16F	21 ± 16	110 ± 27	10S	19 ± 2	9 ± 1	36 ± 6	1	124 ± 53	43 ± 18	81 ± 39	4 (40%)	8/10	502 ± 108	3	3	2.7 ± 0.7	9 (56%)	
Total	70 ± 9/28	24 ± 9	103 ± 28	16S	18 ± 2	9 ± 2	36 ± 6	6 (18%)	131 ± 51	83 ± 36	47 ± 18	9 (50%)	14/17	545 ± 125	6	6	2.8 ± 0.7	18 (64%)	

*Died after mitral valve replacement for mitral regurgitation secondary to papillary muscle dysfunction. Subtotal and total values are presented as mean value ± SD or number (%) of patients. AAA = abdominal aortic aneurysm; AF = atrial fibrillation; APC = atrial premature complex; AT = (multifocal) atrial tachycardia; B = black; BBB = bundle branch block; COPD = chronic obstructive pulmonary disease; EA = ectopic atrial; ECG = electrocardiogram; IVCD = intraventricular conduction delay; J = junctional; LAA = left atrial abnormality; LAFB = left anterior fascicular block; LPFB = left posterior fascicular block; S = sinus; other abbreviations as in Table 1.

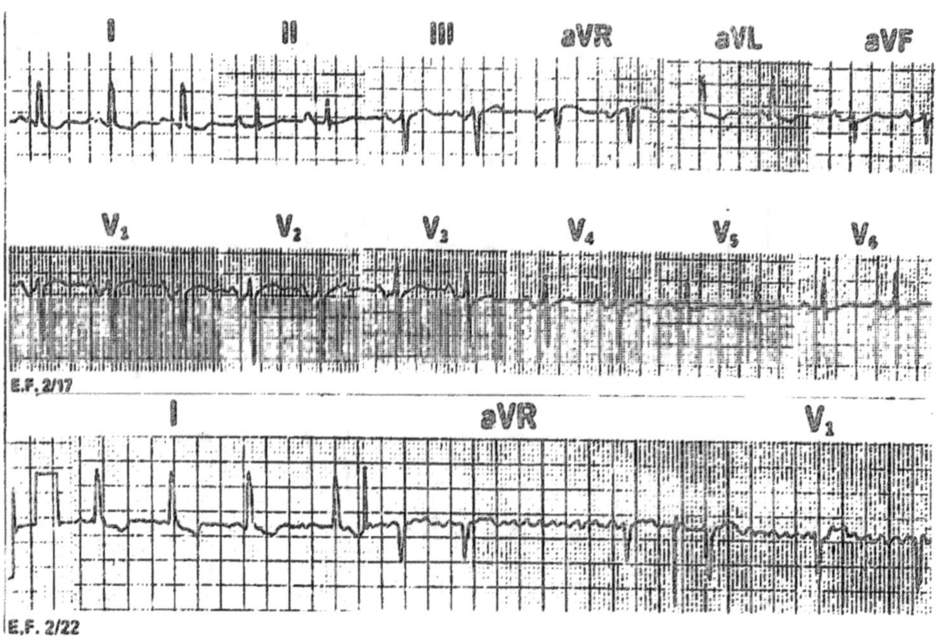

Figure 12. Electrocardiographic recordings obtained 5 days apart in a 74-year old white woman who died of lung cancer. At necropsy, the heart weighed 540 g, the atrial cavities were mildly enlarged and there were no scars in the left ventricular myocardium. The thickness of the atrial septum is 5.4 and 1.4 cm cephalad and caudal, respectively, to the fossa ovalis. Upper two tracings, Typical "dome and dip" P waves in sinus rhythm; Lower tracing, The rhythm is now atrial fibrillation.

pared with only 34% of the patients with an atrial septum 2 to 2.9 cm thick (p < 0.01). Furthermore, in the 31 patients with atrial arrhythmias the atrial septum was thicker than in

Table 6. Comparison of the Clinical and Morphologic Findings in 28 Patients With Small (septal thickness <3 cm) and Large (septal thickness ≥3 cm) Fatty Deposits in the Atrial Septum in Whom a 12-Lead Electrocardiogram Was Available

	Atrial Septal Thickness <3 cm (n = 16)	Atrial Septal Thickness ≥3 cm (n = 12)
Age (yr) (mean)	(69)	(73)
Gender		
Men	7	5
Women	9	7
Systemic hypertension	10 (63%)	9 (75%)
Interval ECG to death (days)	19*	32*
Heart rhythm		
Sinus	13 (82%)*	3 (25%)*
Junctional	1 (6%)	0
Atrial tachycardia	1 (6%)	2 (17%)
Atrial fibrillation	1 (6%)	6 (50)%
Ectopic atrial rhythm	0	1 (8%)
Any atrial rhythm other than sinus	3 (18%)*	9 (75%)*
Conduction abnormality		
QRS voltage		
12-lead	115*	150*
Precordial leads	46	51
Limb leads	69*	99*
Heart weight (g)	515	520
LV fibrosis	3	3
LV necrosis	4	2
Thickness of atrial septum (cm)	2.2*	3.4*
≥1 CA with >75% ↓ in CSA by plaque	12 (75%)	6 (50%)

*p = 0.05. Abbreviations as in Table 1.

patients without these arrhythmias (2.9 vs. 2.3 cm, p < 0.01) (Table 4). Finally, the similar frequency of significant coronary artery disease or myocardial infarction in the patients with and without atrial arrhythmias strongly supports the view that the atrial arrhythmias result in some way from the massive fatty deposits in the atrial septum.

Kluge (2) was the first to mention a possible association between atrial arrhythmias and massive fatty deposits in the atrial septum. He described a 64-year old man with a 3-cm thick atrial septum and atrial tachycardia. The patient also had chronic obstructive pulmonary disease. Hutter and Page (4) described supraventricular arrhythmias in all 10 of their patients with an atrial septal thickness of 1 to 4 cm. Eight had premature atrial complexes that were often multifocal, three had wandering atrial pacemaker, three had multifocal atrial tachycardia and two had paroxysmal atrial tachycardia. One of the 10 patients had sick sinus syndrome and another 2 had atrial fibrillation. In five patients a peculiar P wave configuration (dome and dip P wave) was seen. We found similar P waves in 13 (67%) of our 16 patients in sinus rhythm (Fig. 12); 1 of our 13 patients had P waves suggestive of interatrial conduction block. At necropsy, the left atrium was dilated in only 1 (8%) of the 13 patients with sinus rhythm and an abnormal P wave configuration. Erhardt (15) speculated that the abnormal P waves in these patients result from normal downward activation of the right atrium from the sinus node, whereas the left atrium is electrically activated later in an upward fashion from the AV node. Four of the six patients reported on by Klein and Schaefer (17) with massive atrial septal fat diagnosed at necropsy had ECG abnormalities (intermittent sinoatrial block in two patients and atrial tachycardia and paroxysmal atrial fibrillation in one patient, and incomplete right bundle branch block and first degree

AV block in one). Only one patient had atherosclerotic coronary artery disease.

Other possible effects. Atrial arrhythmias appear to be the only functional consequence of massive fatty infiltrates in the atrial septum. Although other reports (6) have mentioned the possibility of obstruction to blood flow in the superior vena cava, coronary sinus, right pulmonary veins and right atrium, such obstruction has never been proved hemodynamically and none of our patients, even those with the thickest septa, had anatomic evidence of functional compression of adjacent vascular structures.

A potential danger of massive fatty infiltrates in the atrial septum is their confusion with neoplastic infiltration of the septum. Indeed, two patients have been reported (7,8) to have operative excision of the fatty mass in the atrial septum because cancer was suspected.

Diagnosis and nomenclature. In vivo diagnosis of massive fatty deposits in the atrial septum was reported first in 1982 with the use of computed tomography (13). Since then, a number of reports have described the diagnostic usefulness of echocardiography (8–12), computed tomography (11,12) and nuclear magnetic resonance imaging (8,10–12).

The best name for the massive fatty deposits in the atrial septum is still debated. We prefer the simple phrase "massive fatty deposits in the atrial septum" because it best describes the abnormality. The most common phrase is "lipomatous hypertrophy of the atrial septum," but the word "lipomatous" is incorrect because the fatty infiltrates are clearly not lipomas. In our view, the word "hypertrophy" should not be used to describe an infiltrate that should not be there in the first place. Thus, we suggest the simple descriptive phrase "massive fatty deposits in the atrial septum."

References

1. Prior JT. Lipomatous hypertrophy of cardiac interatrial septum: a lesion resembling hibernoma, lipoblastomatosis and infiltrating lipoma. Arch Pathol 1964;78:11–5.
2. Kluge WF. Lipomatous hypertrophy of the interatrial septum. Northwest Med 1969;68:25–30.
3. Page DL. Lipomatous hypertrophy of the cardiac interatrial septum: its development and probable clinical significance. Hum Pathol 1970;1:151–63.
4. Hutter AM, Page DL. Atrial arrhythmias and lipomatous hypertrophy of the cardiac interatrial septum. Am Heart J 1971;82:16–21.
5. McAllister HA, Fenoglio JJ. Tumors of the Cardiovascular System. Fascicle 15, Second Series. Atlas of Tumor Pathology. Armed Forces Institute of Pathology, Washington D.C. 1978:40–4.
6. McNamara RF, Taylor AE, Panner BJ. Superior vena caval obstruction by lipomatous hypertrophy of the right atrium. Clin Cardiol 1987;10:609–10.
7. Tschirkov A, Stegaru B. Lipomatous hypertrophy of interatrial septum presenting as recurring pericardial effusion and mistaken for constrictive pericarditis. Thorac Cardiovasc Surg 1979;27:400–3.
8. Fisher MS, Edmonds P. Lipomatous hypertrophy of the interatrial septum. Diagnosis by magnetic resonance imaging. J Comput Tomogr 1988;12:267–9.
9. Fyke FE III, Tajik AJ, Edwards WD, Seward JB. Diagnosis of lipomatous hypertrophy of the atrial septum by two-dimensional echocardiography. J Am Coll Cardiol 1983;1:1352–7.
10. Applegate PM, Tajik AJ, Ehman RL, Julsrud PR, Miller FA Jr. Two-dimensional echocardiographic and magnetic resonance imaging observations in massive lipomatous hypertrophy of the atrial septum. Am J Cardiol 1987;59:489–91.
11. Kindman LA, Wright A, Tye T, Seale W, Appleton C. Lipomatous hypertrophy of the interatrial septum: characterization by transesophageal and transthoracic echocardiography, magnetic resonance imaging, and computed tomography. J Am Soc Echocardiogr 1988;1:450–4.
12. Levine RA, Weyman AE, Dinsmore RE, et al. Noninvasive tissue characterization: diagnosis of lipomatous hypertrophy of the atrial septum by nuclear magnetic resonance imaging. J Am Coll Cardiol 1986;7:698–92.
13. Isner JM, Swan CS II, Mikus JP, Carter BL. Lipomatous hypertrophy of the interatrial septum: in vivo diagnosis. Circulation 1982;66:470–3.
14. Okel BB. The Wolff-Parkinson-White syndrome: report of a case with fatal arrhythmia and autopsy findings of myocarditis, interatrial lipomatous hypertrophy, and prominent right moderator band. Am Heart J 1968;75:673–8.
15. Erhardt LR. Abnormal atrial activity in lipomatous hypertrophy of the interatrial septum. Am Heart J 1974;87:571–6.
16. Reyes CV, Jablokow VR. Lipomatous hypertrophy of the cardiac interatrial septum: a report of 38 cases and review of the literature. Am J Clin Pathol 1970;72:785–8
17. Klein PJ, Schaefer HE. Das interatriale Lipom des Herzen. Z Krebsforsch 1973;79:11–8.
18. Crocker DW. Lipomatous infiltrates of the heart. Arch Pathol Lab Med 1978;102:69–72.
19. Kindblom LG, Svensson U. Multiple hibernomas of the heart: a case report. Acta Pathol Microbiol Scand 1977;85:122–6.
20. Inove T, Mohri N, Nagahara T, Takanashi R. A case report of "lipomatous hypertrophy of the cardiac interatrial septum," with a proposal for a new term "lipomatous hamartoma of the cardiac atrial septum." Acta Pathol Jpn 1988;38:1583–9.
21. Roberts WC, Roberts JD. The floating heart or the heart too fat to sink: analysis of 55 necropsy patients. Am J Cardiol 1983;52:1286–9.
22. Siegel RJ, Roberts WC. Electrocardiographic observations in severe aortic valve stenosis: correlative necropsy study to clinical hemodynamic and ECG variables demonstrating relation of 12-lead QRS amplitude to peak systolic transaortic pressure gradient. Am Heart J 1982;103:298–301.

The Heart at Necropsy in Massive Obesity (>300 pounds or >136 kilograms)

A 52-year-old African-American man, who weighed 580 pounds (264 kg) and was 72 inches tall (body mass index = 79 kg/m^2!), was hospitalized because of increasing dyspnea. He had been known to have systemic hypertension, sleep apnea, and diabetes mellitus. He never had symptoms or objective evidence of myocardial ischemia. The serum total cholesterol was 142, low-density lipoprotein cholesterol 40, high-density lipoprotein cholesterol 17, and triglycerides 242 mg/dl. An echocardiogram disclosed the left ventricular ejection fraction to be 62%. Twelve days after admission he was found dead in bed. Autopsy disclosed massive pulmonary embolism without pulmonary infarction. The heart weighed 780 g, but did not float in water. The epicardium and the 4 cardiac valves were normal. The walls of the ventricles were devoid of foci of necrosis and fibrosis. The major epicardial coronary arteries were all large and devoid of atherosclerotic plaques. Likewise, the aorta contained few atherosclerotic plaques.

There are relatively few necropsy data on the status of the heart at necropsy in massively obese subjects. Amad et al,[1] in 1965, described findings at necropsy in 6 patients aged 35 to 65 years (mean 47), who weighed from 308 to 495 pounds (140 to 225 kg): the hearts in the 3 women weighed 400, 500, and 620 g and the hearts in the 3 men, 450, 900, and 1,100 g. The weights had been taken from autopsy reports. These authors excluded patients "who had clinical signs or pathologic evidence of coronary atherosclerosis or who had systemic arterial pressures ≥150/90 mm Hg." The number of patients excluded was not described. By gross examination, none of their patients had fatty infiltration into myocardium or grossly visible foci of myocardial necrosis or fibrosis.

Warnes and Roberts,[2] in 1984, described 12 patients at necropsy aged 25 to 59 years (mean 37; 5 women and 7 men) who weighed from 312 to >500 pounds (mean 381). Five patients had died suddenly, 2 of chronic congestive heart failure, 1 of acute myocardial infarction, 1 of aortic dissection, 1 of an intracerebral bleed, 1 of drug overdose, and 1 shortly after ileal bypass. Only 2 of the 12 patients had 1 or more epicardial coronary arteries narrowed >75% in cross-sectional area by atherosclerotic plaque and those 2 were the only 2 with left ventricular foci of either necrosis or fibrosis. Of the 2 patients with narrowing 76% to 100% in cross-sectional area by plaque, each patient had both the right and left anterior descending coronary arteries narrowed to this degree. Of the 48 major epicardial coronary arteries in the 12 patients (4/patient), 4 were narrowed at some point 76% to 100% in cross-sectional area by atheroscle-

rotic plaque. A total of 664 five-mm segments were examined from 11 hearts (mean 60/patient). Only 2 patients had any 5-mm segments narrowed 76% to 100% in cross-sectional area. Of the 664 five-mm coronary segments, 431 (65%) were narrowed 0% to 25% in cross-sectional area; 143 (21%), 26% to 50%; 73 (11%), 51% to 75%; and 17 (3%) were

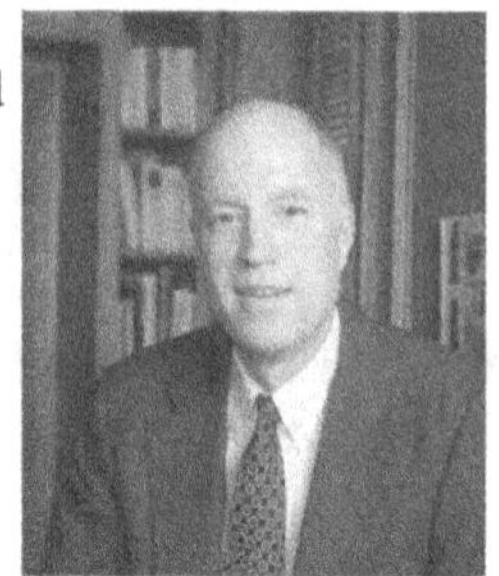

narrowed 76% to 100%. The hearts in the 12 patients were all heavier than normal (380 to 990 g [mean 616]). The subepicardial adipose tissue by visual inspection appeared to be increased in 9 of the 12 patients, but in no patient did the heart float in water.

The average age of death in the 12 patients described by Warnes and Roberts was only 37 and only 1 patient was >50 years of age. That fact may be a major reason for the mild amount of coronary atherosclerosis found in these patients. The 2 with symptomatic fatal coronary disease were aged 42 and 59 years. In none of the 12 patients reported by Warnes and Roberts or in the 6 patients reported by Amad et al were serum cholesterol values available.

No other reports on the heart at necropsy in massively obese persons have appeared since 1984. It appears that the massively obese person usually dies from a noncoronary cause before significant coronary atherosclerosis has had time to develop.

William Clifford Roberts, MD
Editor in Chief
Baylor Heart & Vascular Institute
Baylor University Medical Center
Dallas, Texas

1. Amad KH, Brennan JC, Alexander JK. The cardiac pathology of chronic exogenous obesity. *Circulation* 1965;32:740–745.
2. Warnes CA, Roberts WC. The heart in massive (more than 300 pounds or 136 kilograms) obesity: Analysis of 12 patients studied at necropsy. *Am J Cardiol* 1984;54:1087–1091.

Comparison of Total 12-Lead QRS Voltage in a Variety of Cardiac Conditions and Its Usefulness in Predicting Increased Cardiac Mass

William C. Roberts, MD[a,b,*], Giovanni Filardo, PhD[c,d,e,f], Jong Mi Ko, BA[b], Robert J. Siegel, MD[g], Allen L. Dollar, MD[g], Elizabeth M. Ross, MD[g], and Jamshid Shirani, MD[g]

Echocardiography provides a more accurate method to determine increased cardiac mass than does electrocardiography. Nevertheless, most offices of physicians do not possess echocardiographic machines, but many possess electrocardiographic machines. Many electrocardiographic criteria have been used to determine increased cardiac mass, but few of the criteria have been measured against cardiac weight determined at necropsy or after cardiac transplantation. Such was the purpose of the present study. Cardiac weight at necropsy or after transplantation was determined in 359 patients with 11 different cardiac conditions, and total 12-lead electrocardiographic QRS voltage (from the peak of the R wave to the nadir of either the Q or the S wave, whichever was deeper) was measured in each patient. Even in hearts with massively increased cardiac mass (>1,000 g), the total 12-lead QRS voltage was clearly increased (>175 mm) in only 94%, but this criterion was superior to that of previously described electrocardiographic criteria for "left ventricular hypertrophy." Hearts with excessive adipose tissue infrequently had increased total 12-lead QRS voltage despite increased cardiac weight. Likewise, patients with fatal cardiac amyloidosis had hearts of increased weight but quite low total 12-lead QRS voltage. In conclusion, 12-lead QRS voltage is useful in predicting increased cardiac mass, but that predictability is dependent in part on the cause of the increased cardiac mass. © 2013 Elsevier Inc. All rights reserved. (Am J Cardiol 2013;112:904–909)

Various electrocardiographic criteria have been used to predict left ventricular hypertrophy (LVH), but few have been compared with the actual weight of the heart at necropsy or after cardiac transplantation. Exceptions are the studies by Griep[1] in 1959, and by Allenstein and Hiroyoshi[2] in 1960. The most common criterion used in the past 60 years is that recommended in 1949 by Sokolow and Lyon,[3] who studied 12-lead electrocardiograms in patients who were believed to have LVH on the basis of "a cardiac disorder capable of producing increased strain on the left ventricle (such as hypertension,

aortic valve lesions, coarctation of the aorta, patent ductus arteriosus)." These investigators produced a variety of electrocardiographic criteria for LVH, including among others R in lead V_5 + S_1 in lead V_1 ≥35 mm. A number of other criteria have been suggested subsequently (Table 1).[4–11] Siegel and Roberts[12] in 1982 proposed that measuring the total amplitude (from the peak of the R wave to the nadir of either the Q or the S wave, whichever was deeper) of the QRS complex in all 12 electrocardiographic leads was a better determinant of cardiac mass than the previously reported criteria (Figure 1). Subsequently, several investigators from the same laboratory measured total 12-lead QRS voltage in a variety of cardiac conditions and in each compared it with the heart weight determined by the same investigators.[13–22] Here, we review their findings in 11 different cardiac conditions.

Methods

To be included in this study, a heart had to be studied in the Pathology Branch of the National Heart, Lung, and Blood Institute of the National Institutes of Health (Bethesda, Maryland). An accurate heart weight and a 12-lead electrocardiogram had to be available in all cases to be included in this study. The patients were divided into 11 groups (Table 2). The electrocardiographic QRS voltage was measured in each of the 12 leads, as demonstrated in Figure 1. In patients with >1 twelve-lead electrocardiogram available, the one measured was the one recorded closest to the patient's death or closest to cardiac transplantation. The medical records were reviewed in all cases to provide pertinent clinical information. All hearts were examined and classified morphologically by one investigator (WCR). The QRS measurements were

aDepartments of Internal Medicine and Pathology; bBaylor Heart and Vascular Institute, Dallas, Texas; cInstitute for Health Care Research and Improvement, Baylor Health Care System; dCardiovascular Epidemiology, Baylor University Medical Center, Dallas, Texas; eCardiovascular Epidemiology, The Heart Hospital Baylor, Plano, Texas; fSouthern Methodist University, Dallas, Texas; and gPathology Branch, National Heart, Lung, and Blood Institute, National Institutes of Health, Bethesda, Maryland. Manuscript received April 3, 2013; revised manuscript received and accepted April 23, 2013.

Present address (RJS): Cedars-Sinai Medical Center, Division of Cardiology, 8700 Beverly Boulevard, Suite 5623, Los Angeles, CA 90048.

Present address (ALD): Emory University School of Medicine (Cardiology), 49 Jesse Hill Drive, Atlanta, GA 30303.

Present address (EMR): 2021 K Street, NW, Suite 315, Washington, DC 20006.

Present address (JS): St. Luke's University Health Network Cardiology, 801 Ostrum Street, Bethlehem, PA 18015.

This work was supported by grants from Baylor Health Care System Foundation.

See page 909 for disclosure information.

*Corresponding author: Tel: (214) 820-7911; fax: (214) 820-7533.

E-mail address: wc.roberts@baylorhealth.edu (W.C. Roberts).

Table 1

Recommended or modified electrocardiographic criteria for determining left ventricular hypertrophy as to 17 patients with hearts at necropsy weighing >1,000 grams*

No.	QRS Complex Measured	Value Considered Upper Limit of Normal (mm)	No. (%) of 17 Patients Above Normal Limit
1a	$SV_1 + RV_5$ or V_6 (larger)	35	12 (71%)
1b	$SV_1 + RV_5$ or V_6 (larger)	40	11 (65%)
2a	SV_1 or V_2 (larger) + RV_5 or V_6 (larger)	35	15 (88%)
2b	SV_1 or V_2 (larger) + RV_5 or V_6 (larger)	40	14 (82%)
3a	SV_1 or V_2 (larger) + RV_6	35	15 (88%)
3b	SV_1 or V_2 (larger) + RV_6	40	13 (76%)
4a	$SV_2 + RV_5$	35	14 (82%)
4b	$SV_2 + RV_5$	40	14 (82%)
5a	Deepest $SV_1 - V_3$ + tallest $RV_4 - V_6$	35	14 (82%)
5b	Deepest $SV_1 - V_3$ + tallest $RV_4 - V_6$	40	13 (76%)
5c	Deepest $SV_1 - V_3$ + tallest $RV_4 - V_6$	45	13 (76%)
5d	Deepest $SV_1 - V_3$ + tallest $RV_4 - V_6$	50	13 (76%)
6a	Tallest R + deepest S in any V lead	35	14 (82%)
6b	Tallest R + deepest S in any V lead	40	14 (82%)
7a	Deepest $SV_1 - V_3$	25	14 (82%)
7b	Deepest $SV_1 - V_3$	30	12 (71%)
8a	Tallest $RV_4 - V_6$	25	9 (53%)
8b	Tallest $RV_4 - V_6$	30	8 (27%)
9a	Deepest $SV_1 - V_2$	25	14 (82%)
9b	Deepest $SV_1 - V_2$	30	12 (71%)
10a	Tallest RV_5 or V_6	25	9 (53%)
10b	Tallest RV_5 or V_6	30	8 (27%)
11	$RV_6 > RV_5$	≤1	13 (76%)
12a	Tallest limb-lead R + deepest limb-lead S	15	15 (88%)
12b	Tallest limb-lead R + deepest limb-lead S	20	12 (71%)
13a	$R_1 + S_3$	15	12 (71%)
13b	$R_1 + S_3$	20	10 (59%)
14a	Tallest limb-lead R	10	14 (82%)
14b	Tallest limb-lead R	15	6 (35%)
15a	Deepest limb-lead S	10	10 (59%)
15b	Deepest limb-lead S	15	6 (35%)
16	R_1	10	11 (65%)
17	S_3	10	7 (41%)
18a	Total 12-lead QRS voltage	175	16 (94%)
18b	Total 12-lead QRS voltage	200	15 (88%)
18c	Total 12-lead QRS voltage	225	13 (76%)
18d	Total 12-lead QRS voltage	250	13 (76%)

* From Roberts and Podolak.[13]

performed by the first author of each study and "spot checked" by WCR when not the first author.

Means, SDs, and percentages were calculated to describe the study cohort (n = 359). A multivariate linear regression model was used to assess the adjusted association between patients' heart weight (grams) and 12-lead QRS voltage (millimeters).[23] Covariates included gender, age, and cardiac condition. Restricted cubic splines were used for all continuous variables.[24] Adjusted p values and plots of the association between patient's heart weight and 12-lead QRS voltage were also estimated.

Results

A total of 359 patients, 208 men (58%) and 151 women (42%), were included and divided into 11 groups (Table 2). Their ages ranged from 14 to 85 years; of the 359 patients, 8 (2%) were aged ≤20 years, including 1 aged 20 years, 5 aged 19 years, 1 aged 16 years, and 1 aged 14 years. The heart weights in the 359 patients ranged from 150 to 1,360 g, and the mean heart weights were of increased mass (heart weight >350 g in women and >400 g in men) in 8 of the 11 groups in men and in 10 of the 11 groups in women. Total 12-lead QRS voltage (measured with normal [10 mm] standardization [10 mm = 1 mV]) ranged from 58 to 601 mm. In 8 of the 11 groups, the mean total 12-lead QRS voltage was lower in male than in female patients; in contrast, the mean heart weight was higher in male than in female patients in 9 of the 11 groups. Additionally, the ratio of total 12-lead QRS voltage (millimeters) to heart weight (grams) was lower in male than in female patients in all 11 groups. Figure 2 depicts the adjusted (by age and gender) association between heart weight and total 12-lead QRS voltage in the 10 patient groups and in the normal group. (Individual patient-level data in the aortic stenosis patient group were not available.) The electrocardiograms obtained in the patients who underwent

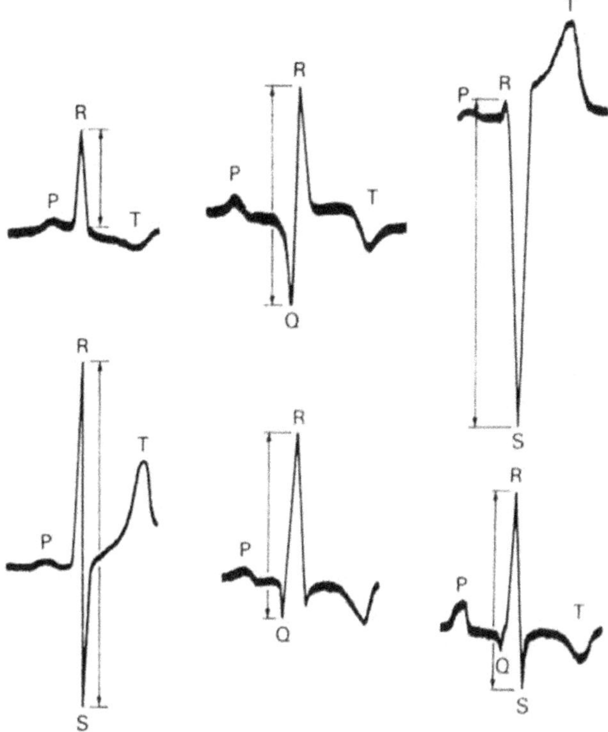

Figure 1. Various QRS complexes showing how each was measured. Reproduced from Siegel and Roberts[12] with permission of the publisher.

cardiac operations were the ones recorded immediately preoperatively.

Hearts weighing >1,000 g[13]: Of these 17 patients, 16 (94%) were men aged 29 to 64 years (mean 42). The one woman's heart weighed 1,250 g (3.6 times the upper limit of normal), and her total 12-lead QRS voltage, 601 mm, was the largest of any of the 359 patients. The cause of the massive cardiomegaly in these 17 patients was isolated pure aortic regurgitation (5 patients), combined pure aortic regurgitation and pure mitral regurgitation (4 patients), pure aortic regurgitation plus ventricular septal defect (2 patients), aortic stenosis and regurgitation (2 patients), aortic regurgitation plus mitral stenosis with regurgitation (1 patient), hypertrophic cardiomyopathy (2 patients), and ventricular septal defect with mitral stenosis (1 patient). The total 12-lead QRS voltage was highest in this group than in any of the others.

Aortic valve stenosis[12]: These 50 patients, aged 16 to 65 years (mean 48), had peak systolic transvalvular pressure gradients ranging from 52 to 180 mm Hg (mean 98) and peak left ventricular systolic pressures ranging from 149 to 270 mm Hg (average 210). All had anatomically normal mitral valves. Aortic valve replacement had been done in 38 patients (76%), and all died <6 weeks after the operation; 2 others died during anesthesia induction. The aortic valve was unicuspid unicommissural in 5 patients (12%), congenitally bicuspid in 29 patients (58%), and tricuspid in 15 patients (30%). Because the total 12-lead QRS amplitude (millimeters) roughly equaled the peak left ventricular systolic pressure (millimeters of mercury), Siegel and Roberts[13] suggested that the total 12-lead QRS voltage (millimeters) minus the systemic arterial systolic pressure (millimeters of mercury) roughly equaled the peak systolic pressure gradient (millimeters of mercury) between the left ventricle and the systemic artery.

Aortic regurgitation[14]: These 30 patients, aged 19 to 65 years (mean 45), all had chronic pure (no element of aortic stenosis) severe aortic regurgitation secondary to infective endocarditis that had healed (8 patients), syphilis (6 patients), ankylosing spondylitis (5 patients), Marfan syndrome (5 patients), and uncertain or other causes (6 patients). Nineteen patients (63%) had undergone aortic valve replacement, and all died <60 days after the operation. Only 2 of these 30 hearts weighed >1,000 g (1,010 and 1,100 g).

Mitral regurgitation[15]: These 24 patients, aged 21 to 84 years (mean 42), all had chronic isolated severe pure (no element of stenosis) mitral regurgitation. The cause of the regurgitation was attributed to rheumatic disease (14 patients), mitral valve prolapse (7 patients), and infective endocarditis that had healed (3 patients). Nine patients (30%) had undergone mitral valve replacement.

Hypertrophic cardiomyopathy (studied at necropsy)[16]: These 57 patients ranged in age from 14 to 87 years (mean 49). Cardiac catheterization data within 2 years of death were available in 42 patients: left ventricular to systemic arterial peak pressure gradient at rest >10 mm Hg was present in 32 patients (77%) and with provocation in 35 patients (85%). The resting peak systolic gradients ranged from 12 to 162 mm Hg (mean 79) and the provoked gradients, from 40 to 190 mm Hg (mean 104). There were no differences between patients with and without outflow pressure gradients with regard to heart weight, ventricular septal thickness, total 12-lead QRS amplitude, and Romhilt-Estes score.[6] The mean Sokolow-Lyon index was insignificantly different: 37 in the obstructive group and 28 in the nonobstructive group.

Hypertrophic cardiomyopathy (studied after cardiac transplantation)[17]: These 10 patients, aged 19 to 46 years (mean 35), all had severe chronic heart failure, and only 1 had left ventricular outflow obstruction. Nine had dilated left ventricular cavities, and 8 had extensive left ventricular wall scarring without narrowing of the epicardial coronary arteries. Six of the 9 had left ventricular ejection fractions <50%.

Idiopathic dilated cardiomyopathy[18]: These 49 patients, aged 19 to 75 years (mean 45), had typical clinical and morphologic cardiac features of this condition.

Lipomatous hypertrophy of the atrial septum[19]: The thickness of the atrial septum cephalad to the fossa ovalis is these 28 patients ranged from 2.0 to 5.0 cm (mean 2.8). The 12 men ranged in age from 48 to 84 years (mean 67) and the 16 women, from 59 to 83 years (mean 74). The total 12-lead QRS voltage in the men ranged from 93 to 241 mm (mean 140) and in the women from 59 to 266 mm (mean 124). The heart weights in the men averaged 576 g and in the women, 502 g.

Carcinoid syndrome[20]: Of these 36 patients, 21 (57%) had carcinoid heart disease and 15 (43%) did not. The 2 groups were similar in mean age (54 vs 55 years), duration of clinical illness (4.7 vs 6.3 years), body weight (50 vs 52 kg), and systemic blood pressure (117/77 vs 128/77 mm Hg). The 2 groups were different in the frequency of the presence

Table 2

Total 12-lead QRS voltage, heart weight, and age of groups of 331 patients with various cardiac conditions

Condition	Gender	Number of Cases	Ages (yrs), Range (Mean)	Total 12-Lead QRS Voltage (mm), Mean	Patients With 12-Lead QRS Voltage >175 mm	Heart Weight (g), Range (Mean)	Total 12-Lead QRS Voltage (mm)/Heart Weight (g)	Year of Publication	Authors (Reference Number)
Hearts weighing >1,000 g	M	16	29−64 (42)	140−414 (306)	16	1,005−1,360 (1,102)	0.28	1985	Roberts and Podolak[13]
	F	1	20	601	(94%)	1,250	0.48		
Aortic valve stenosis	M	36	16−64 (48)	144−417 (249)	47	440−880 (639)	0.39	1982	Siegel and Roberts[12]
	F	14	16−65 (47)	193−376 (277)	(94%)	380−700 (521)	0.53		
Aortic regurgitation	M	22	19−59 (44)	109−428 (271)	27	430−1,100 (717)	0.38	1985	Roberts and Day[14]
	F	8	35−56 (48)	169−384 (275)	(90%)	375−950 (638)	0.43		
Mitral regurgitation	M	11	24−84 (47)	111−364 (245)	17	400−775 (629)	0.39	1992	Glick and Roberts[15]
	F	13	21−64 (37)	114−290 (199)	(71%)	350−675 (472)	0.42		
Hypertrophic cardiomyopathy without cardiac transplantation	M	21	14−68 (46)	107−339 (190)	30	325−1,070 (671)	0.28	1989	Dollar and Roberts[16]
	F	36	19−87 (51)	68−327 (201)	(53%)	290−1,230 (547)	0.38		
Hypertrophic cardiomyopathy with cardiac transplantation	M	6	19−46 (35)	109−201 (142)	4	310−480 (393)	0.36	1993	Shirani et al[17]
	F	4	24−45 (35)	172−378 (241)	(40%)	290−650 (408)	0.59		
Idiopathic dilated cardiomyopathy	M	35	19−73 (46)	74−281 (147)	20	400−940 (620)	0.24	1987	Roberts et al[18]
	F	14	22−75 (54)	75−243 (167)	(41%)	400−860 (602)	0.28		
Lipomatous hypertrophy of the atrial septum	M	12	48−84 (67)	93−24 (140)	3	410−795 (576)	0.24	1993	Shirani and Roberts[19]
	F	16	59−83 (74)	59−266 (124)	(11%)	330−680 (502)	0.25		
Carcinoid syndrome With carcinoid heart disease	M	11	39−72 (56)	58−227 (120)	2	220−480 (350)	0.34	1985	Ross and Roberts[20]
	F	8	28−64 (54)	58−128 (84)	(11%)	200−290 (245)	0.34		
Without carcinoid heart disease	M	10	42−75 (55)	89−129 (137)	2	240−570 (350)	0.39		
	F	5	28−67 (50)	102−135 (121)	(13%)	150−270 (230)	0.53		
Cardiac amyloidosis	M	15	32−69 (52)	60−197 (99)	2	410−850 (570)	0.17	1983	Roberts and Waller[21]
	F	15	21−93 (69)	58−199 (109)	(7%)	370−900 (494)	0.22		
Cardiac adiposity	M	13	51−73 (64)	73−159 (114)	1	320−795 (485)	0.24	1995	Shirani et al[22]
	F	17	40−85 (70)	77−210 (124)	(3%)	250−575 (395)	0.31		

of precordial murmurs consistent with tricuspid regurgitation and/or pulmonary stenosis (95% vs 13%), cardiomegaly by chest x-ray (38% vs 0%), low voltage on electrocardiography (47% vs 0%), and location of the primary carcinoid neoplasm. Total 12-lead QRS voltage was similar in each group (105 vs 132 mm; 10 mm = 1 mV). Of those with carcinoid heart disease, 43% died of cardiac causes, whereas in those without carcinoid heart disease, none died of a cardiac cause.

Cardiac amyloidosis[21]: All 30 patients, aged 32 to 92 years (mean 59), died from amyloidosis that involved the heart extensively and also multiple other organs. The peak systemic arterial systolic pressure in the 9 patients with hemodynamic studies was ≤110 mm Hg.

Cardiac adiposity (cor adiposum)[22]: These 30 patients died from noncardiac causes. The heart weights ranged from 250 to 795 g (mean 435) and were increased (>350 g in women, >400 g in men) in 17 (57%). Adipose tissue constituted 4% to 52% (mean 22%) of the total heart weight (mean weight of adipose tissue = 105 g). No heart had grossly visible evidence of myocardial fibrosis or necrosis. Total 12-lead QRS voltage decreased significantly as the quantity of cardiac adipose tissue increased. As the ratio of adipose tissue to heart weight × 100 increased from 12 ± 3 to 20 ± 4 to 32 ± 9 mm/100 g, the ratio of total 12-lead QRS voltage to heart weight × 100 decreased significantly from 36 ± 9 to 34 ± 9 to 21 ± 6 mm/100 g. The amount of subepicardial fat increased with increasing body weight. Simple visual assessment of the extent of cardiac adiposity and the degree of buoyancy of the heart when placed in a container of water estimated well the amounts of subepicardial fat. If the amount of subepicardial fat was considered normal by visual

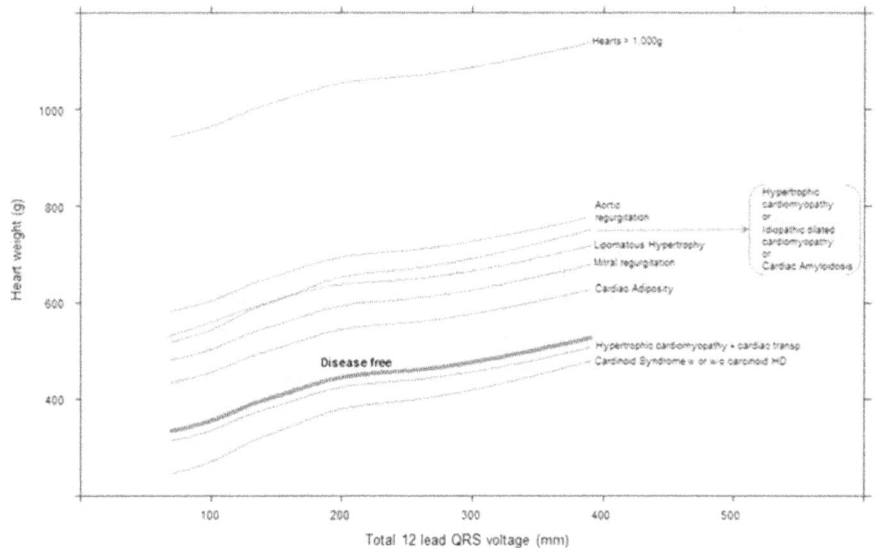

Figure 2. Adjusted (by gender and age) association between patient's heart weight and 12-lead QRS voltage by cardiac condition. HD = heart disease; transp = transplantation.

inspection, then the adipose tissue constituted a mean of 12% (range 4% to 14%) of the heart weight; if the subepicardial tissue was increased but the heart did not float in water, then fat constituted a mean of 20% (range 15% to 28%) of the heart weight; in the 12 hearts that floated in water, a mean of 32% (range 21% to 52%) of the heart weight was composed of adipose tissue.

Discussion

This study summarizes 11 previously published studies on total 12-lead QRS voltage in 11 different cardiac conditions and compares that voltage with heart weight. The best cut-off point for total 12-lead QRS voltage separating hearts with increased weight compared with those of normal weight has not been fully established. Odom et al[25] determined heart weight in 30 men free of cardiopulmonary disease and found that total 12-lead QRS voltage ranged from 80 to 185 mm (mean 127; 10 mm = 1 mV). These authors considered 175 mm as the best upper range of normal 12-lead QRS voltage. Rodríguez Padial[26] studied M-mode and 2-dimensional echocardiograms and 12-lead electrocardiograms in 74 consecutive patients with systemic hypertension and calculated left ventricular mass. This author found a total 12-lead QRS voltage >120 mm to be a good electrocardiographic criterion and "better than those most frequently used."[27] Yang et al[28] studied total 12-lead QRS voltage in 120 adults free of cardiopulmonary disease and 114 patients with LVH by echocardiography. They found >190 mm to be a good criterion for LVH, with sensitivity of 77%, specificity of 96%, and accuracy of 87%, and suggested that total 12-lead QRS voltage had a relatively high reliability for diagnosing LVH. Pelliccia et al[29] studied total 12-lead QRS voltage in 67 patients with idiopathic dilated cardiomyopathy and found that total 12-lead QRS voltage (also the sum of T/R wave ratios) was the only independent predictor of left ventricular mass determined by either angiography or echocardiography.

In the present study of patients with clear increased cardiac mass at autopsy (>350 g in women, >400 g in men) total 12-lead QRS voltage in 118 men averaged 239 mm (range 107 to 428). These 118 men included 16 with hearts weighing >1,000 g, 36 with aortic stenosis, 22 with pure aortic regurgitation, 11 with pure mitral regurgitation, and 21 with hypertrophic cardiomyopathy (without cardiac transplantation). The upper limit for total 12-lead QRS voltage in women without cardiopulmonary disease has not been established. As listed in Table 2, 12-lead QRS voltage generally was slightly higher in women than men with the same cardiac condition, although heart weight on average was lower in the women than in the men. Clearly, total 12-lead QRS voltage is not perfect in diagnosing increased cardiac mass, but as listed in Table 1, it is more reliable in predicting increased cardiac mass than are previously recommended electrocardiographic criteria for LVH.

There is some variation in the relation of total 12-lead QRS voltage to heart weight depending on the underlying cardiac condition. As listed in Table 2, all 49 patients with idiopathic dilated cardiomyopathy had hearts weighing ≥400 g, and yet the mean total 12-lead QRS voltage in men and women was relatively low (147 and 167 mm, respectively). Wilensky et al[30] showed that QRS voltage in patients with this condition diminishes with time, and therefore, electrocardiograms recorded shortly before death show lower QRS voltages than those recorded at earlier times. Additionally, all 30 patients with fatal cardiac amyloidosis had hearts of increased mass, but mean total 12-lead QRS voltage in them averaged only 104 mm. Possibly as much as half or more of their cardiac mass, however, was contributed by the amyloid deposits in the heart and not by cardiac myocardium. The patients with excessive cardiac adiposity, with or without lipomatous hypertrophy of the atrial septum, also usually had hearts of increased mass with relatively low total 12-lead QRS voltages.

Lanti et al[31] studied electrocardiograms in 154 men without clinical evidence of heart disease and compared electrocardiographic findings in 67 who died suddenly to the 87 who had nonsudden death. They found that 12-lead QRS voltage had a significant and independent relation to sudden death and helped identify subjects at increased risk for sudden coronary death. These investigators also found that the Sokolow-Lyon index was inversely related to nonsudden death.

The strong features of the present study are the following: (1) the 12-lead QRS voltage was determined in a variety of cardiac conditions, and (2) heart weights in all patients studied were available and accurately determined. Relatively few previous studies on electrocardiographic determination of LVH actually compared the electrocardiographic criteria with actual heart weight, and those that did acquired those data from autopsy protocols produced by a variety of prosecutors with varying expertise in cardiovascular disease.

Disclosures

The authors have no conflicts of interest to disclose.

1. Griep AH. Pitfalls in the electrocardiographic diagnosis of left ventricular hypertrophy: a correlative study of 200 autopsied patients. *Circulation* 1959;20:30−34.
2. Allenstein BJ, Hiroyoshi M. Evaluation of electrocardiographic diagnosis of ventricular hypertrophy based on autopsy comparison. *Circulation* 1960;21:401−412.
3. Sokolow M, Lyon TP. The ventricular complex in left ventricular hypertrophy as obtained by unipolar precordial and limb leads. *Am Heart J* 1949;37:161−186.
4. Holt DH, Spodick DH. The Rv_6:Rv_5 voltage ratio in left ventricular hypertrophy. *Am Heart J* 1962;63:65−66.
5. Carter WA, Estes EH Jr. Electrocardiographic manifestations of ventricular hypertrophy; a computer study of ECG-anatomic correlations in 319 cases. *Am Heart J* 1964;68:173−182.
6. Romhilt DW, Estes WH Jr. A point-score system for the ECG diagnosis of left ventricular hypertrophy. *Am Heart J* 1968;75:752−758.
7. Romhilt DW, Bove KE, Norris RJ, Conyers E, Conradi S, Rowlands DT, Scott RC. A critical appraisal of the electrocardiographic criteria for the diagnosis of left ventricular hypertrophy. *Circulation* 1969;40:185−195.
8. Bennett DH, Evans DW. Correlation of left ventricular mass determined by echocardiography with vectorcardiographic and electrocardiographic voltage measurements. *Br Heart J* 1974;36:981−987.
9. Casale PN, Devereux RB, Alonso DR, Camp E, Kligfield P. Improved sex-specific criteria of left ventricular hypertrophy for clinical and computer interpretation of electrocardiograms: validation with autopsy findings. *Circulation* 1987;3:565−572.
10. Koito H, Spokick DH. Accuracy of the RV_6:RV_5 voltage ratio for increased left ventricular mass. *Am J Cardiol* 1988;62:985−987.
11. Velury S, Spodick DH. Increased left ventricular mass in patients with lateral low voltage electrocardiograms. *Am J Cardiol* 1992;69:707−708.
12. Siegel RJ, Roberts WC. Electrocardiographic observations in severe aortic valve stenosis: correlative necropsy study to clinical, hemodynamic, and ECG variables demonstrating relation of 12-lead QRS amplitude to peak systolic transaortic pressure gradient. *Am Heart J* 1982;103:210−221.
13. Roberts WC, Podolak MJ. The king of hearts: analysis of 23 patients with hearts weighing 1000 grams or more. *Am J Cardiol* 1985;55:485−494.
14. Roberts WC, Day PJ. Electrocardiographic observations in clinically isolated, pure, chronic, severe aortic regurgitation: analysis of 30 necropsy patients aged 19 to 65 years. *Am J Cardiol* 1985;55:431−438.
15. Glick BN, Roberts WC. Usefulness of total 12-lead QRS voltage in diagnosing left ventricular hypertrophy in clinically isolated, pure, chronic, severe mitral regurgitation. *Am J Cardiol* 1992;70:1088−1092.
16. Dollar AL, Roberts WC. Usefulness of total 12-lead QRS voltage compared with other criteria for determining left ventricular hypertrophy in hypertrophic cardiomyopathy: analysis of 57 patients studied at necropsy. *Am J Med* 1989;87:377−381.
17. Shirani J, Maron BJ, Cannon RO III, Shahin S, Roberts WC. Clinicopathologic features of hypertrophic cardiomyopathy managed by cardiac transplantation. *Am J Cardiol* 1993;72:434−440.
18. Roberts WC, Siegel RJ, McManus BM. Idiopathic dilated cardiomyopathy: analysis of 152 necropsy patients. *Am J Cardiol* 1987;60:1340−1355.
19. Shirani J, Roberts WC. Clinical, electrocardiographic and morphologic features of massive fatty deposits ("lipomatous hypertrophy") in the atrial septum. *J Am Coll Cardiol* 1993;22:226−238.
20. Ross EM, Roberts WC. The carcinoid syndrome: comparison of 21 necropsy subjects with carcinoid heart disease to 15 necropsy subjects without carcinoid heart disease. *Am J Heart* 1985;79:339−354.
21. Roberts WC, Waller BF. Cardiac amyloidosis causing cardiac dysfunction: analysis of 54 necropsy patients. *Am J Cardiol* 1983;52:137−146.
22. Shirani J, Berezowski K, Roberts WC. Quantitative measurement of normal and excessive (cor adiposum) subepicardial adipose tissue, its clinical significance, and its effect on electrocardographic QRS voltage. *Am J Cardiol* 1995;76:414−418.
23. Harrell FE Jr. Regression Modeling Strategies: With Application to Linear Models, Logistic Regression, and Survival Analysis. New York: Springer-Verlag, 2001.
24. Filardo G, Hamilton C, Hamman B, Ng HK, Grayburn P. Categorizing BMI may lead to biased results in studies investigating in-hospital mortality after isolated CABG. *J Clin Epidemiol* 2007;60:1132−1139.
25. Odom H II, Davis JL, Dinh H, Baker BJ, Roberts WC, Murphy ML. QRS voltage measurements in autopsied men free of cardiopulmonary disease: a basis for evaluating total QRS voltage as a index of left ventricular hypertrophy. *Am J Cardiol* 1986;58:801−804.
26. Rodríguez Padial L. Usefulness of total 12-lead QRS voltage for determining the presence of left ventricular hypertrophy in systemic hypertension. *Am J Cardiol* 1991;68:261−262.
27. Rodríguez Padial L, Navarro A, Sánchez J. RVG: RV_5 voltage ratio in systemic hypertension. *Am J Cardiol* 1990;66:869−871.
28. Yang TH, Deng SY, Cai YC. The normal values of total 12-lead QRS voltage and its significance in diagnosing left ventricular hypertrophy. *Chinese J Cardiol* 1988;16:353−355.
29. Pelliccia F, Critelli G, Cianfrocca C, Nigri A, Reale A. Electrocardiographic correlates with left ventricular morphology in idiopathic dilated cardiomyopathy. *Am J Cardiol* 1991;68:642−647.
30. Wilensky RL, Yudelman P, Cohen A, Fletcher RD, Atkinson J, Virmani R, Roberts WC. Serial electrocardiographic changes in idiopathic dilated cardiomyopathy confirmed at necropsy. *Am J Cardiol* 1988;62:276−283.
31. Lanti M, Puddu PE, Menotti A. Voltage criteria of left ventricular hypertrophy in sudden and nonsudden coronary artery disease mortality: the Italian section of the seven countries study. *Am J Cardiol* 1990;66:1181−1185.

Two causes in one patient for extremely low voltage on the electrocardiogram

William C. Roberts, MD, Melody Joy Sherwood, MD, and Paul A. Grayburn, MD

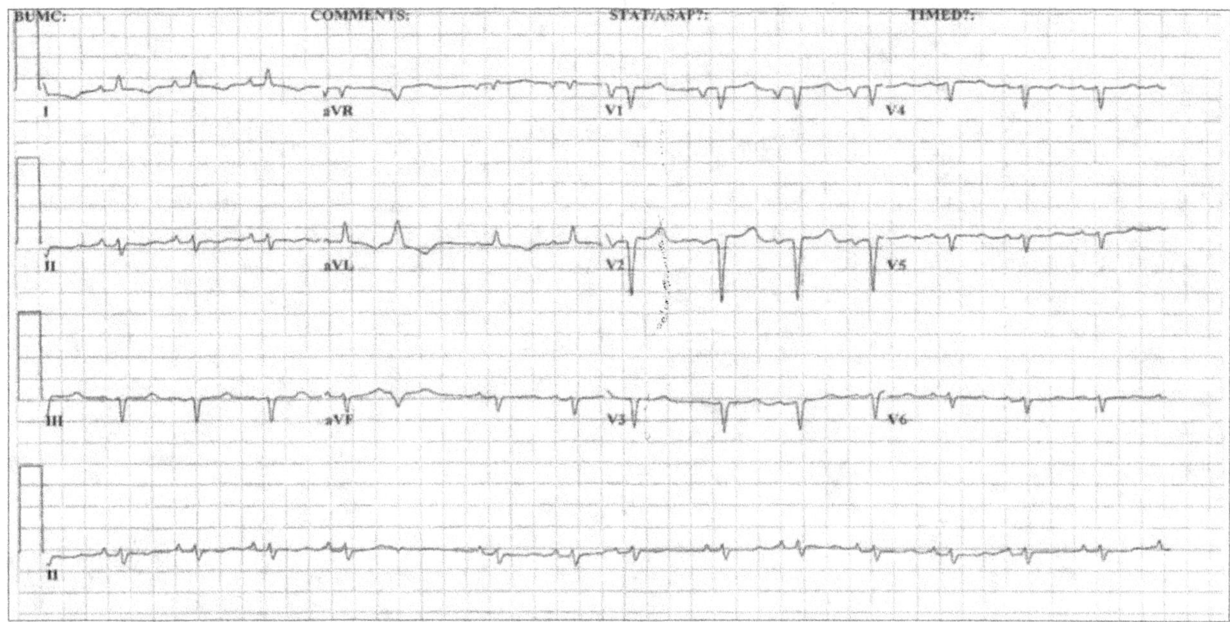

Figure 1. Electrocardiogram in the patient described. The standard is 20 mm, rather than the usual 10 mm.

An 80-year-old woman is described with two different causes (pericardial effusion and cardiac amyloidosis) for low QRS voltage on the electrocardiogram. Total 12-lead QRS voltage (from the peak of the R wave to the nadir of either the Q or the S wave, whichever is deeper) was only 34 mm (10 mm standard in all leads), the lowest we have encountered among 331 previously reported patients with 10 different cardiac conditions.

A mong the causes of extremely low voltage on the electrocardiogram are large pericardial effusions and cardiac amyloidosis. The occurrence of both conditions in the same patient can lead to extremely low voltage on the electrocardiogram. The occurrence of such a situation prompted this report.

CASE DESCRIPTION

An 80-year-old woman with dementia was hospitalized because of worsening confusion and lower leg edema. She was known to have systemic hypertension and diabetes mellitus. She was in no acute distress. Her blood pressure was 85/60 mm Hg. Her body mass index was 18 kg/m^2. No abdominal organs or subcutaneous

lymph nodes were palpated. The electrocardiogram showed total 12-lead QRS voltage of 17 mm (standard $\approx$ 20 mm; double standard) *(Figure 1)*. An echocardiogram disclosed pericardial effusion, thickened right and left ventricular walls, and low ($\approx$20%) ejection fraction *(Figure 2)*. Both ventricular cavities were of normal size.

DISCUSSION

Total 12-lead QRS voltage was introduced in 1982 as a means to predict the presence of left ventricular hypertrophy (1) *(Figure 3)*. Subsequently, total 12-lead QRS voltage has been described in 10 different disease states involving 331 patients and compared in all to heart weight (2). It has been found to be a better predictor of left ventricular hypertrophy than any previous criteria.

The concept of low QRS voltage was described initially when only three electrocardiographic leads were available. The 12-lead

From the Baylor Heart and Vascular Institute and the Department of Internal Medicine, Division of Cardiology, Baylor University Medical Center at Dallas, Texas.

Corresponding author: William C. Roberts, MD, Baylor Heart and Vascular Institute, Baylor University Medical Center at Dallas, 3500 Gaston Avenue, Dallas, TX 75246 (e-mail: william.roberts1@bswhealth.org).

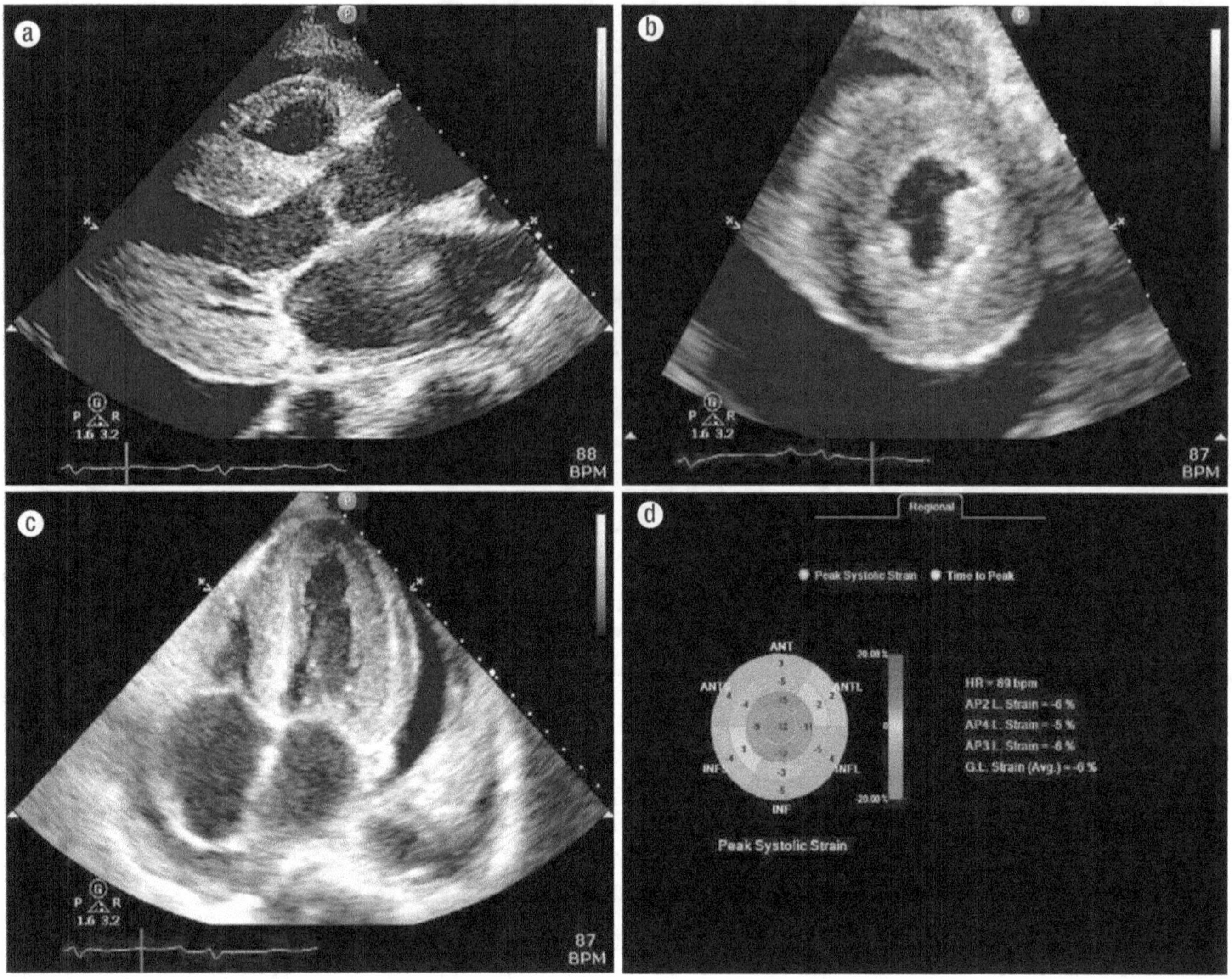

Figure 2. Transthoracic echocardiographic views—**(a)** parasternal short-axis view, **(b)** short-axis parasagittal view, and **(c)** apical four-chamber view—showing a brightly echogenic myocardium, thickened right ventricular and left ventricular walls, thickened valve leaflets, dilated right atrium, dilated left atrium, and a pericardial effusion. **(d)** A "bulls-eye" map of peak systolic longitudinal strain showing the characteristic "cherry-on-top" pattern of myocardial amyloidosis with preserved strain at the apex (dark red center) and abnormal strain elsewhere (pink or blue).

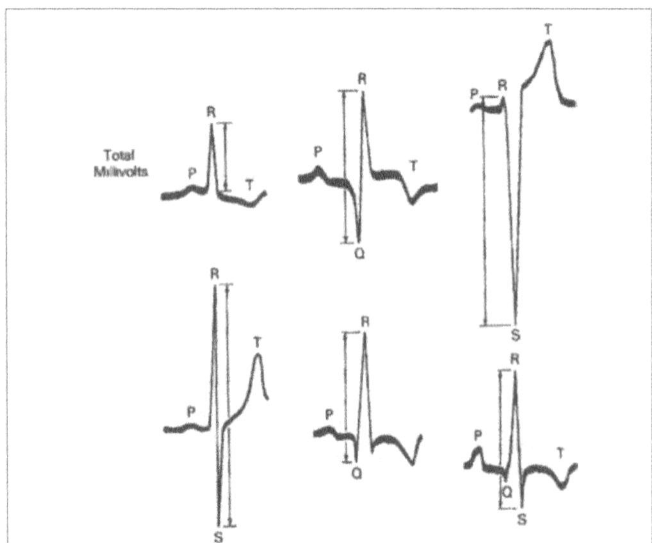

Figure 3. Various QRS complexes showing how each was measured. Reproduced from Siegel and Roberts (1) with permission of the authors and the publisher.

total QRS voltage has rarely been employed as an indicator of low QRS voltage. Among the 10 conditions in which total QRS voltage was measured and reported, those with the lowest voltage included cardiac amyloidosis, 58–199 mm (mean 104); cardiac adiposity, 73–210 mm (mean 120); and the carcinoid syndrome, 48–227 mm (mean 117). The lowest total 12-lead QRS voltage among the previously described 331 patients was 58 mm. Thus, to have an electrocardiographic total 12-lead QRS voltage of only 34 mm, as in the present patient, is indeed unusual.

A limitation of the present report is the lack of anatomic confirmation of cardiac amyloidosis. The echocardiogram, however, is virtually diagnostic of extensive cardiac amyloidosis.

1. Siegel RJ, Roberts WC. Electrocardiographic observations in severe aortic valve stenosis: correlative necropsy study to clinical, hemodynamic, and ECG variables demonstrating relation of 12-lead QRS amplitude to peak systolic transaortic pressure gradient. *Am Heart J* 1982;103(2):210–221.
2. Roberts WC, Filardo G, Ko JM, Siegel RJ, Dollar AL, Ross EM, Shirani J. Comparison of total 12-lead QRS voltage in a variety of cardiac conditions and its usefulness in predicting increased cardiac mass. *Am J Cardiol* 2013;112(6):904–909.

Usefulness of Total 12-Lead QRS Voltage as a Clue to Diagnosis of Patients With Cardiac Sarcoidosis Severe Enough to Warrant Orthotopic Heart Transplant

William C. Roberts, MD; Tiffany M. Becker, BS; Shelley A. Hall, MD

IMPORTANCE Severe heart failure caused by cardiac sarcoidosis is difficult to diagnosis without biopsy.

OBJECTIVE To assess whether total electrocardiographic 12-lead QRS voltage may be a clue to diagnosis.

DESIGN, SETTING, PARTICIPANTS Case-series study with cases collected at Baylor University Medical Center at Dallas, Dallas, Texas, from January 13, 2005, to January 24, 2017. The clinical records of 16 patients with severe heart failure caused by cardiac sarcoidosis were studied. Examination of total 12-lead electrocardiographic QRS voltage (peak of the R wave to the nadir of either the Q or S wave, whichever was deeper) was performed prior to orthotopic heart transplant (OHT). Gross and microscopic pathologic specimens of the native hearts were studied.

MAIN OUTCOMES AND MEASURES The primary outcome was to correlate the total 12-lead QRS voltage measurement with various morphologic features in the native diseased heart.

RESULTS The 16-patient study group consisted of 8 men and 8 women; 12 (75%) were white and 4 (25%) were black. At the time of OHT, patient age ranged from 50 to 67 years (mean, 57 years). Cardiac sarcoidosis was diagnosed by pre-OHT biopsy results in 2 (13%) patients and by examination of the native heart after OHT in 14 (87%) patients. Total nonpaced 12-lead QRS voltage mean was 117 mm (range, 52-155 mm) for 8 patients and total paced 12-lead QRS voltage was 90 mm (range, 67-161 mm) for 12 patients. These low mean values were similar to those of patients with carcinoid heart disease (mean [SD], 105 [40] mm), cardiac amyloidosis (104 [35] mm), and severe cardiac adiposity (120 [31] mm) studied at necropsy or after OHT. In contrast, mean (SD) values were 323 (109) mm in patients with massive cardiomegaly, 257 mm in patients with severe aortic stenosis, 272 (86) mm in patients with severe pure aortic regurgitation, 220 (67) mm in patients with severe pure mitral regurgitation, 197 (64) mm in patients with hypertrophic cardiomyopathy, and 153 (40) mm in patients with idiopathic dilated cardiomyopathy.

CONCLUSIONS AND RELEVANCE Most patients diagnosed with cardiac sarcoidosis causing severe heart failure and warranting OHT had low total 12-lead QRS voltage measurements despite having native hearts of increased weight. This finding may provide a clue to the diagnosis of this disease.

Author Affiliations: Baylor Heart and Vascular Institute, Baylor University Medical Center at Dallas, Dallas, Texas (Roberts, Becker, Hall); Department of Pathology, Baylor University Medical Center, Dallas, Texas (Roberts, Becker, Hall); Department of Internal Medicine, Baylor University Medical Center, Dallas, Texas (Roberts, Becker, Hall).

Corresponding Author: William C. Roberts, MD, Baylor Heart and Vascular Institute, 621 N Hall St, Ste H030, Dallas, TX 75226 (william.roberts1@bswhealth.org).

JAMA Cardiol. 2018;3(1):64-68. doi:10.1001/jamacardio.2017.4172
Published online November 15, 2017.

The first study of the utility of total 12-lead electrocardiographic QRS voltage was published in 1982 and reported findings for patients with aortic valve stenosis.[1] Subsequently, total 12-lead QRS voltage has been reported in a number of other conditions.[2] In each of those studies, the total 12-lead QRS voltage was compared with the weight of the native diseased heart at necropsy or after orthotopic heart transplant (OHT). The present report describes total 12-lead QRS voltage of 16 patients undergoing OHT because of severe heart failure due to cardiac sarcoidosis.

Methods

From January 13, 2005, through January 24, 2017, 16 patients at Baylor University Medical Center at Dallas (BUMC), Dallas, Texas, had OHT because of cardiac sarcoidosis. The study was approved by the Baylor Research Institute Institutional Review Board, which also waived the need for informed patient consent.

Each patient's native heart was examined by one of us (W.C.R.), and he prepared the final report. Accurate scales were used to weigh the native heart after fixation in formaldehyde for several days. The aorta and pulmonary trunk were excised about 2 cm above the sinotubular junction; all extraneous tissue was removed before weighing. Prior to weighing, the heart was opened and excessive water or formaldehyde was removed from its surfaces by gentle patting with paper towels. Clinical records and all electrocardiograms recorded at BUMC were reviewed and examined. The total 12-lead QRS voltage (defined as the distance in millimeters from the peak of the R wave to the nadir of either the Q or S wave, whichever was deeper) was measured by 2 of us (W.C.R. and T.M.B.). The statistics performed were limited to the calculation of the mean and SD. No statistical package or system was required for these calculations.

Results

The 16-patient study group consisted of 8 men and 8 women; 12 were white and 4 were black. Pertinent morphologic and electrocardiographic findings for the 16 patients are detailed in the **Table** and illustrated in **Figure 1** and **Figure 2**. At the time of OHT, the patient age ranged from 50 to 67 (mean, 57) years. Cardiac sarcoidosis was diagnosed by biopsy in 2 patients (13%) and by examination of the native heart after OHT in 14 patients (87%). The body mass index (calculated as the weight in kilograms divided by height in meters squared) ranged from 18.8 to 32.9 (mean, 27.1). Before OHT, 6 of the 16 patients (37%) had atrial fibrillation; 12 (75%) had bundle branch block (4 with left bundle branch block and 8 with right bundle branch block), and 7 (44%) had complete heart block. The low-density lipoprotein cholesterol levels before OHT ranged from 52 to 147 mg/dL (mean, 93 mg/dL) (to convert to millimoles per liter, multiply by 0.0259). Only patient 12 (Table) had greater than 75% in cross-sectional area narrowing of 1 or more major epicardial coronary arteries (defined as the right, left main, left anterior descending, and left circumflex).

Key Points

Question Is total 12-lead electrocardiographic QRS voltage a diagnostic clue for patients with cardiac sarcoidosis severe enough to warrant orthotopic heart transplant?

Findings In this case-series study, the mean total 12-lead QRS voltage in 16 patients with severe heart failure caused by extensive cardiac sarcoidosis (101 mm) was similar to that determined in patients with cardiac amyloidosis, carcinoid heart disease, and severe cardiac adiposity. In contrast, patients with fatal idiopathic dilated cardiomyopathy had a mean total 12-lead QRS voltage (153 mm).

Meaning The low total 12-lead QRS voltage measurement on electrocardiogram in patients with cardiac sarcoidosis, despite increased weight of the native heart, may be a clue to its correct diagnosis before orthotopic heart transplant.

The native heart weighed from 420 to 605 g (mean, 509 g) for the 8 men and from 370 to 600 g (mean, 442 g) for the 8 women. The quantity of cardiac adipose tissue was excessive such that the heart floated in a container of formaldehyde in 7 of the 11 hearts (64%) in which that determination was made. (Cardiac adipose tissue weighs less than myocardium.) Typical sarcoid granulomas were found in the walls of the right and left ventricles and in the ventricular spectrum in all patients. In 1 patient, however, granulomas were seen in the left ventricular wall ("button") removed for insertion of a left ventricular assist device but were not seen in the heart specimen after OHT. The number of granulomas and extent of ventricular wall scarring were subjectively quantified on a scale of 1+ (mild scarring) to 3+ (severe scarring). The distribution of sarcoid lesions is shown in the gross pathologic heart specimens for 3 of the 16 patients (Figure 2).

QRS voltage was measured using a 10-mm standard scale (10 mm = 1 mV) in all 12 leads of an electrocardiogram for all 16 patients. Mean total nonpaced 12-lead QRS voltage was 117 mm (range, 52-155 mm) for 8 patients: 3 men (mean, 137 mm [range, 121-155 mm]) and 5 women (mean, 105 mm [range, 52-144 mm]). Mean total paced 12-lead QRS voltage was 90 mm (range, 67-161 mm) for 12 patients: 6 men (mean, 81 mm [range, 47-103 mm]) and 6 women (mean, 98 mm [range, 67-161 mm]).

Discussion

Described herein are findings from measurement of total 12-lead electrocardiographic QRS voltage and findings from the examination of the native heart in 16 patients who underwent OHT because of severe heart failure due to cardiac sarcoidosis. These low total 12-lead nonpaced (mean, 117 mm) and paced (mean, 90 mm) QRS voltage values are similar to those values previously reported in patients with a variety of other conditions after OHT or necropsy.[2] The mean (SD) total 12-lead QRS voltage for several cardiac diseases is as follows: 105 (40) mm in 19 patients with carcinoid heart disease,[3] 104 (35) mm in 30 patients with cardiac amyloidosis,[4] and 120 (31) mm in 30 patients with severe cardiac adiposity.[5] In contrast, mean (SD) total 12-lead QRS voltage was 323 (109) mm in 17 patients with massive cardiomegaly (weight of native heart, >1000 g),[6] 257 mm in 50 patients with

Table. Pertinent Clinical and Morphological Findings in 16 Patients Who Underwent Heart Transplant for Cardiac Sarcoidosis

Patient No.	Age at HT, y	ECG Paced[a]	QRS Amplitude in Each ECG Lead												Total 12-Lead QRS Voltage, mm	Interval to ECG and HT, mo	BBB (Side)[b]	CHB[b]	LDL-C, mg/dL	SA Pressure, s/d, mm Hg	CI, L/min/m^2	HW, g	Location of Granulomas and Scar			Heart Floated[c]
			I	II	III	aVR	aVL	aVF	V$_1$	V$_2$	V$_3$	V$_4$	V$_5$	V$_6$									RV	VS	LV	
Men																										
1	50	0	7	11	14	5	9	12	6	14	19	7	10	7	121	31	+ (L)	0	119	130/89	1.7	605	0	1+	3+	NA
2	52	0	14	12	8	13	11	7	12	8	8	18	22	22	155	32	+ (R)	0	108	98/58 (I)	1.6	440	1+	2+	1+	NA
3	53	+	7	7	10	4	8	9	5	7	5	6	7	6	81	5	0	+	120	116/66 (I)	1.9	535	3+	3+	3+	NA
4	53	+	4	12	9	6	3	9	7	7	3	7	10	9	86	0.1	+ (R)	+	112	104/70 (I)	1.6	555	3+	3+	3+	+
5	58	+	9	9	6	4	4	6	5	3	8	8	8	7	77	1	+ (L)	0	64	88/55 (I)	1.2	420	3+	3+	3+	0
6	63	+	5	12	8	8	5	10	8	9	14	10	9	5	103	9	+ (L)	+	52	126/78	1.6	470	3+	3+	3+	+
7	63	0	8	6	3	6	6	4	9	10	13	18	22	29	134	34	+ (R)	0	86	120/84 (I)	1.7	540	3+	3+	3+	+
		+	5	8	11	5	6	11	2	4	12	17	11	3	95	2										
8	67	+	4	5	7	2	5	5	2	2	6	5	3	1	47	3	0	+	70	96/59	1.6	510	3+	3+	3+	+
Women																										
9	50	0	6	15	7	9	3	10	7	10	16	16	17	16	132	40	0	+	74	100/60 (I)	–	440	1+	3+	3+	0
		+	2	23	13	6	7	28	4	12	16	20	18	12	161	1										
10	52	+	5	5	5	5	2	8	6	7	7	5	5	7	67	3	+ (L)	0	64	115/79	2.3	440	1+	3+	2+	0
11	56	+	4	7	8	5	6	8	4	8	4	5	7	7	73	0.5	0	0	118	92/64	–	450	1+	3+	3+	+
12	57	0	5	1	6	3	6	4	5	9	5	4	2	2	52	18	+ (R)	0	94	101/58 (I)	1.4	380	3+	3+	3+	NA
13	58	0	8	8	15	3	11	12	5	7	4	4	6	6	89	49	+ (R)	0	147	102/57 (I)	2.2	560	3+	3+	3+	+
		+	3	3	4	2	3	3	3	7	3	3	4	4	69	2										
14	59	0	11	11	17	8	14	13	9	5	9	12	16	19	144	36	+ (R)	+	69	124/92	1.3	370	1+	2+	1+	NA
		+	10	12	19	8	14	15	8	9	10	13	15	14	147	35										
15	61	+	4	4	5	3	6	4	4	10	5	7	7	8	72	0.5	+ (R)	+	60	95/61 (I)	1.2	300	3+	3+	3+	+
16	62	0	10	11	10	7	7	7	10	9	7	9	10	10	107	1	+ (R)	0	129	109/68 (I)	1.5	600	1+	1+	3+	0

Abbreviations: a, augmented; BBB, bundle branch block; CHB, complete heart block; CI, cardiac index; ECG, electrocardiogram; HT, heart transplant; HW, weight of native heart; I, indirect; L, left (or left arm for ECG leads); LDL-C, low-density lipoprotein cholesterol; LV, left ventricle; NA, no information available; R, right (or right arm for ECG leads); RV, right ventricle; SA, systemic artery; s/d, systolic/diastolic; V, voltage; VS, ventricular septum.

SI conversion factor: To convert LDL-C to millimoles per liter, multiply by 0.0259.

[a] + Indicates paced; 0, nonpaced.

[b] + Indicates present; 0, not present.

[c] + Indicates present; 0, not present; and NA, no information available.

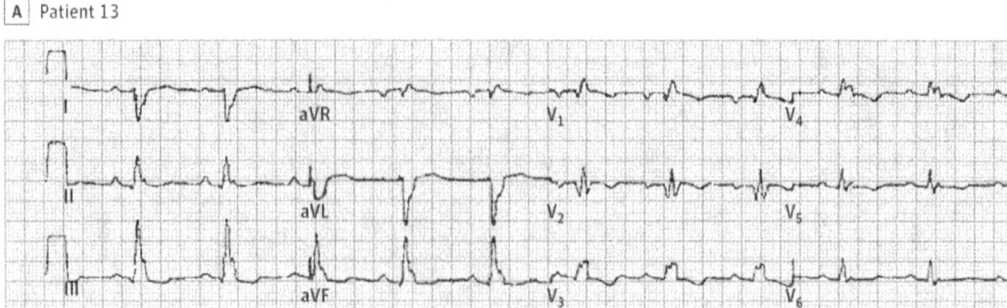

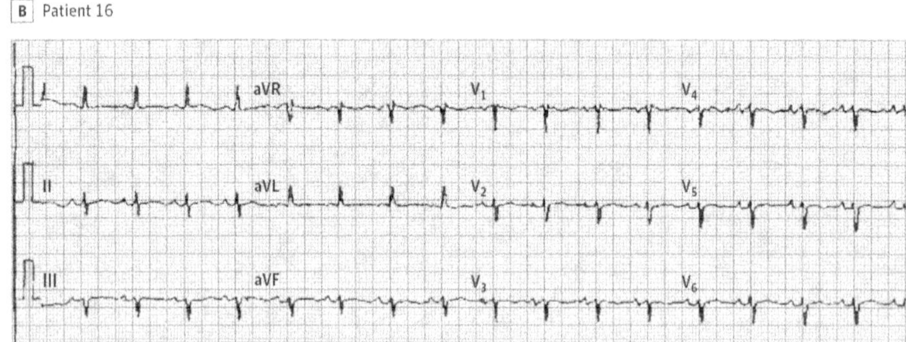

A, Patient 13: total 12-lead QRS voltage is 89 mm; weight of native heart, 560 g. B, Patient 16: total 12-lead QRS voltage is 107 mm; weight of native heart = 600 g. Leads (recording electrodes) are designated as follows: standard (bipolar) leads, I, II, and III; precordial (unipolar) leads, V_1, V_2, V_3, V_4, V_5, and V_6; and augmented limb leads/unipolar extremity leads, aVR, aVL, and aVF (a, augmented; V, voltage; R, right arm; L, left arm; and F, foot).

severe aortic stenosis,[1] 272 (86) mm in 30 patients with severe pure aortic regurgitation,[7] 220 (67) mm in 24 patients with pure mitral regurgitation,[8] 197 (64) mm in 57 patients with hypertrophic cardiomyopathy,[9,10] and 153 (40) mm in 49 patients with idiopathic dilated cardiomyopathy.[11] Thus, most of our patients (15 of 16 [94%]) with severe cardiac sarcoidosis, despite having native hearts of increased weight (>350 g in women and >400 g in men), had low total 12-lead QRS voltages.

Limitations and Strengths

A limitation of the present report is that the time interval between the recording of the electrocardiogram tracing and the OHT procedure was rather long for some patients. It is likely, however, as described previously in patients with idiopathic dilated cardiomyopathy,[12] that the total 12-lead QRS voltage would decrease as the time interval increases

between initially developing cardiac sarcoidosis and OHT procedure.[12]

The strong features of the present report are that both the weight of the native heart and the extent of the cardiac sarcoid lesions were known for all 16 patients. To our knowledge, electrocardiographic QRS voltage has not been described previously in patients with cardiac sarcoidosis.[12]

Conclusions

Most patients diagnosed with cardiac sarcoidosis causing severe heart failure and warranting OHT had low total 12-lead QRS voltage measurements despite having native hearts of increased weight. This finding may provide a clue to the diagnosis of this disease.

ARTICLE INFORMATION

Accepted for Publication: September 19, 2017.

Published Online: November 15, 2017.
doi:10.1001/jamacardio.2017.4172

Author Contributions: Dr Roberts and Ms Becker had full access to all of the data in the study and take responsibility for the integrity of the data and the accuracy of the data analysis.
Study concept and design: Roberts, Becker.
Acquisition, analysis, or interpretation of data: All authors.
Drafting of the manuscript: Roberts.
Critical revision of the manuscript for important intellectual content: Roberts.

Administrative, technical, or material support: Hall.
Study supervision: Roberts.

Conflict of Interest Disclosures: All authors have completed and submitted the ICMJE Form for Disclosure of Potential Conflicts of Interest and none were reported.

REFERENCES

1. Siegel RJ, Roberts WC. Electrocardiographic observations in severe aortic valve stenosis: correlative necropsy study to clinical, hemodynamic, and ECG variables demonstrating relation of 12-lead QRS amplitude to peak systolic transaortic pressure gradient. *Am Heart J.* 1982;103 (2):210-221.

2. Roberts WC, Filardo G, Ko JM, et al. Comparison of total 12-lead QRS voltage in a variety of cardiac conditions and its usefulness in predicting increased cardiac mass. *Am J Cardiol.* 2013;112(6): 904-909.

3. Ross EM, Roberts WC. The carcinoid syndrome: comparison of 21 necropsy subjects with carcinoid heart disease to 15 necropsy subjects without carcinoid heart disease. *Am J Med.* 1985;79(3): 339-354.

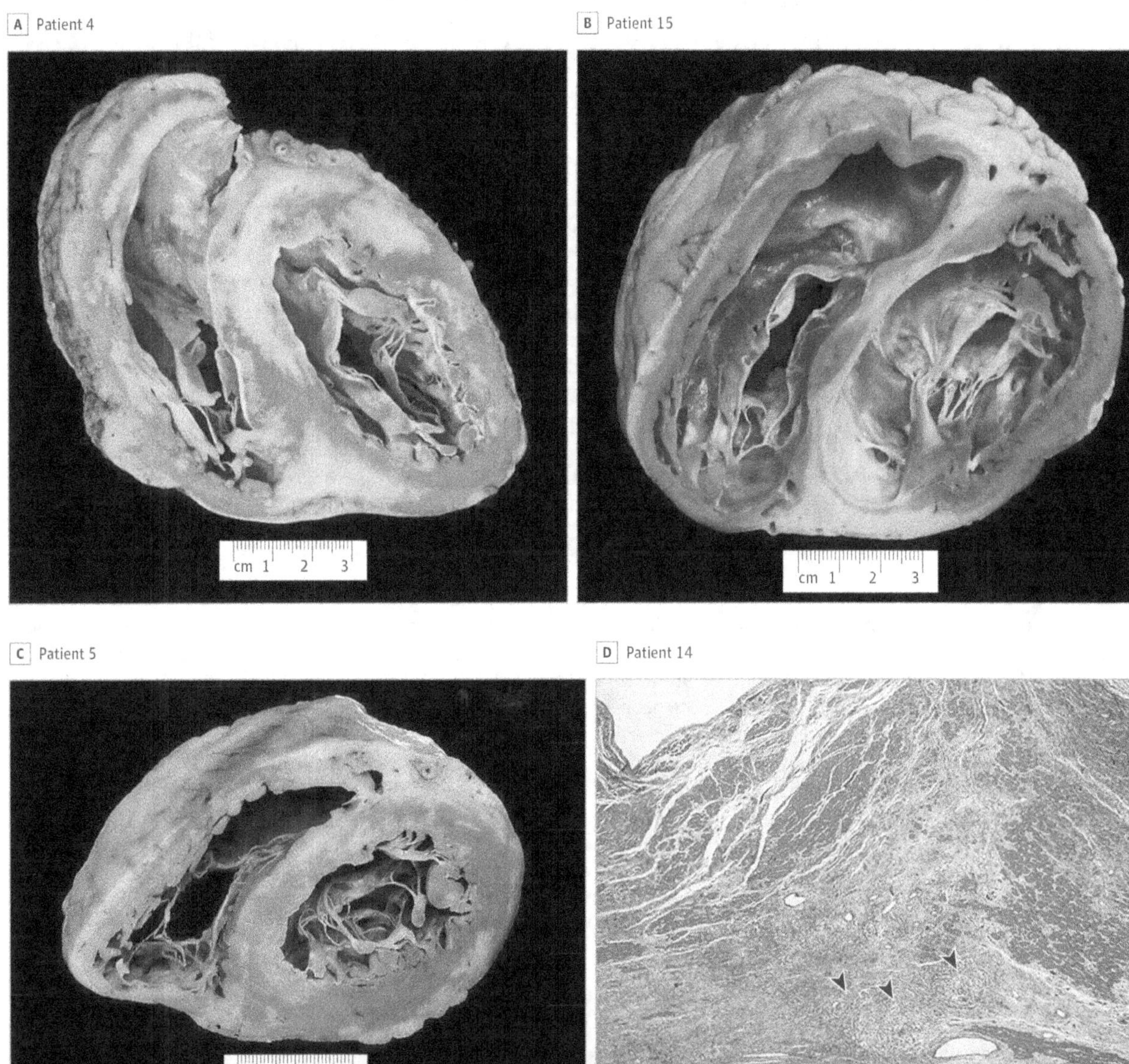

Basal portions of the heart exposing the tricuspid and mitral values. The ventricular septal and left ventricular free wall and a portion of right ventricular free wall contain white lesions; these represent scar tissue within which are sarcoid granulomas. All ventricular cavities are largely dilated. D, Photomicrograph of a portion of the left ventricular free wall of patient 14. The myocardial wall is partially, but extensively replaced by dense fibrous tissue that stains blue and contains several sarcoid granulomas (arrowheads) (trichrome stain, original magnification ×100). Scale bars in A through C are in centimeters.

4. Roberts WC, Waller BF. Cardiac amyloidosis causing cardiac dysfunction: analysis of 54 necropsy patients. *Am J Cardiol*. 1983;52(1):137-146.

5. Shirani J, Roberts WC. Clinical, electrocardiographic and morphologic features of massive fatty deposits ("lipomatous hypertrophy") in the atrial septum. *J Am Coll Cardiol*. 1993;22(1):226-238.

6. Roberts WC, Podolak MJ. The king of hearts: analysis of 23 patients with hearts weighing 1,000 grams or more. *Am J Cardiol*. 1985;55(4):485-494.

7. Roberts WC, Day PJ. Electrocardiographic observations in clinically isolated, pure, chronic,

severe aortic regurgitation: analysis of 30 necropsy patients aged 19 to 65 years. *Am J Cardiol*. 1985;55(4):432-438.

8. Glick BN, Roberts WC. Usefulness of total 12-lead QRS voltage in diagnosing left ventricular hypertrophy in clinically isolated, pure, chronic, severe mitral regurgitation. *Am J Cardiol*. 1992;70(11):1088-1092.

9. Dollar AL, Roberts WC. Usefulness of total 12-lead QRS voltage compared with other criteria for determining left ventricular hypertrophy in hypertrophic cardiomyopathy: analysis of 57 patients studied at necropsy. *Am J Med*. 1989;87(4):377-381.

10. Shirani J, Maron BJ, Cannon RO III, Shahin S, Roberts WC. Clinicopathologic features of hypertrophic cardiomyopathy managed by cardiac transplantation. *Am J Cardiol*. 1993;72(5):434-440.

11. Roberts WC, Siegel RJ, McManus BM. Idiopathic dilated cardiomyopathy: analysis of 152 necropsy patients. *Am J Cardiol*. 1987;60(16):1340-1355.

12. Wilensky RL, Yudelman P, Cohen AI, et al. Serial electrocardiographic changes in idiopathic dilated cardiomyopathy confirmed at necropsy. *Am J Cardiol*. 1988;62(4):276-283.

Usefulness of Total 12-Lead QRS Voltage for Diagnosis of Arrhythmogenic Right Ventricular Cardiomyopathy in Patients With Heart Failure Severe Enough to Warrant Orthotopic Heart Transplantation and Morphologic Illustration of Its Cardiac Diversity

William C. Roberts, MD*, Nitin Kondapalli, MBBS, and Shelley A. Hall, MD

Although several electrocardiographic features of arrhythmogenic right ventricular cardiomyopathy (ARVC) (also called dysplasia) have been described, total 12-lead QRS voltage is not one of them. This report describes total 12-lead QRS voltage in 11 patients with ARVC who underwent orthotopic heart transplantation (OHT) because of progressively severe heart failure. Additionally, it illustrates the varied morphologic features of ARVC. The total 12-lead nonpaced QRS voltages before OHT ranged from 28 to 118 mm (mean 74 ± 32), and those in the paced tracings, from 33 to 129 mm (62 ± 32). The voltages are the lowest we have encountered among 12 previously reported cardiovascular conditions. The heart weights among the 11 ARVC patients ranged from 285 to 670 g (mean 448 ± 125). Very low 12-lead QRS voltage is characteristic of patients with ARVC with heart failure severe enough to warrant OHT, and thus may serve as a clue to its diagnosis. © 2018 Elsevier Inc. All rights reserved. (Am J Cardiol 2018;122:1051−1061)

Although recognized by morphologic studies earlier,[1] the present concepts of arrhythmic right ventricular cardiomyopathy (ARVC) were introduced by Marcus et al in 1982.[2] Several reports have described various electrocardiographic features of ARVC but none have described total 12-lead QRS voltage or its potential diagnostic usefulness.[3–13] Such is one purpose of this report. Another is to illustrate several hearts of patients with ARVC to demonstrate the morphologic variability of this condition.

Methods

From 2009 to 2017, 11 adults at Baylor University Medical Center at Dallas had orthotopic heart transplantation (OHT) because of ARVC. The study was approved by the Baylor Research Institute's Institutional Review Board, which also waived the need for informed patient consent.

One of us (WCR) examined each patient's native heart and also prepared the final report. Accurate scales were used to weigh the native heart after fixation in formaldehyde for several days. The ascending aorta and pulmonary trunk were excised about 2 cm above the sinotubular junction; all extraneous tissues were removed before weighing. Before weighing, the heart was opened and excessive water or formaldehyde was removed from its surfaces by gentle patting with paper towels. Clinical records and all

From the Baylor Scott & White Heart and Vascular Institute, the Departments of Pathology and Internal Medicine (Division of Cardiology), Baylor University Medical Center, Part of Baylor Scott & White Health, Dallas, Texas. Manuscript received May 30, 2018; revised manuscript received and accepted June 6, 2018.

*Corresponding author: Tel: (214) 820-7911; fax: (214) 820-7533.

E-mail addresses: ajc@baylorhealth.edu, William.Roberts1@bswhealth.org (W.C. Roberts).

electrocardiograms recorded at Baylor University Medical Center were reviewed and examined. The total 12-lead QRS voltage (defined as the distance in millimeters from the peak of the R wave to the nadir of either the Q or S wave, whichever was deeper, with 10 mm standard [=1 mV]) was measured by 2 of us (WCR and NK). The statistics performed was limited to the calculation of the means and standard deviations.

Results

Pertinent clinical, morphologic, and electrocardiographic data are displayed in Tables 1 and 2. At the time of OHT, the patients' ages ranged from 21 to 70 years (mean 49 ± 17); 8 were men and 3 were women. ARVC was diagnosed before OHT in 3 patients and from examination of the operatively excised heart in the other 8 patients. All 11 patients had clinical evidence of heart failure, especially severe right-sided heart failure; by electrocardiogram, 8 had documented runs of ventricular tachycardia, 3 had epsilon waves (small amplitude distinct potentials between the end of the QRS complex and the beginning of the T wave), and 5 had inverted T waves in 1 or more precordial leads; all 11 had low QRS voltage, and 5 had right bundle branch block; by echocardiogram or computed tomography, all 11 patients had very dilated right ventricular cavities and 10 had dilated, but less so, left ventricular cavities. The body mass indexes ranged from 22 to 37 kg/m^2 (mean 29 ± 5). The progression of heart failure to class III or IV prompted the OHT.

The electrocardiographic findings before OHT are tabulated in Table 2. Six nonpaced and 7 paced electrocardiographic tracings were available for analysis. The nonpaced total 12-lead QRS voltages ranged from 28 to 118 mm (mean 74 ± 32), and those in paced tracings, from

Table 1
Arrhythmogenic right ventricular cardiomyopathy—Clinical and morphologic features

Patient no (figure no)	Age at OHT (yrs)	Family history of SD/VT	BMI (kg/m^2)	TC (mg/dl)	LDL-C (mg/dl)	HDL-C (mg/dl)	TG (mg/dl)	LVEF (%)	CI (L/min/m^2)	ARVC diagnosed clinically	Pressures (mm Hg) (s/d) SA	RV	PA	HW (g)	Coronary artery narrowing (>75% CSA) by plaque	Heart floated in formalin	LV involvement Scar	Fat	Associated Condition
MEN																			
1(3)	21	0	27	147	72	65	62	5	1.1	0	144/96*	21/14	17/11	490	0	0	0	0	0
2	26	0	35	204	134	56	149	10	0.8	0	180/100*	-	50/30	595	0	0	0	0	Gilbert's syndrome
3(4)	34	0	27	154	73	80	65	3	1.3	0	75/55*	48/12	20/14	515	0	0	+	0	Rheumatoid arthritis
4	44	+	22	175	112	50	87	25	1.9	0	95/60*	19/12	22/11	315	0	0	0	0	Hypothyroidism
5(5)	54	+	26	145	68	62	74	30	1.5	+	75/50*	31/4	25/10	670†	+	+	+	+	0
6(1&6)	62	0	35	173	86	82	94	20	1.4	0	100/70*	25/10	21/12	420	0	+	0	0	Guillain Barre syndrome
7(7)	66	0	29	235	107	94	184	15	1.5	0†	80/55*	18/9	16/3	450	0	+	+	+	Hypothyroidism
8(8)	68	0	28	165	97	32	296	30	1.4	0	155/80*	26/7	24/16	460	+‡	+	+	0	0
WOMEN																			
9(9)¶	44	+	37	204	149	44	119	10	1.5	0	125/85*	40/-1	42/13	420	0	+	0	0	Limb-girdle muscular dystrophy
10(10)	49	0	27	237	112	100	200	56	1.5	+	85/40*	22/12	20/13	305	0	+	0	0	0
11(2&11)	70	+	26	254	149	68	297	55	1.7	+	185/100*	17/5	17/3	285	0	+	0	0	Hypothyroidism

ARVC = arrhythmogenic right ventricular cardiomyopathy; BMI = body mass index; CABG = coronary artery bypass grafting; CI = cardiac index; CSA = cross-sectional area; g = gram(s); Hg = hydrargyrum (Mercury); HW = heart weight; ICD = Implantable Cardioverter Defibrillator; kg = kilogram(s); L = Liter(s); LDL-C = low-density lipoprotein cholesterol; LVAD = left ventricular assist device; LVEF = left ventricular ejection fraction; m = meter(s); min = minute(s); OHT = orthotopic heart transplantation; PA = pulmonary artery; RV = right ventricle; s/d = peak systole/end-diastole; SD = sudden death; SA = systemic artery; TC = total cholesterol; VT = ventricular tachycardia; Yrs = year(s).

* Indirect pressure (cuff).
† An LVAD was inserted 34 months before the OHT.
‡ The result of performed biopsy was negative for ARVC changes.
§ Patient had CABG 25 years before the OHT.
¶ Patient died 48 days after the OHT.

Table 2
Electrocardiographic features of arrhythmogenic right ventricular cardiomyopathy

Patient no. (figure no.)	Age at OHT (yrs)	ECG Paced	QRS amplitude in each electrocardiographic lead(mm)												Total 12-lead QRS voltage (mm)	ECG to OHT interval (mos)	HW (g)	ECG changes before OHT							
			I	II	III	aVR	aVL	aVF	V1	V2	V3	V4	V5	V6				AF	VPCs	VT	Epsilon wave	Inverted T waves	Right BBB	LAFB	CHB
MEN																									
1(3)	21	0	5	3	3	3	3	2	6	11	14	14	8	19	91	8.0	490	0	+	0	0	+	0	0	0
2	26	0	3	3	6	2	5	5	4	5	10	8	7	9	67	0.2	595	0	+	+	0	+	+	+	0
		+	4	3	8	2	7	5	4	5	8	8	7	7	68	3.0									
3(4)	34	+	3	4	4	3	4	5	6	6	4	7	11	8	65	0.7	515	0	+	0	0	0	0	0	+
4	44	+	1	4	4	3	2	5	2	3	6	8	9	5	52	0.5	315	+	0	+	0	0	+	0	0
5(5)	54	+	3	8	9	5	4	10	8	13	23	20	16	10	129	15.5	670*	0	+	+	0	0	0	0	0
6(1&6)	62	0	6	6	10	5	8	9	7	9	6	7	10	7	90	170.0	420	+	+	+	+	+	+	+	0
		+	3	3	5	2	4	4	2	6	2	3	3	4	41	5.0									
7(7)	66	+	3	2	3	1	3	3	1	3	3	5	4	2	33	0.3	450	+	0	+	0	0	0	0	0
8(8)	68	+	3	3	2	3	2	1	2	9	7	6	5	4	47	0.3	460	+	+	+	0	0	0	0	0
WOMEN																									
9(9)	44	0	10	10	10	10	8	9	11	12	10	10	9	9	118	23.0	420	+	+	+	0	+	+	0	0
10(10)	49	0	2	3	3	2	2	3	2	2	3	2	2	2	28	3.5	305	+	+	0	+	0	+	0	0
11(2&11)	70	0	8	3	7	4	7	3	2	5	2	2	4	5	52	1.0	285	+	+	+	+	+	0	+	0

AF = atrial fibrillation; BBB = bundle branch block; CHB = complete heart block; ECG = electrocardiogram; LAFB = left anterior fascicular block; mm = millimeter(s); OHT = orthotopic heart transplantation; VPCs = ventricular premature complexes; VT = ventricular tachycardia; Yrs = year(s).

* A left ventricular assist device was inserted 34 months before the OHT.

Table 3
Total 12-lead QRS voltage in different cardiovascular conditions[*]

Condition	Gender	No. of cases	Age in years (mean)	Total 12-Lead QRS voltage in mm (mean)	Patients with 12-Lead QRS voltage >175mm	Heart weight (g)	Total 12-lead QRS voltage (mm)/heart weight (g)	Year of Publication	Authors (reference Number)
Hearts weigh >1000 g	M	16	29-64 (42)	140-414 (306)	16 (94%)	1005-1360 (1102)	0.28	1985	Roberts and Podolak[14]
	F	1	20	601		1250	0.48		
Aortic valve stenosis	M	36	16-64 (48)	144-417 (249)	47 (94%)	440-880 (639)	0.39	1982	Siegel and Roberts[15]
	F	14	16-65 (47)	193-376 (277)		380-700 (521)	0.53		
Aortic regurgitation	M	22	19-59 (44)	109-428 (271)	27 (90%)	430-1100 (717)	0.38	1985	Roberts and Day[16]
	F	8	35-56 (48)	169-384 (275)		375-950 (638)	0.43		
Mitral regurgitation	M	11	24-84 (47)	111-364 (245)	17 (71%)	400-775 (629)	0.39	1992	Glick and Roberts[17]
	F	13	21-64 (37)	114-290 (199)		350-675 (472)	0.42		
Hypertrophic cardiomyopathy without cardiac transplantation	M	21	14-68 (46)	107-339 (190)	30 (53%)	325-1070 (671)	0.28	1989	Dollar and Roberts[18]
	F	36	19-87 (51)	68-327 (201)		290-1230 (547)	0.38		
Hypertrophic cardiomyopathy with cardiac transplantation	M	6	19-46 (35)	109-201 (142)	4 (40%)	310-480 (393)	0.36	1993	Shirani et al[19]
	F	4	24-45 (35)	172-378 (241)		290-650 (408)	0.59		
Idiopathic dilated cardiomyopathy	M	35	19-73 (46)	74-281 (147)	20 (41%)	400-940 (620)	0.24	1987	Roberts et al[20]
	F	14	22-75 (54)	75-243 (167)		400-860 (602)	0.28		
Lipomatous hypertrophy of the atrial septum	M	12	48-84 (67)	93-241 (140)	3 (11%)	410-795 (576)	0.24	1993	Shirani and Roberts[21]
	F	16	59-83 (74)	59-266 (124)		330-680 (502)	0.25		
Carcinoid syndrome with carcinoid heart disease	M	11	39-72 (56)	58-227 (120)	2 (11%)	220-480 (350)	0.34	1985	Ross and Roberts[22]
	F	8	28-64 (54)	58-128 (84)		200-290 (245)	0.34		
Carcinoid syndrome without carci-noid heart disease	M	10	42-75 (55)	89-129 (137)	2 (13%)	240-570 (350)	0.39		
	F	5	28-67 (50)	102-135 (121)		150-270 (230)	0.53		
Aortic syphilis	M	11	33-84 (28)	57-161 (120)	0	-	-	2015	Roberts et al[23]
	F	13	58-83 (28)	64-146 (106)		-	-		
Cardiac adiposity	M	13	51-73 (64)	73-159 (114)	1 (3%)	320-795 (485)	0.24	1995	Shirani et al[24]
	F	17	40-85 (70)	77-210 (124)		250-575 (395)	0.31		
Cardiac amyloidosis	M	15	32-69 (52)	60-197 (99)	2 (7%)	410-850 (570)	0.17	1983	Roberts and Waller[25]
	F	15	21-93 (69)	58-199 (109)		370-900 (494)	0.22		
Cardiac sarcoidosis (Nonpaced)	M	3	50,52,63 (55)	121,155,134 (137)	0	605,440,540 (528)	0.26	2018	Roberts et al[26]
	F	5	50-62 (57)	52-144 (105)		370-600 (470)	0.22		
Cardiac sarcoidosis (Paced)	M	6	53-67 (59)	47-103 (82)	0	420-555 (505)	0.16		
	F	6	50-61 (56)	67-161 (98)		300-560 (427)	0.23		
Arrhythmogenic right ventricular cardiomyopathy (Nonpaced)	M	3	21,26,62 (36)	91,67,90 (83)	0	490,595,420 (502)	0.17	2018	Roberts et al
	F	3	44,49,70 (54)	28,61,118 (69)		420,305,285 (337)	0.2		
Arrhythmogenic right ventricular cardiomyopathy (Paced)	M	7	26-68 (51)	33-129 (62)	0	315-670 (489)	0.13		
	F	0	-	-		-	-		

[*] Parts of this table have been published previously in the following reports: Roberts WC, Filardo G, Ko JM, Siegel RJ, Dollar AL, Ross EM, Shirani J. Comparison of total 12-lead QRS voltage in a variety of cardiac conditions and its usefulness in predicting increased cardiac mass. *Am J Cardiol* 2013; 112(6):904-909. Permission to republish this updated table is granted by the authors and the publisher, Elsevier.

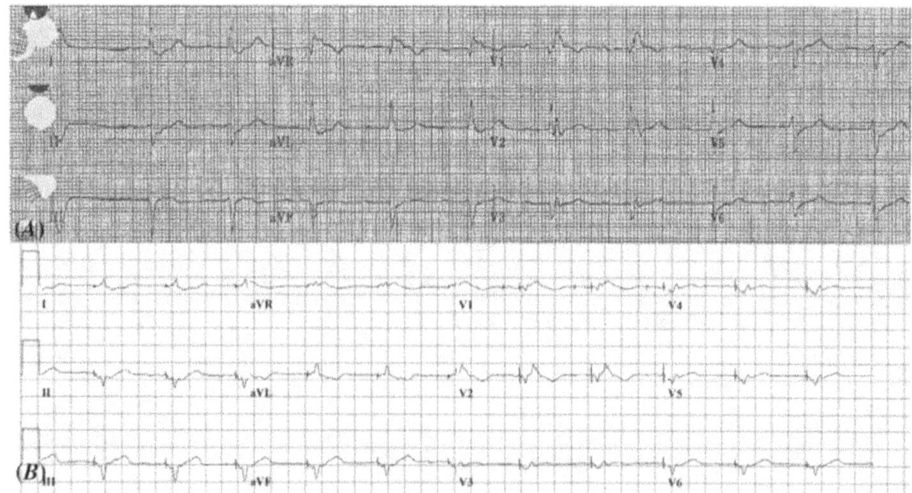

Figure 1. Case #6, Tables 1 and 2. Electrocardiograms nonpaced *(upper)* and paced *(lower)*. The total 12-lead QRS voltage in the upper tracing is 90 mm and in the lower tracing, 41 mm with 10 mm standard. Prominent epsilon waves are present in 1 or more precordial leads in the two patients.

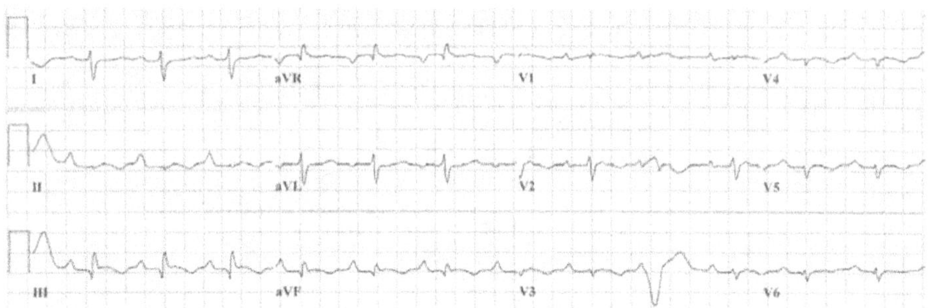

Figure 2. Case #11, Tables 1 and 2. Nonpaced electrocardiogram with total 12-lead QRS voltage of 52 mm. The PR interval is prolonged (236 ms), many T waves are inverted, and an occasional ventricular premature complex is present.

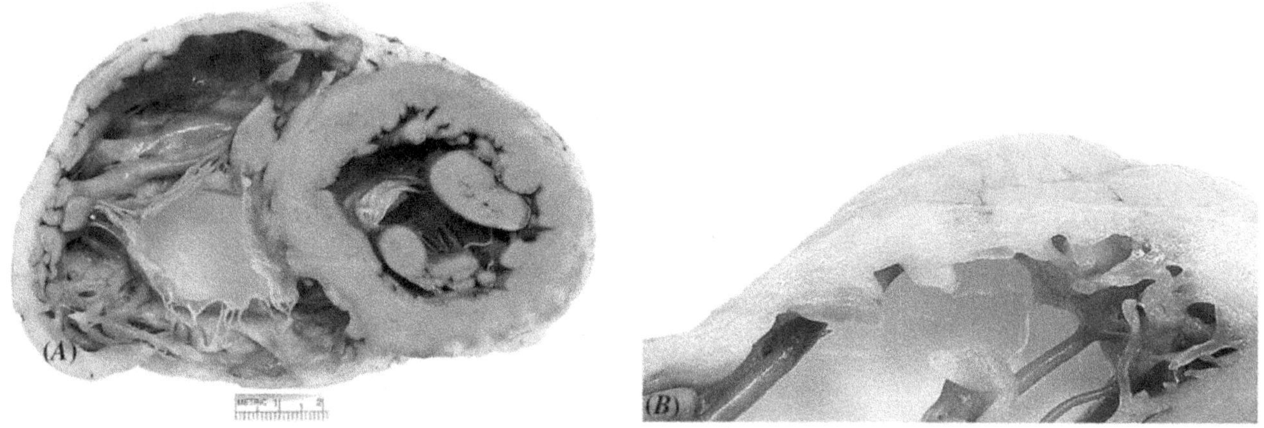

Figure 3. Case #1, Tables 1 and 2. Shown here are 2 photographs of the heart in a 21-year-old man. (*A*) Shown here is the basal portion of the heart showing marked dilatation of the right ventricular cavity and dilatation but less so of the left ventricular cavity. Most of the right ventricular wall is replaced by adipose tissue. There is some infiltration of fat in the subepicardial portion of left ventricular wall and some small scars in the subepicardial portion of left ventricular wall. (*B*) A close-up of the right ventricular outflow tract showing the right ventricular wall to be focally replaced by adipose tissue. Total nonpaced 12-lead QRS voltage in this patient was 91 mm and the heart weighed 490 g.

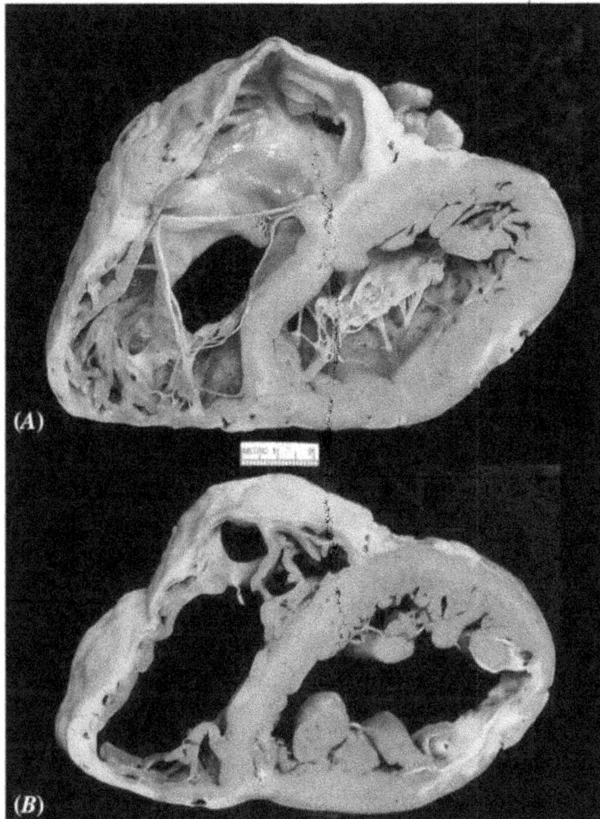

Figure 4. Case #3, Tables 1 and 2. Shown here is the basal portion of the ventricular walls in a 34-year-old man. The two ventricular cavities are dilated but the right one far more than the left. (*A*) The right ventricular free wall is replaced focally by either adipose tissue or fibrous tissue or both. (*B*) This cut of the ventricular walls not only shows the thinning of the right ventricular free wall focally but also a scar in the lateral wall of left ventricular between the two papillary muscles. The epicardial coronary arteries were wide open. Total paced 12-lead QRS voltage was 65 mm, and the heart weighed 515 g.

33 to 129 mm (mean 62 ± 32). Before OHT, atrial fibrillation was present in 7 patients, and occasional ventricular premature complexes in 9 patients, 5 of whom also had runs of ventricular tachycardia.

The hearts of the 8 men ranged in weight from 315 to 670 g (mean 489 ± 108), and in the 3 women, from 285 to 420 g (mean 337 ± 73). The quantity of adipose tissue in the heart was huge in 7 of 11 patients causing their hearts to float in a container of formaldehyde (adipose tissue is lighter than myocardium). Two patients had narrowing of 1 or more major epicardial coronary arteries, one of whom had undergone coronary arterial bypass grafting 25 years before the OHT. All patients had dilated right ventricular cavities and all but 1 also had dilated left ventricular cavities but in all cases the right ventricular cavity was much more dilated than the left one. The right ventricular wall was focally replaced mainly by adipose tissue in which some scar tissue usually also was present. Focal scars replaced portions of the left ventricular free wall and/or ventricular septum in 4 patients, 2 of whom had narrowing >75% in cross-sectional

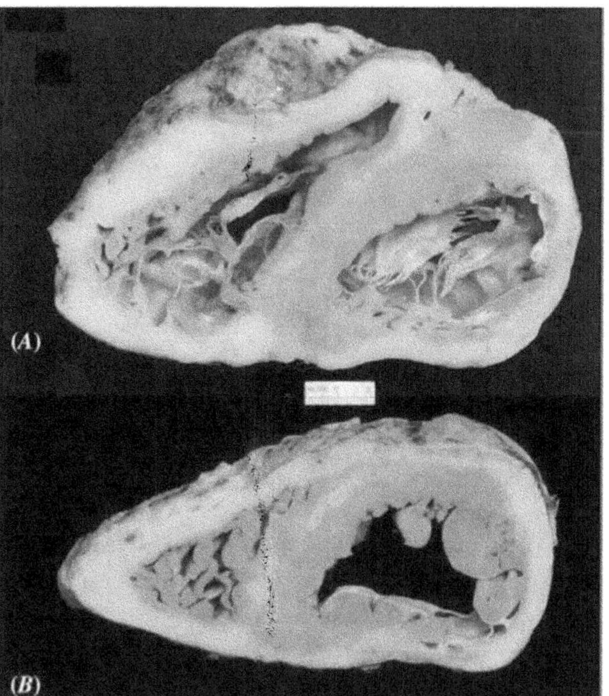

Figure 5. Case #5, Tables 1 and 2. Shown here is the basal portion of the ventricles in *A* and another portion more apically located in *B*. (*A*) The two ventricular cavities are dilated. Most of the right ventricular wall is replaced by adipose tissue. (*B*) Much of the entire left ventricular free wall, particularly the subepicardial region, is replaced by adipose tissue making the wall much thinner than the ventricular septum. The lumen of the right coronary artery was considerably narrowed by atherosclerotic plaque. Total paced 12-lead QRS voltage was 129 mm and the heart weighed 670 g. This patient had a left ventricular assist device in place for 34 months before the OHT.

area by plaques of 1 or more major epicardial coronary arteries. Two of 4 patients with left ventricular scars also had focal fatty replacement of these walls by adipose tissue.

Discussion

Described herein are findings from measurement of total 12-lead QRS voltage and findings from the examination of the native hearts in 11 patients who underwent OHT because of severe heart failure due to ARVC. These total 12-lead nonpaced QRS voltages (mean 74 ± 32) and paced (mean 62 ± 32) are the lowest found in any of the 12 previously reported conditions we have studied (summarized in Table 3).[14–26] The total 12-lead QRS voltage was lower in the 7 paced electrocardiograms than in the 6 nonpaced electrocardiograms.

A limitation of the present report is that the time interval between the recording of the electrocardiogram and the OHT procedure was rather long in 3 of 11 patients. It is likely, however, as described previously in patients with idiopathic dilated cardiomyopathy that the total 12-lead QRS voltage would decrease as the time interval increased

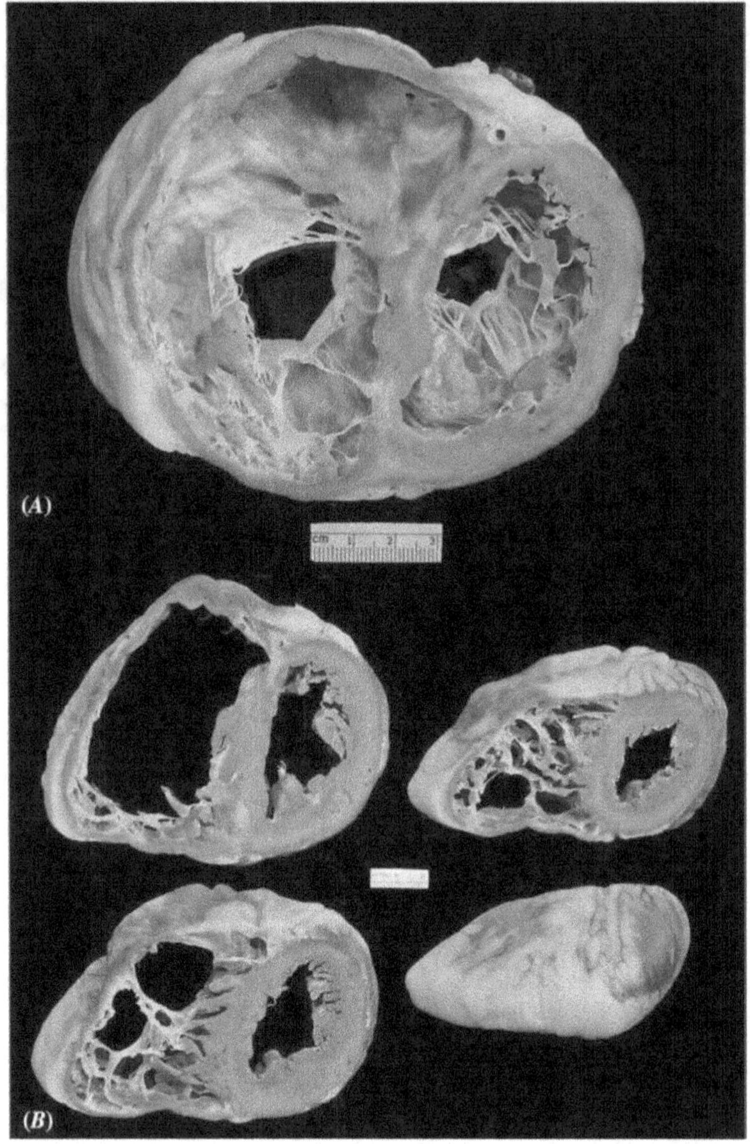

Figure 6. Case #6, Tables 1 and 2. Shown here are portions of a heart in a 63-year-old man. (*A*) The two ventricular cavities are greatly dilated, the right much more than the left. The right ventricular free wall is focally replaced, mainly by adipose tissue. Focal scars are also present in the ventricular septum. (*B*) These are transverse cuts of the ventricles caudal to the view shown in *A*. These views show scarring in the right ventricular pectinate muscles as well as focally in the ventricular septum. The right ventricular cavity is much larger than the left. Total nonpaced 12-lead QRS voltage was 90 mm and paced, 41 mm, and the heart weighed 420 g.

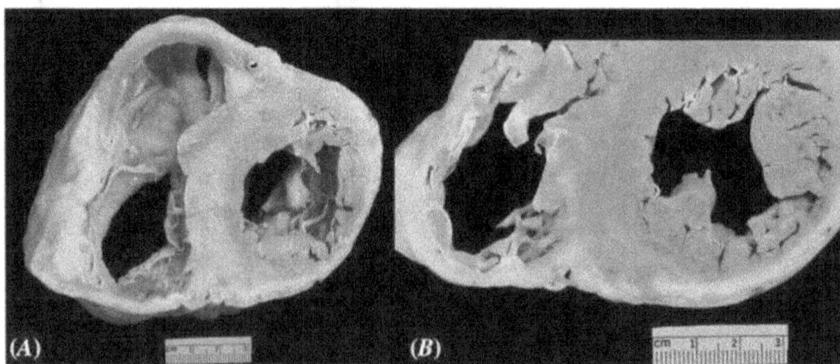

Figure 7. Case #7, Tables 1 and 2. Shown in *A* is the basal portion of the heart showing replacement of much of the walls of the two ventricles by adipose tissue. The lateral wall of the left ventricle is much thinner than the ventricular septum due to replacement of myocardium by both adipose tissue and fibrous tissue. (*B*) A closer view more apically better showing the fatty infiltration of the myocardial walls. The quantity of fat was such that the heart floated in a container of formaldehyde (adipose tissue is lighter than myocardium). The total paced 12-lead QRS voltage was only 33 mm, and the heart weighed 450 g.

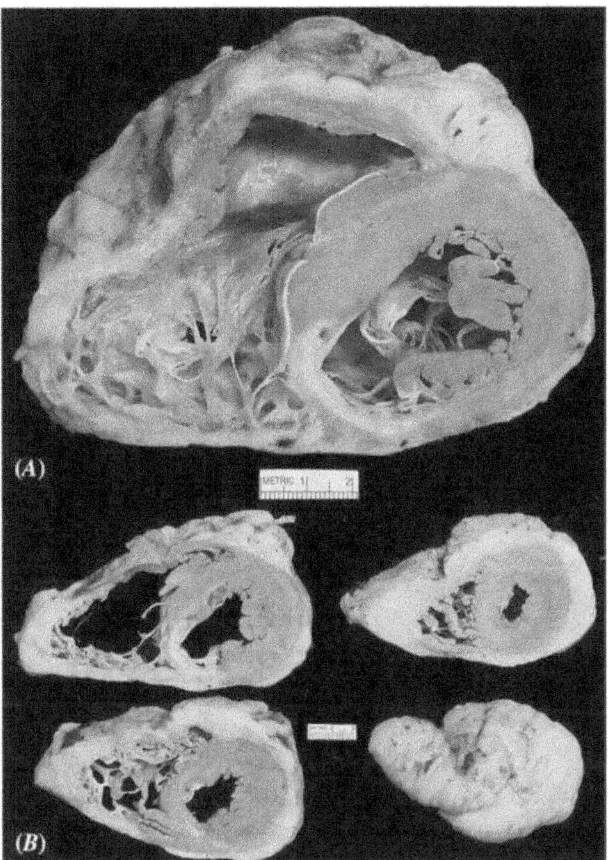

Figure 8. Case #8, Tables 1 and 2. Shown here are views of the cardiac ventricles on various levels in a 68-year-old man. The two ventricular cavities are dilated but the right far more than the left. The right ventricular cavity posteriorly and laterally is replaced by mainly adipose tissue but some scar tissue is present. The posterior portion of the ventricular septum and the posterior left ventricular free wall is replaced by scar tissue. (*B*) Photographs of the ventricular slices caudal to the view shown in *A*. The quantity of subepicardial adipose tissue is excessive such that the heart floated in a container of formaldehyde. Total paced 12-lead QRS voltage was 47 mm, and the heart weighed 460 g.

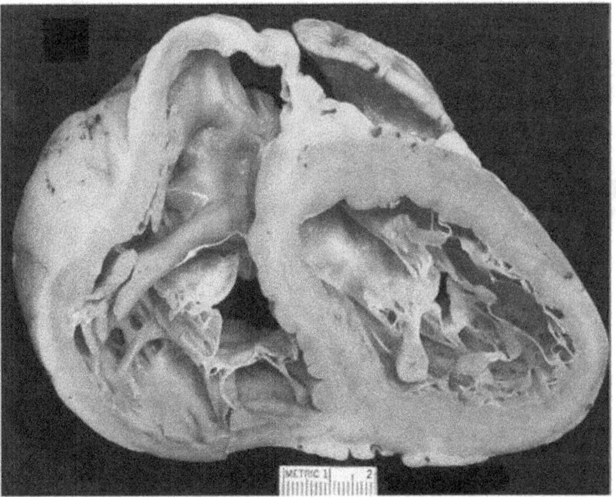

Figure 9. Case #9, Tables 1 and 2. Shown here is the basal portion of the heart in a 44-year-old woman who had limb-girdle muscular dystrophy. This photograph shows marked dilatation of the two ventricular cavities. The right ventricular free wall anteriorly adjacent to the septum is replaced by adipose tissue. The lateral wall of left ventricle between the two papillary muscles is thinner than other portions of the left ventricular free wall. Total nonpaced 12-lead QRS voltage in this patient was 118 mm, and the heart weighed 420 g.

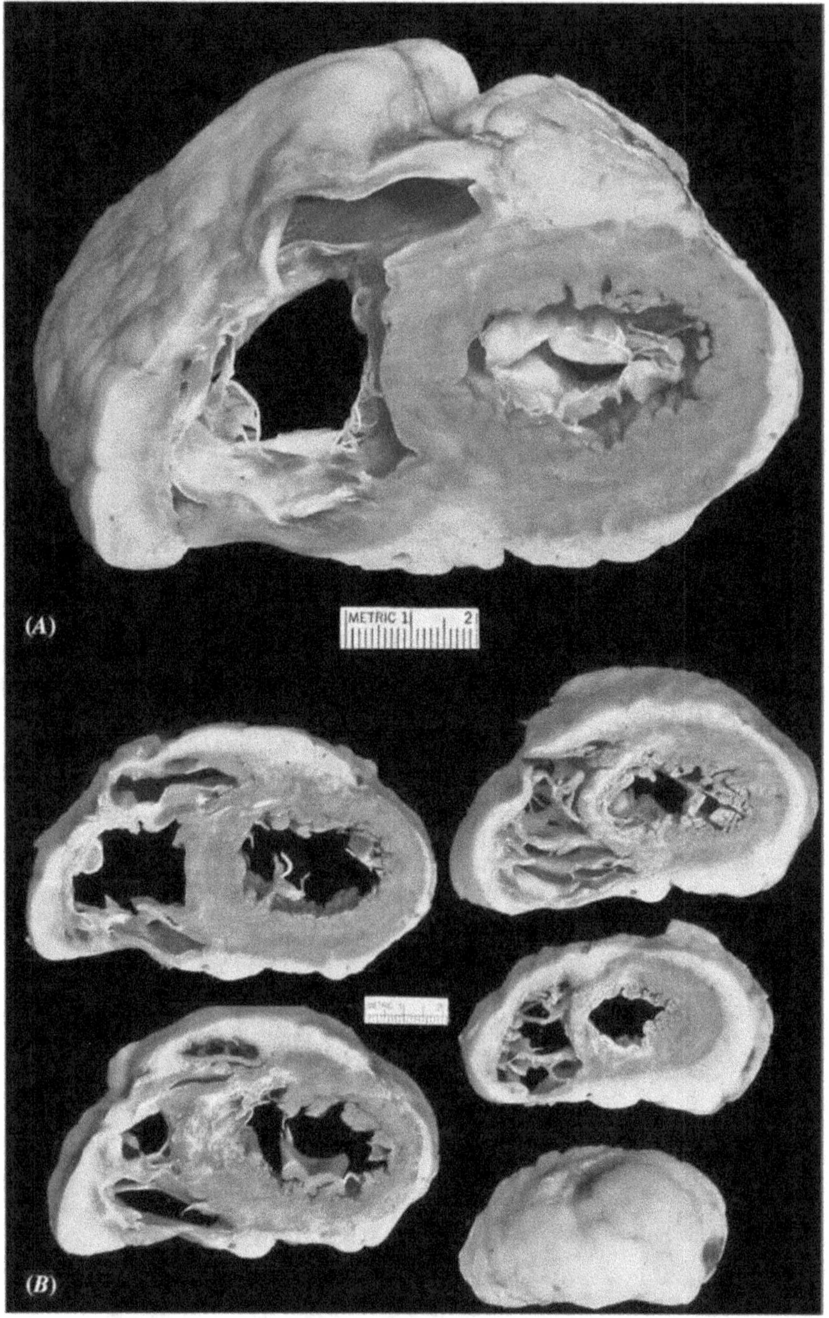

Figure 10. Case #10, Tables 1 and 2. Shown here is the heart in a 49-year-old woman. (A) Shown is the basal portion of the ventricles. The right ventricular cavity is considerably dilated and the left, minimally so. Portions of the endocardium of right ventricle are thickened by fibrous tissue and portions of the right ventricular free wall are replaced by fibrous tissue. No definite lesions are noted in the left ventricular free wall at the base. (B) Shown here are more apical cuts of the ventricular wall. The ventricular septum and the right ventricular free wall are extensively scarred. The epicardial coronary arteries were wide open. The total nonpaced 12-lead QRS voltage was 118 mm, and the heart weighed only 305 g. The heart floated in a container of formaldehyde.

between initially developing ARVC and the OHT procedure.[27] Strong features of the present report are that both the weight of the native heart and the extent of the cardiac lesions were known in all 11 patients. To our knowledge, total 12-lead electrocardiographic QRS voltage has not been described previously in patients with ARVC, and gross differing features of the hearts have not been well illustrated previously. The electrocardiographic findings may provide a clue to the diagnosis of ARVC (Figures 1–11).

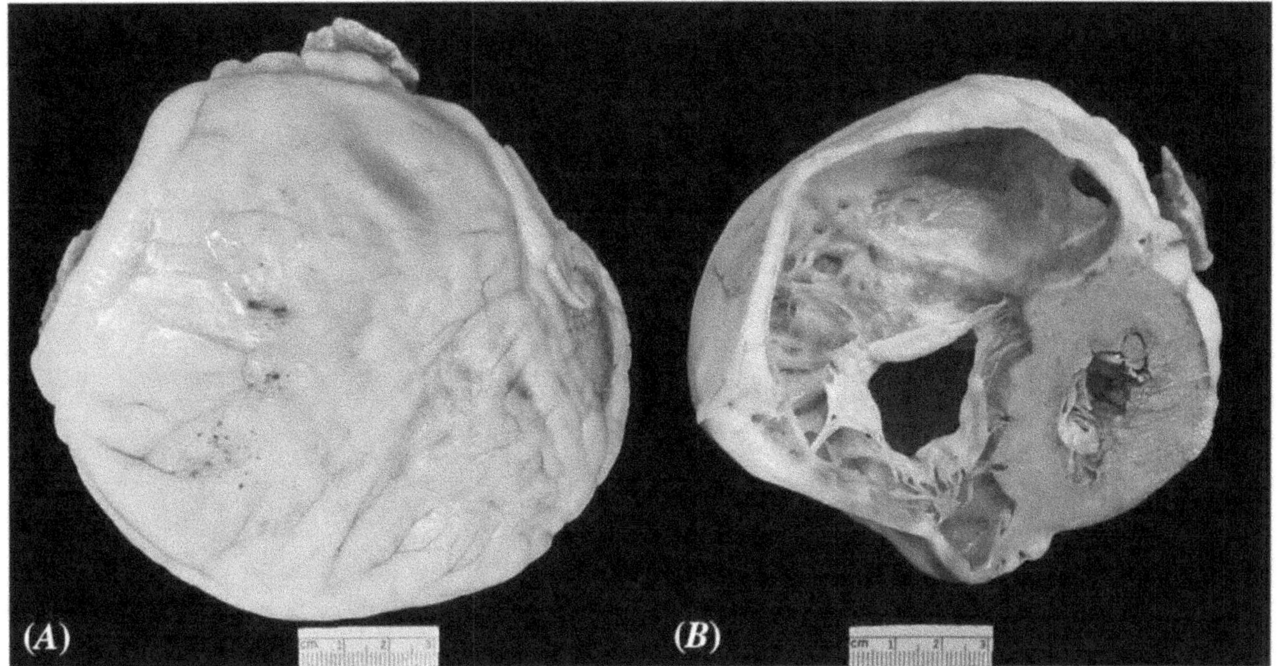

Figure 11. Case #11, Tables 1 and 2. Shown in *A* is the outside of the heart anteriorly. The right ventricular cavity is greatly dilated and totally covered by adipose tissue. (*B*) A photograph of the basal portion of the ventricles showing the enormously dilated right ventricular cavity and a normal-sized left ventricular cavity. About 90% of the right ventricular free wall is replaced by adipose tissue. The tricuspid valve annulus is greatly dilated. In contrast, no lesions are noted in the left ventricular free wall or in the ventricular septum. This patient was 70 years of age at the time of the OHT. ARVC was diagnosed clinically and the patient was found to have the nonsense mutation PKP2 c.235 C ->T (p.Arg79*), one of the mutations specific for ARVC. The same mutation was found in the patient's son and grandson, but neither had signs or symptoms of ARVC. The total nonpaced 12-lead QRS voltage was 52 mm, and the heart, which floated in formaldehyde, weighed only 285 g.

1. Roberts WC, Ko JM, Kuiper JJ, Hall SA, Meyer DM. Some previously neglected examples of arrhythmic right ventricular dysplasia/cardiomyopathy and frequency of its various reported manifestations. *Am J Cardiol* 2010;106:268–2074.
2. Marcus FI, Fontaine GH, Guiraudon G, Frank R, Laurenceau JL, Malergue C, Grosgogeat Y. Right ventricular dysplasia: a report of 24 adult cases. *Circulation* 1982;65:384–398.
3. Blomström-Lundqvist C, Sabel KG, Olsson SB. A long-term follow-up of 15 patients with arrhythmogenic right ventricular dysplasia. *Br Heart J* 1987;58:477–488.
4. Lemery R, Brugada P, Janssen J, Cheriex E, Dugernier T, Wellens HJ. Nonischemic sustained ventricular tachycardia: clinical outcome in 12 patients with arrhythmogenic right ventricular dysplasia. *J Am Coll Cardiol* 1989;14:96–105.
5. Pinamonti B, Sinagra G, Salvi A, Di Lenarda A, Morgera T, Silvestri F, Bussani R, Camerini F. Left ventricular involvement in right ventricular dysplasia. *Am Heart J* 1992;12:711–724.
6. Corrado D, Basso C, Thiene G, McKenna WJ, Davies MJ, Fontaliran F, Nava A, Silvestri F, Blomstrom-Lundqvist C, Wlodarska EK, Fontaine G, Camerini F. Spectrum of clinicopathologic manifestations of arrhythmogenic right ventricular cardiomyopathy/dysplasia: a multicenter study. *J Am Coll Cardiol* 1997;30:1512–1520.
7. Hulot JS, Jouven X, Empana JP, Frank R, Fontaine G. Natural history and risk stratification of arrhythmogenic right ventricular dysplasia/cardiomyopathy. *Circulation* 2004;110:1879–1884.
8. Dalal D, Nasir K, Bomma C, Prakasa K, Tandri H, Piccini J, Roguin A, Tichnell C, James C, Russell SD, Judge DP, Abraham T, Spevak PJ, Bluemke DA, Calkins H. Arrhythmogenic right ventricular dysplasia: a United States experience. *Circulation* 2005;112:3823–3832.
9. Marcus FI, Zareba W. The electrocardiogram in right ventricular cardiomyopathy/dysplasia. How can the electrocardiogram assist in understanding the pathologic and functional changes of the heart in this disease? *J Electrocardiol* 2009;42, 136.e1-136.e5.
10. Marcus FI, McKenna WJ, Sherrill D, Basso C, Bauce B, Bluemke DA, Calkins H, Corrado D, Cox MG, Daubert JP, Fontaine G, Gear K, Hauer R, Nava A, Picard MH, Protonotarios N, Saffitz JE, Sanborn DM, Steinberg JS, Tandri H, Thiene G, Towbin JA, Tsatsopoulou A, Wichter T, Zareba W. Diagnosis of arrhythmogenic right ventricular cardiomyopathy/dysplasia: proposed modification of the task force criteria. *Circulation* 2010;121:1533–1541.
11. Hauer RN, Cox MG, Groeneweg JA. Impact of new electrocardiographic criteria in arrhythmogenic cardiomyopathy. *Front Physiol* 2012;3:352.
12. Mast TP, James CA, Calkins H, Teske AJ, Tichnell C, Murray B, Loh P, Russell SD, Velthuis BK, Judge DP, Dooijes D, Tedford RJ, van der Heijden JF, Tandri H, Hauer RN, Abraham TP, Doevendans PA, Te Riele AS, Cramer MJ. Evaluation of structural progression in arrhythmogenic right ventricular dysplasia/cardiomyopathy. *JAMA Cardiol* 2017;2:293–302.
13. Corrado D, Link MS, Calkins H. Arrhythmogenic right ventricular cardiomyopathy. *N Engl J Med* 2017;376:61–72.
14. Roberts WC, Podolak MJ. The king of hearts: analysis of 23 patients with hearts weighing 1000 grams or more. *Am J Cardiol* 1985;55:485–494.
15. Siegel RJ, Roberts WC. Electrocardiographic observations in severe aortic valve stenosis: correlative necropsy study to clinical, hemodynamic, and ECG variables demonstrating relation of 12-lead QRS amplitude to peak systolic transaortic pressure gradient. *Am Heart J* 1982;103:210–221.
16. Roberts WC, Day PJ. Electrocardiographic observations in clinically isolated, pure, chronic, severe aortic regurgitation: analysis of 30 necropsy patients aged 19 to 65 years. *Am J Cardiol* 1985;55:432–438.
17. Glick BN, Roberts WC. Usefulness of total 12-lead QRS voltage in diagnosing left ventricular hypertrophy in clinically isolated, pure, chronic, severe mitral regurgitation. *Am J Cardiol* 1992;70:1088–1092.
18. Dollar AL, Roberts WC. Usefulness of total 12-lead QRS voltage compared with other criteria for determining left ventricular hypertrophy in hypertrophic cardiomyopathy: analysis of 57 patients studied at necropsy. *Am J Med* 1989;87:377–381.
19. Shirani J, Maron BJ, Cannon RO III, Sheyda S, Roberts WC. Clinicopathologic features of hypertrophic cardiomyopathy managed by cardiac transplantation. *Am J Cardiol* 1993;72:434–440.

20. Roberts WC, Siegel RJ, McManus BM. Idiopathic dilated cardiomyopathy: analysis of 152 necropsy patients. *Am J Cardiol* 1987;60:1340–1355.
21. Shirani J, Roberts WC. Clinical electrocardiographic and morphologic features of massive fatty deposits ("lipomatous hypertrophy") in the atrial septum. *J Am Coll Cardiol* 1993;22:226–238.
22. Ross EM, Roberts WC. The carcinoid syndrome: comparison of 21 necropsy subjects with carcinoid heart disease to 15 necropsy subjects without carcinoid heart disease. *Am J Med* 1985;79:339–354.
23. Roberts WC, Barbin CM, Weissenborn MR, Ko JM. Electrocardiographic total 12-lead QRS voltage in patients having operative resection of syphilitic aortic aneurysm. *Am J Cardiol* 2015;116:973–976.
24. Shirani J, Berezowski K, Roberts WC. Quantitative measurement of normal and excessive (cor adiposum) subepicardial adipose tissue, its clinical significance, and its effect on electrocardiographic QRS voltage. *Am J Cardiol* 1995;76:414–418.
25. Roberts WC, Waller BF. Cardiac amyloidosis causing cardiac dysfunction: analysis of 54 necropsy patients. *Am J Cardiol* 1983;52:137–146.
26. Roberts WC, Becker TM, Hall SA. Usefulness of total 12-lead QRS voltage as a clue to diagnosis of patients with cardiac sarcoidosis severe enough to warrant orthotopic heart transplant. *JAMA Cardiol* 2018;3:64–68.
27. Wilensky RL, Yudelman P, Cohen AI, Fletcher RD, Atkinson J, Virmani R, Roberts WC. Serial electrocardiographic changes in idiopathic dilated cardiomyopathy confirmed at necropsy. *Am J Cardiol* 1988;62:276–283.

Total 12-Lead QRS Voltage in Patients Having Orthotopic Heart Transplantation for Heart Failure Caused by Adriamycin-Induced Cardiomyopathy

William C. Roberts[a, b]   Sarah Haque[c]   Shelley A. Hall[b]

[a]Baylor Scott and White Heart and Vascular Institute, Baylor University Medical Center, Dallas, TX, USA; [b]Division of Cardiology, Departments of Pathology and Internal Medicine, Baylor University Medical Center, Dallas, TX, USA; [c]Austin College, Sherman, TX, USA

Keywords
Adriamycin cardiomyopathy · Cardiotoxicity · Orthotopic heart transplantation

Abstract
Objective: Although several studies have described the effects of adriamycin on the heart, electrocardiographic total 12-lead QRS voltage (distance in millimeters from the peak of the R wave to the nadir of either the Q or S wave, whichever was deeper, with 10 mm [1 mV] being standard) both before and after orthotopic heart transplantation (OHT) has not been reported. This study describes the total 12-lead QRS voltage in 8 patients studied at Baylor University Medical Center at Dallas, from 1994 to June 2018, who underwent OHT for severe heart failure caused by anthracycline-induced cardiomyopathy. *Method:* Prior to OHT, the total 12-lead non-paced QRS voltages ranged from 86 to 189 mm (mean 125 ± 56) and for paced QRS voltages from 82 to 113 mm (mean 97 ± 15). The total 12-lead QRS voltages post-OHT ranged from 100 to 190 mm (mean 130 ± 30). Total 12-lead QRS voltages were lower in patients with a pacemaker than without. *Results/Conclusion:* These low voltages are like those found in patients with carcinoid syndrome, severe cardiac adiposity, cardiac amyloidosis, and cardiac sarcoidosis.

© 2019 S. Karger AG, Basel

Introduction

Orthotopic heart transplantation (OHT) has proven to be a useful therapy for patients with heart failure (HF) secondary to adriamycin cardiotoxicity [1]. Little electrocardiographic data are available in patients with HF secondary to adriamycin toxicity severe enough to warrant OHT. To fill this void, we measured the total 12-lead QRS voltage in 8 patients who underwent OHT for severe HF secondary to adriamycin cardiotoxicity.

Materials and Methods

Review of all OHT cases performed at Baylor University Medical Center at Dallas from 1994 through June 2018, a 24-year period, yielded 8 patients who had received anthracycline therapy. The native hearts for all 8 patients were examined and described by one of us (W.C.R.). The clinical records and all available electrocardiograms recorded between the onset of HF and OTH for each patient were reviewed. The total 12-lead QRS voltage was measured by S.H. and confirmed by W.C.R.

Results

The pertinent clinical, electrocardiographic, and morphologic findings are summarized in Table 1. Three patients had non-Hodgkin lymphoma, 3 had breast cancer, and 2 had leukemia. At the time of cancer diagnosis and treatment, the patients ranged in age from 6 to 64 years (mean 36 ± 20),

Table 1. Pertinent clinical and morphological findings in 8 patients with adriamycin-induced cardiomyopathy

| Case No. | Age at cancer Dx and Rx, years | Age at OHT, years | Year of OHT | Type of cancer | Rad Rx | Height, in | Body weight, lb | BMI | EF, % | Paced | QRS amplitude in each electrocardiographic lead | | | | | | | | | | | | Total 12-lead QRS voltage, mm | HW, g | Floating heart | Alive in 6/2018 | Intervals, days | |
											I	II	III	aVR	aVL	aVF	V1	V2	V3	V4	V5	V6					P or NP ECG to OHT	OHT to PHT ECG
Men																												
1	8	26	4/2015	Leukemia	no	70	183	26	10	NP	11	7	10	7	9	9	20	36	24	15	19	22						
										PHT	12	9	13	8	11	9	6	13	14	8	9	9	121					
2	6	30	9/2008	Leukemia	no	71	185	27	15	P	2	5	5	2	5	4	11	14	18	6	5	5	82	365	no	no	109	14
										PHT	7	7	7	6	6	5	16	35	49	32	12	8	190					
3	50	55	5/2011	Lymphoma[1]	no	68	220	33	15	P	4	12	10	5	5	8	5	5	5	7	10	8	84	525	yes	yes	46	135
										PHT	11	7	5	9	8	3	9	16	15	16	15	10	124					
Women																												
4	30	37	5/2017	Lymphoma[1]	yes	62	180	33	15	NP	4	7	12	4	8	10	9	14	10	8	7	6	99	260	yes	yes	252	32
										PHT	9	1	9	5	10	5	8	23	7	8	8	7	100					
5	38	50	5/2007	Breast	yes	64	180	31	10	NP	5	3	5	2	4	4	5	9	18	12	11	8	86	405	yes	yes	16	27
										PHT	12	5	11	7	11	4	8	9	10	10	12	10	109					
6	41	64	5/2004	Breast	yes	63	135	24	10	P	7	6	7	6	6	6	5	2	28	18	11	9	111	325	no	no	47	14
										PHT	9	10	8	10	6	6	9	20	24	21	17	11	151					
7	49	65	3/2011	Lymphoma[1]	yes	61	146	28	–	P	8	10	16	8	4	16	6	6	13	5	14	7	113	560	yes	yes	74	184
										PHT	12	8	11	10	14	6	8	7	8	8	9	12	113					
8	64	68	9/2011	Breast	no	64	155	27	15	P	4	5	8	2	6	5	3	5	20	18	11	8	95	500	yes	yes	98	14
										PHT	10	5	7	7	9	3	5	14	18	23	20	14	135					

AF, atrial fibrillation; BMI, body mass index; CI, cardiac index; Dx, diagnosis; ECG, electrocardiogram; EF, ejection fraction; HW, heart weight; LV, left ventricular; NP, non-paced; OHT, orthotopic heart transplant; P, paced; PHT, post-OHT; Rad, radiation; Rx, treatment; –, no information available. [1] Non-Hodgkin lymphoma.

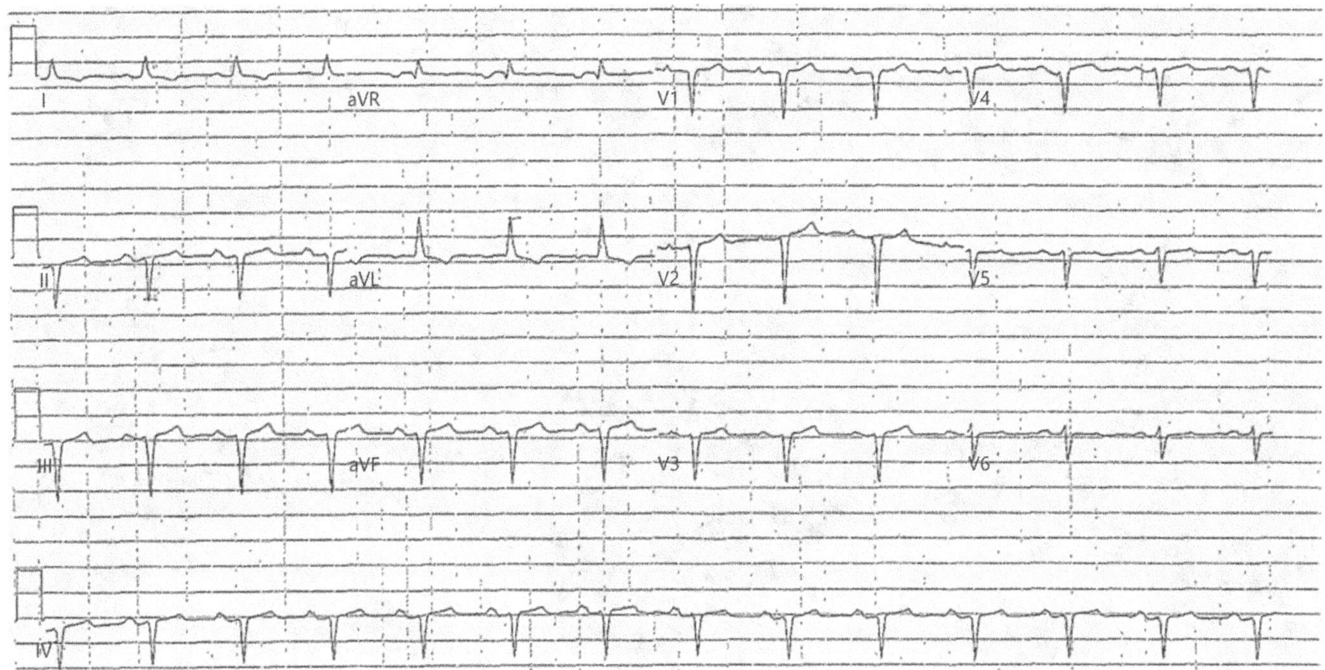

Fig. 1. Case No. 4. Pre-OHT non-paced electrocardiogram. The total 12-lead QRS voltage was 99 mm.

and at OHT from 26 to 68 years (mean 49 ± 17). The interval from the start of anthracycline treatment to OHT ranged from 4 to 24 years (mean 14 ± 8). Of the 8 patients, 3 were men and 5 were women. The body mass index ranged from 24 to 33 (mean 29 ± 3). The heart weights ranged from 260 to 558 g (mean 414 ± 105). Four patients were known to have received mediastinal irradiation at some point during chemotherapy. Adriamycin-induced cardiomyopathy was diagnosed prior to OHT in all 8 patients.

We obtained 3 non-paced and 5 paced pre-OHT electrocardiographic tracings and all 8 post-transplant tracings (Fig. 1). The total 12-lead QRS voltages prior to OHT ranged from 82 to 189 mm (mean 107 ± 49). Tracings for pre-OHT non-paced patients ranged from 86 to 189 mm (mean 125 ± 56), while pre-OHT paced voltages ranged from 82 to 113 mm (mean 97 ± 15). The total 12-lead QRS voltage post-OHT ranged from 100 to 190 mm (mean 130 ± 30). The basal portions of the cardiac ventricles in 4 of the 8 patients are shown in Figure 2.

Discussion and Conclusion

Described herein are total 12-lead electrographic QRS voltages and characteristics of the native hearts of 8 patients who underwent OHT for HF caused by adri-

amycin-induced cardiomyopathy. The total paced and non-paced (means 97 ± 15 and 125 ± 56 mm, respectively) 12-lead QRS voltages seen in these 8 patients are similar to those found in carcinoid syndrome (mean 117 mm), cardiac adiposity (mean 120 mm), cardiac amyloidosis (mean 104 mm), and cardiac sarcoidosis (mean 117 mm) [2]. The native hearts had no grossly visible myocardial lesions in any of the 8 patients [3, 4].

A positive feature of this report is that it is the first to describe total 12-lead electrocardiographic QRS voltages in patients with HF secondary to adriamycin-induced cardiomyopathy severe enough to warrant OHT. A limitation of the present report is the small number of patients studied and particularly the small number of electrocardiograms available before pacemaker insertion. Also, the amount of adriamycin administered years before the OHT is not known.

Acknowledgements

We thank Saba Ilyas for her excellent photographic work.

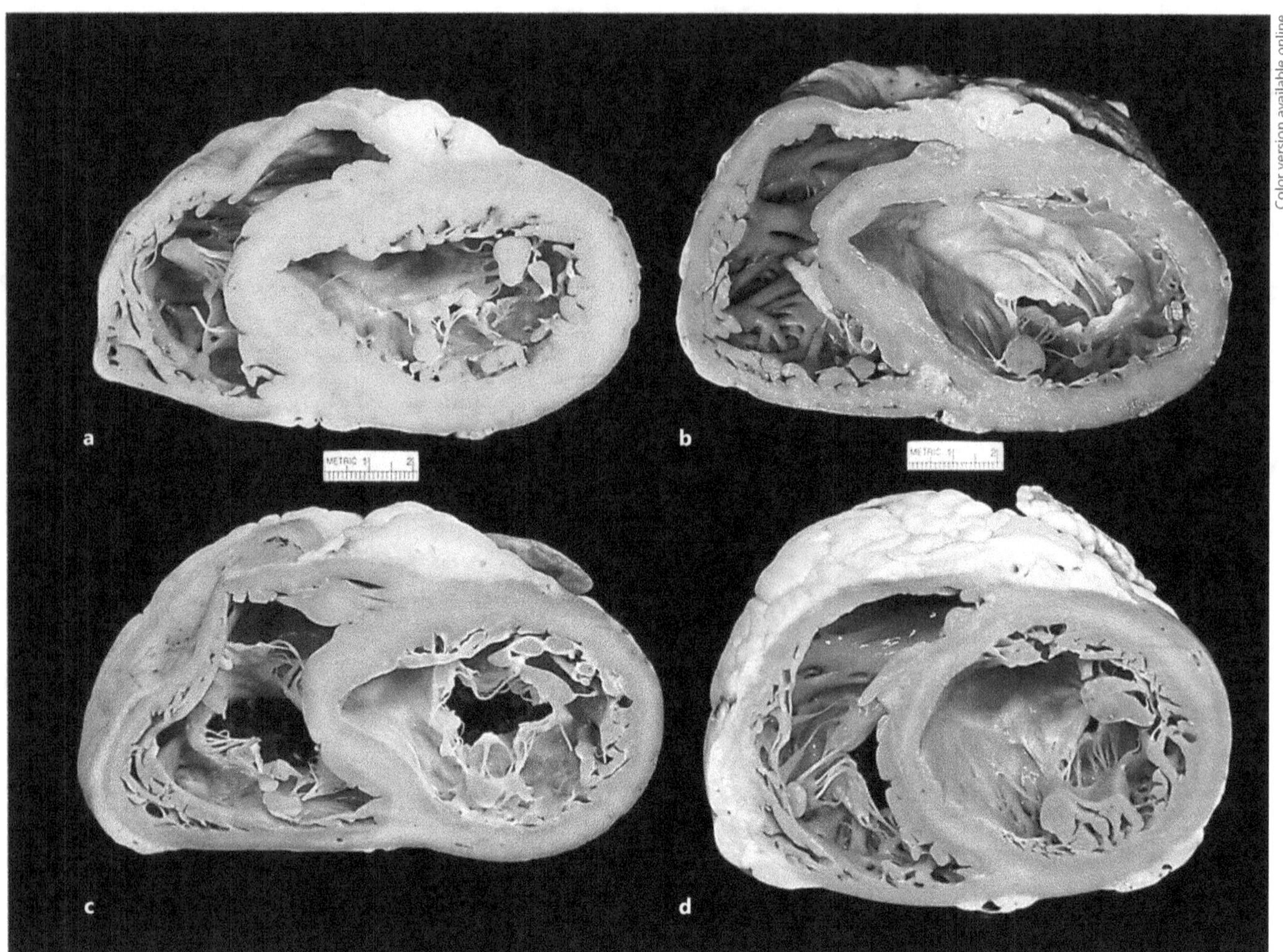

Fig. 2. Views of the basal portion of the ventricles in 4 patients having OHT for adriamycin cardiotoxicity. **a** Case No. 1. The total non-paced 12-lead QRS voltage prior to OHT was 189 mm and the heart weighed 370 g. **b** Case No. 2. The total non-paced 12-lead QRS voltage prior to OHT was 82 mm and the heart weighed 365 g. **c** Case No. 4. The total non-paced 12-lead QRS voltage prior to OHT was 99 mm and the heart weighed 260 g. **d** Case No. 5. The total non-paced 12-lead QRS voltage prior to OHT was 86 mm and the heart weighed 405 g.

Statement of Ethics

The authors have no ethical conflicts to disclose.

Disclosure Statement

The authors have no conflicts of interest to declare.

References

1 Lenneman AJ, Wang L, Wigger M, Frangoul H, Harrell FE, Silverstein C, et al. Heart transplant survival outcomes for adriamycin-dilated cardiomyopathy. Am J Cardiol. 2013 Feb; 111(4):609–12.

2 Roberts WC, Filardo G, Ko JM, Siegel RJ, Dollar AL, Ross EM, et al. Comparison of total 12-lead QRS voltage in a variety of cardiac conditions and its usefulness in predicting increased cardiac mass. Am J Cardiol. 2013 Sep; 112(6):904–9.

3 Lefrak EA, Pitha J, Rosenheim S, Gottlieb JA. A clinicopathologic analysis of adriamycin cardiotoxicity. Cancer. 1973 Aug;32(2):302–14.

4 Isner JM, Ferrans VJ, Cohen SR, Witkind BG, Virmani R, Gottdiener JS, et al. Clinical and morphologic cardiac findings after anthracycline chemotherapy. Analysis of 64 patients studied at necropsy. Am J Cardiol. 1983 Apr; 51(7):1167–74.

Total 12-lead QRS voltage in patients with spontaneous acute aortic dissection with an initiating tear in the ascending aorta

William C. Roberts, MD[a,b], Shaffin Siddiqiquiz[a,c], and Charles S. Roberts, MD[a,d]

[a]Baylor Scott & White Heart and Vascular Institute, Baylor University Medical Center, Dallas, Texas; [b]Division of Cardiology, Department of Medicine, Baylor University Medical Center, Dallas, Texas; [c]Princeton University, Princeton, New Jersey; [d]Department of Cardiac Surgery, Baylor University Medical Center, Dallas, Texas

ABSTRACT

Because nearly all patients with acute aortic dissection have systemic hypertension, we examined electrocardiograms (ECGs) in 21 patients with spontaneous acute type A aortic dissection. An earlier study had shown that total 12-lead QRS voltage was the best criterion for determining left ventricular hypertrophy from the ECG. We measured total 12-lead QRS voltage in 21 patients with spontaneous (no previous cardiac or aortic operation) acute type A aortic dissection and operative repair. Using >175 mm as evidence of left ventricular hypertrophy, only 8 patients (38%) had hearts of increased mass. Total 12-lead QRS voltage corresponded slightly with age but not with body mass index. In conclusion, total 12-lead QRS voltage is not useful for diagnostic purposes in patients with acute type A aortic dissection undergoing operative repair.

KEYWORDS Aortic dissection; body mass index; left ventricular hypertrophy; operative repair

Total 12-lead QRS voltage has now been measured and reported in a number of cardiac conditions[1] *(Table 1)*. In general, the higher the total 12-lead QRS voltage, the greater the cardiac mass. This criterion appears to be better than others proposed through the years for left ventricular hypertrophy.[1] Since patients with acute aortic dissection nearly always have systemic hypertension, we theorized that patients with acute aortic dissection would have electrocardiographic evidence of left ventricular hypertrophy. Accordingly, we measured total 12-lead QRS voltage in 21 patients with spontaneous aortic dissection with tears in the ascending aorta.

METHODS

From July 24, 2018, to July 31, 2020 (26 months), 45 patients of a single surgeon at Baylor University Medical Center at Dallas underwent repair of spontaneous acute ascending aortic type A dissection with a tear originating in the ascending aorta. Electrocardiograms (ECGs) before the aortic operation were available for examination in 21 (47%) of the 45 patients: 18 (86%) were done on the day of the operation; 2 within a day or two, and 1 (patient 21), 60 days before the aortic operation. Twelve patients had >1 ECG recorded before operative repair of the acute dissection. The total 12-lead QRS voltage (defined as the distance in milliliters from the peak of the R wave to the nadir of either the Q or S wave, whichever was deeper) was measured in each ECG with 10-mm standard for all measurements *(Figure 1)*.

RESULTS

The results of the ECG measurements are tabulated for each patient in *Table 2*. In the 6 women, the average 12-lead QRS voltage was 157 mm and the median was 133 mm; in the 15 men, the mean was 148 mm and the median was 152 mm. The relation of the total 12-lead QRS voltage to age is displayed in *Figure 2* and the relation to body mass index in

Corresponding author: William C. Roberts, MD, Baylor Scott & White Heart and Vascular Institute, 621 N. Hall Street, Suite H-030, Dallas, TX 75226 (e-mail: William.Roberts1@bswhealth.org.org)

The authors have no conflicts of interests to disclose.

Received January 7, 2021; Revised February 22, 2021; Accepted February 23, 2021.

Table 1. Total 12-lead QRS voltage, heart weight, and age of groups of 331 patients with various cardiac conditions

Condition	Sex	Number of cases	Age (years): range (mean)	Total 12-lead QRS voltage (mm) (mean)	QRS voltage >175 mm	Heart weight (g): range (means)	Year of publication
Aortic valve stenosis	M	36	16-64 (48)	144-417 (249)	47 (94%)	440-880 (639)	1982
	F	14	16-65 (47)	193-376 (277)		380-700 (521)	
Hearts weighing >1000 g	M	16	29-64 (42)	140-414 (306)	16 (94%)	1005-1360 (1102)	1985
	F	1	20	601		1250	
Aortic regurgitation	M	22	19-59 (44)	109-428 (271)	27 (90%)	430-1100 (717)	1985
	F	8	35-56 (48)	169-384 (275)		375-950 (638)	
Mitral regurgitation	M	11	24-84 (47)	111-364 (245)	17 (71%)	400-775 (629)	1992
	F	13	21-64 (37)	114-290 (199)		350-675 (472)	
Hypertrophic cardiomyopathy without cardiac transplantation	M	21	14-68 (46)	107-339 (190)	30 (53%)	325-1070 (671)	1989
	F	36	19-87 (51)	68-327 (201)		290-1230 (547)	
Hypertrophic cardiomyopathy with cardiac transplantation	M	6	19-46 (35)	109-201 (142)	4 (40%)	310-480 (393)	1993
	F	4	24-45 (35)	172-378 (241)		290-650 (408)	
Idiopathic dilated cardiomyopathy	M	35	19-73 (46)	74-281 (147)	20 (41%)	400-940 (620)	1987
	F	14	22-75 (54)	75-243 (167)		400-860 (602)	
Lipomatous hypertrophy of the atrial septum	M	12	48-84 (67)	93-24 (140)	3 (11%)	410-795 (576)	1993
	F	16	59-83 (74)	59-266 (124)		330-680 (502)	
Carcinoid syndrome							1985
With carcinoid HD	M	11	39-72 (56)	58-227 (120)	2 (11%)	220-480 (350)	
	F	8	28-64 (54)	58-128 (84)		200-290 (245)	
Without carcinoid HD	M	10	42-75 (55)	89-129 (137)	2 (13%)	240-570 (350)	
	F	5	28-67 (50)	102-135 (121)		150-270 (230)	
Cardiac amyloidosis	M	15	32-69 (52)	60-197 (99)	2 (7%)	410-850 (570)	1983
	F	15	21-93 (69)	58-199 (109)		370-900 (494)	
Cardiac adiposity	M	13	51-73 (64)	73-159 (114)	1 (3%)	320-795 (485)	1995
	F	17	40-85 (70)	77-210 (124)		250-575 (395)	
Adriamycin cardiotoxicity	M	3	26-55 (37)	82-182 (116)	1 (13%)	365-525 (445)	2018
	F	5	30-64 (57)	30-64 (101)		260-560 (410)	

HD indicates heart disease.

Table 2. Total 12-lead QRS voltage before operation for acute type A aortic dissection in the 21 patients studied

Patient number	Age (years)	Race	BMI (kg/m^2)	SH	I	II	III	aVR	aVL	aVF	V1	V2	V3	V4	V5	V6	T 12-lead QRS voltage (mm)
Women																	
1	35	B	40	+ (Hx)	20	27	13	23	7	18	27	19	31	40	37	30	292
2	57	W	21	+ (Hx)	6	20	14	12	2	10	9	15	25	27	25	22	187
3	64	W	17	+ (Rx)	2	11	9	6	4	11	11	12	22	17	13	7	125
4	72	W	24	+ (Rx)	9	12	6	10	5	10	6	10	19	21	17	10	135
5	78	W	22	+ (Rx)	11	8	10	8	9	7	14	10	11	21	15	8	132
6	93	W	23	0	6	4	3	4	5	2	3	4	8	14	11	7	71
Mean	67		24.5		9	14	9	11	5	10	12	12	19	23	20	14	157
Median																	133.5
Men																	
7	33	B	33	+ (Rx)	5	6	4	6	4	4	5	7	13	13	10	9	86
8	34	W	33	+ (Hx)	13	21	8	16	7	16	15	17	16	14	20	17	180
9	39	W	28	+ (Rx)	15	12	7	13	10	5	12	10	9	14	21	24	152
10	41	W	33	+ (Hx)	11	9	3	10	8	4	19	29	27	17	20	21	178
11	42	W	24	+ (Rx)	17	12	15	12	15	9	14	16	25	26	22	15	198
12	43	W	45	+ (Rx)	14	9	11	11	13	8	7	11	9	10	8	8	119
13	45	B	22	+ (Rx)	6	15	14	9	7	14	10	14	25	31	32	18	195
14	45	W	34	+ (Rx)	7	13	6	9	3	10	8	6	17	14	20	12	125
15	52	W	34	+ (Rx)	12	19	10	14	7	15	23	20	17	20	8	11	176
16	57	W	26	+ (Rx)	13	5	10	9	12	5	9	17	16	14	16	16	142
17	58	B	31	+	7	9	6	6	5	8	4	20	27	26	22	16	156
18	60	W	29	+ (Rx)	8	5	4	6	6	2	11	11	11	10	13	11	98
19	61	W	28	+ (Rx)	9	6	4	8	6	2	2	16	19	17	18	10	117
20	65	B	28	+ (Rx)	13	14	6	12	6	8	10	27	23	25	18	15	177
21	67	W	29	+ (Rx)	6	8	5	7	3	6	3	5	16	22	22	13	116
Mean	49		30.5		10	11	8	10	7	8	10	15	18	18	18	14	148
Median																	152

B indicates black; BMI, body mass index; ECG, electrocardiogram; Hx, history; Rx, treatment; SH, systemic hypertension; T, total; W, white.

Figure 3. ECGs with the highest and lowest total 12-lead QRS voltage for both men and women are shown in *Figures 4 and 5.* In 12 (57%) of the 21 patients >1 ECG before the aortic operation was available for examination. The total 12-lead QRS voltage in some patients increased over time, in others it decreased, and in a few it did not change.

DISCUSSION

Examination of the 46 ECGs in the 21 patients with type A acute aortic dissection disclosed no particular trends to help in diagnosis. The initial purpose of the study was to determine the frequency of left ventricular hypertrophy by the ECG in this patient group. All but one of the patients had hypertension before the aortic dissection. One potential problem in using total 12-lead QRS voltage as a surrogate for cardiac mass is that the total 12-lead QRS voltage in persons with hearts of normal mass ($\leq$350 g in women and $\leq$400 g in men) has not been definitely established. If total 12-lead QRS voltage >175 mm is used as the upper limit of normal, only 8 (38%) of the 21 patients had left ventricular

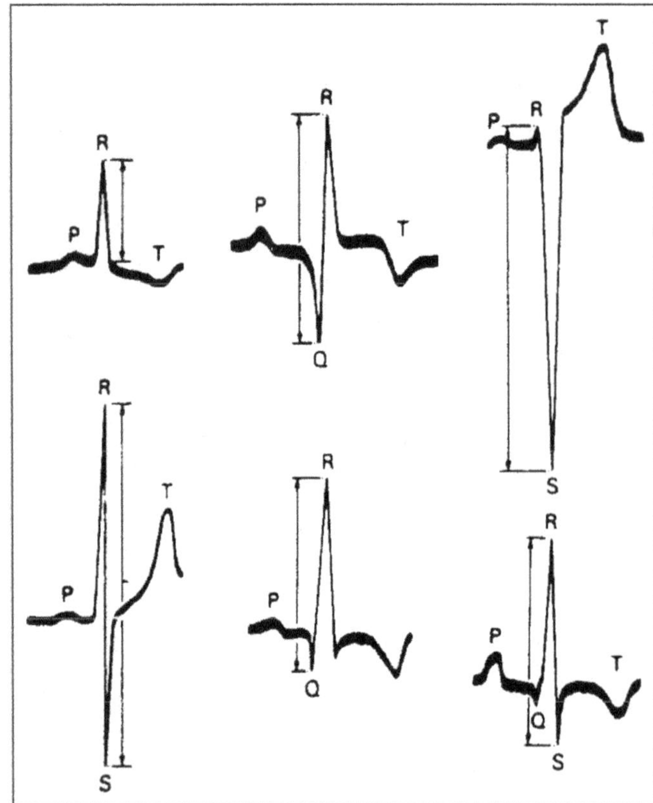

Figure 1. Various QRS complexes showing how each was measured. Reproduced with permission from the authors (Roberts WC, Podolak MJ. *Am J Cardiol* 1985;55:485-494) and the publisher (Elsevier).

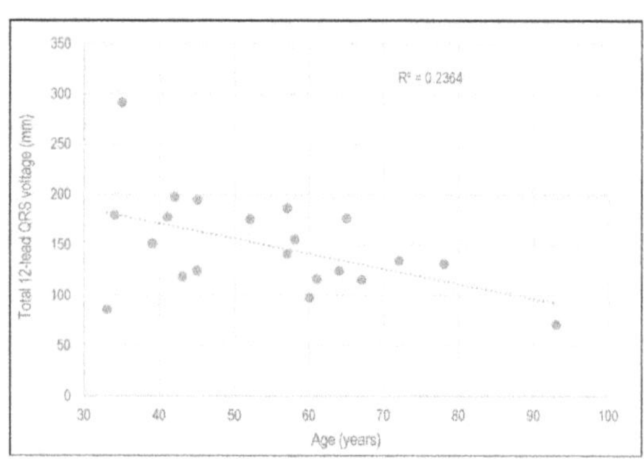

Figure 2. Relation of total 12-lead QRS voltage to age.

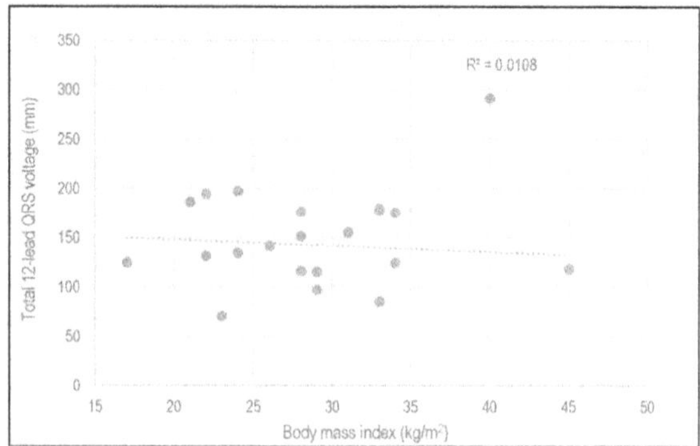

Figure 3. Relation of total 12-lead QRS voltage to body mass index.

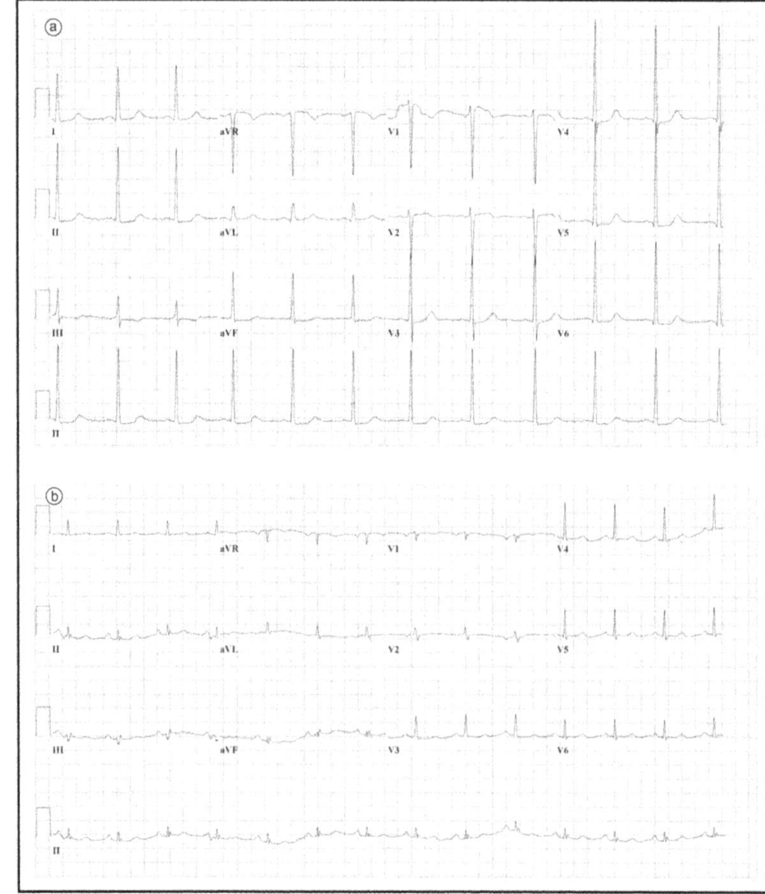

Figure 4. Electrocardiograms of two women showing the maximal and minimal total 12-lead QRS voltage occurring in the six women listed in *Table 2*: **(a)** Patient 1, 292 mm, and **(b)** Patient 6, 71 mm.

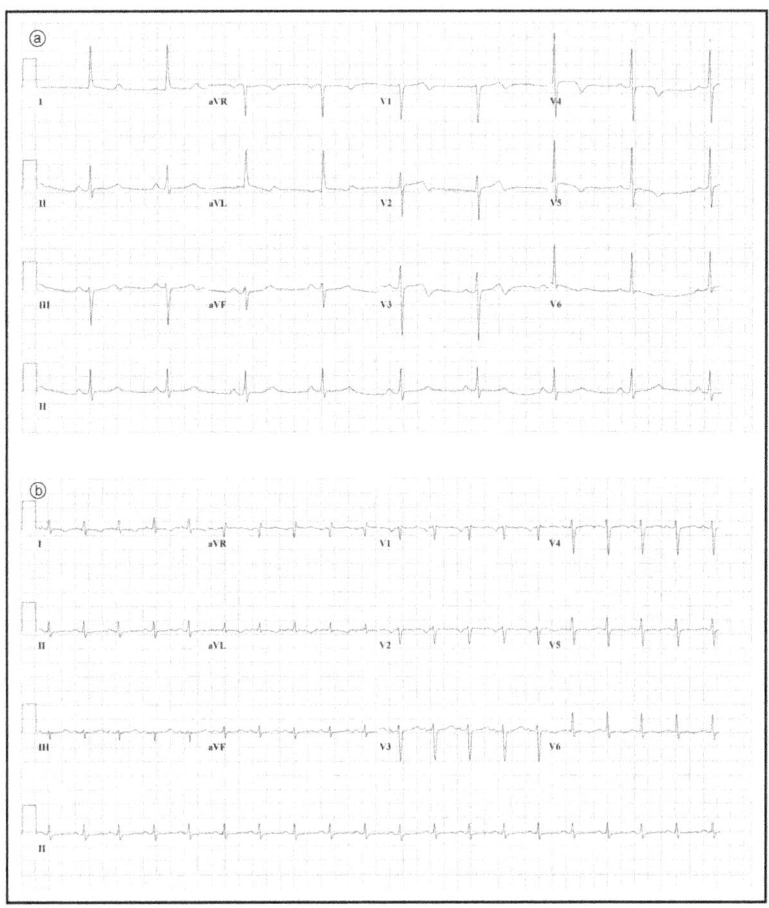

Figure 5. Electrocardiograms of two men showing the maximal and minimal total 12-lead QRS voltage occurring in the 15 men listed in *Table 2*: **(a)** Patient 11, 198 mm, and **(b)** Patient 7, 86 mm.

hypertrophy by this criterion.[2] A deficiency of the present study is the lack of cardiac weights in these patients. A previous publication, however, compared total 12-lead QRS voltage to cardiac mass (heart weight), and patients with increased cardiac mass usually had total 12-lead QRS voltage >175 mm.[2]

We found only three previously reported publications of ECGs in patients with type A acute aortic dissection.[3–5] None measured total 12-lead QRS voltage. All three discussed the usefulness of the ECG in predicting the prognosis of acute type A aortic dissection.

1. Roberts WC, Filardo G, Ko JM, et al. Comparison of total 12-lead QRS voltage in a variety of cardiac conditions and its usefulness in predicting increased cardiac mass. *Am J Cardiol.* 2013;112(6): 904–909. doi:10.1016/j.amjcard.2013.04.061.
2. Odom H, 2nd, Davis JL, Dinh H, Baker BJ, Roberts WC, Murphy ML. QRS voltage measurements in autopsied men free of cardiopulmonary disease: a basis for evaluating total QRS voltage as an index of left ventricular hypertrophy. *Am J Cardiol.* 1986;58(9):801–804. doi: 10.1016/0002-9149(86)90357-7.
3. Pourafkari L, Tajlil A, Ghaffari S, et al. Electrocardiography changes in acute aortic dissection-association with troponin leak, coronary anatomy, and prognosis. *Am J Emerg Med.* 2016;34(8):1431–1436. doi:10.1016/j.ajem.2016.04.024.
4. Kalkan AK, Cakmak HA, Kalkan ME, et al. The predictive value of admission fragmented QRS complex for in-hospital cardiovascular mortality of patients with type 1 acute aortic dissection. *Ann Noninvasive Electrocardiol.* 2015;20(5):454–463. doi:10.1111/anec. 12232.
5. Zhang R, Chen S, Zhang H, et al. Biomarkers investigation for in-hospital death in patients with Stanford type A acute aortic dissection. *Int Heart J.* 2016;57(5):622–626. doi:10.1536/ihj.15-484.